T0344672

Ureteric Stenting

Ureteric Stenting

Edited by Ravi Kulkarni

Ashford and St Peter's Hospitals NHS Foundation Trust, UK

WILEY Blackwell

This edition first published in 2017
© 2017 by John Wiley & Sons Ltd

Registered Office
John Wiley & Sons Ltd, The Atrium, Southern Gate, Chichester, West Sussex, PO19 8SQ, UK

Editorial Offices
9600 Garsington Road, Oxford, OX4 2DQ, UK
The Atrium, Southern Gate, Chichester, West Sussex, PO19 8SQ, UK.
111 River Street, Hoboken, NJ 07030-5774, USA

For details of our global editorial offices, for customer services and for information about how to apply for
permission to reuse the copyright material in this book please see our website at
www.wiley.com/wiley-blackwell

The right of Ravi Kulkarni to be identified as the editor of this work has been asserted in accordance with the UK Copyright,
Designs and Patents Act 1988.

Library of Congress Cataloging-in-Publication Data

Names: Kulkarni, Ravi, 1953– author.
Title: Ureteric stenting / Ravi Kulkarni.
Description: Chichester, West Sussex ; Hoboken, NJ : John Wiley & Sons Inc., 2017. |
    Includes bibliographical references and index.
Identifiers: LCCN 2016044215 | ISBN 9781119085683 (cloth) | ISBN 9781119085690 (Adobe PDF) |
    ISBN 9781119085706 (epub)
Subjects: | MESH: Ureter–surgery | Stents | Ureteral Obstruction–surgery | Drainage–methods |
    Urologic Diseases–prevention & control
Classification: LCC RD578 | NLM WJ 26 | DDC 617.4/62–dc23
LC record available at https://lccn.loc.gov/2016044215

A catalogue record for this book is available from the British Library.

Wiley also publishes its books in a variety of electronic formats. Some content that appears in print may not be available in
electronic books.

Cover image courtesy of macroworld/Gettyimages
Cover design by Wiley

Set in 10/12pt Warnock by SPi Global, Pondicherry, India
Printed and bound in Malaysia by Vivar Printing Sdn Bhd

10 9 8 7 6 5 4 3 2 1

Contents

List of Contributors

Husain Alenezi
Endourology Fellow
Division of Urology, Department of
Surgery
Schulich School of Medicine & Dentistry-
Western University
London, Ontario
Canada

Justin Chan
Department of Urologic sciences,
The Stone Centre at Vancouver General
Hospital, Jack Bell Research Center
Vancouver, British Columbia
Canada

Alex Chapman
Consultant Radiologist
Ashford and St Peter's Hospitals
NHS Foundation Trust
Chertsey, Surrey
UK

Ben H. Chew
Assistant Professor of Urology
University of British Columbia
Vancouver, British Columbia
Canada
Director of Clinical Research, The Stone
Centre at Vancouver General Hospital,
Vancouver, Canada

Robin Cole
Consultant Urological Surgeon
Ashford and St Peter's Hospitals
NHS Foundation Trust
Chertsey, Surrey, UK

Jonathan Cloutier
Consultant Urologist, Department of
Urology
University Hospital Center of Quebec City
Saint-François d'Assise Hospital
Quebec City
Canada

John D. Denstedt
Professor of Urology
Division of Urology, Department of
Surgery
Schulich School of Medicine & Dentistry-
Western University
London, Ontario
Canada

Steeve Doizi
Research Fellow, Endourology and Stone
Disease, Department of Urology
University of Texas Southwestern
Medical Center
Dallas, Texas
USA

Rami Elias
Laparoscopy and Endourology Fellow
Division of Urology, McMaster University
Hamilton, Ontario
Canada

Helena Gresty
Department of Academic Surgery
The Royal Marsden NHS Foundation
Trust,
London, UK

Chad M. Gridley
Department of Urology
The Ohio State University Wexner
Medical Center
Ohio, USA

David I. Harriman
Department of Urologic Sciences
University of British Columbia
Vancouver, BC
Canada

Alexander P. Jay
Clinical Fellow
The Royal Marsden NHS Foundation
Trust, London
UK

Navroop Johal
Department of Academic Surgery
The Royal Marsden NHS Foundation
Trust,
London, UK

Hrishi B. Joshi
Consultant Urological Surgeon and
Honorary Lecturer, Department of Urology
University Hospital of Wales and School
of Medicine, Cardiff University
Wales
UK

Panagiotis Kallidonis
Urology Specialist
Department of Urology
University Hospital of Patras
Patras
Greece

Wissam Kamal
Department of Urology
University Hospital of Patras
Patras
Greece

Bodo E. Knudsen
Interim Chair, Program Director
Associate Professor and Henry A. Wise II
Professorship in Urology
Department of Urology
The Ohio State University Wexner
Medical Center
USA

Ravi Kulkarni
Consultant Urological Surgeon
Ashford and St Peter's Hospitals
NHS Foundation Trust
Chertsey, Surrey, UK

Pardeep Kumar
Consultant Urological Surgeon
Department of Academic Surgery
The Royal Marsden NHS Foundation
Trust, London
UK

Dirk Lange
Director of Basic Science Research,
Assistant Professor of Urology
The Stone Centre at Vancouver General
Hospital, Jack Bell Research Center
Vancouver, British Columbia
Canada

David A. Leavitt
The Smith Institute for Urology
Hofstra-North Shore-LIJ Health System
New Hyde Park, NY
USA

Evangelos Liatsikos
Professor of Urology
Department of Urology
University Hospital of Patras
Patras, Greece

Stuart Nigel Lloyd
Consultant Urological Surgeon
Hinchingbrooke Park, Huntingdon
UK

Edward D. Matsumoto
Professor of Urology
Division of Urology
Department of Surgery
DeGroote School of Medicine
McMaster University
Hamilton, Ontario
Canada

Piruz Motamedinia
The Smith Institute for Urology
Hofstra-North Shore-LIJ School of
Medicine

New Hyde Park, NY
USA

David L. Nicol
Chief of Surgery/Consultant Urologist
The Royal Marsden NHS Foundation
Trust, London
UK
Professor of Surgical Oncology
Institute of Cancer Research, UK
Professor of Surgery
University of Queensland
Australia

Zeph Okeke
The Smith Institute for Urology
Hofstra-North Shore-LIJ School of
Medicine
New Hyde Park, NY
USA

Vasilis Panagopoulos
Department of Urology
University Hospital of Patras
Patras, Greece

Margaret S. Pearle
Professor of Urology and Internal
Medicine
University of Texas Southwestern
Medical Center
Dallas, Texas,
USA

Stephen Perrio
Ashford and St Peter's Hospitals
NHS Foundation Trust
Chertsey, Surrey
UK

Aditya Raja
Research Fellow in Urology
University Hospital of Wales and School
of Medicine, Cardiff University
Cardiff, Wales
UK

Ravindra Sabnis
Professor of Urology
Department of Urology
Muljibhai Patel Urological Hospital

Nadiad, Gujarat
India

Arthur D. Smith
Professor of Urology
The Smith Institute for Urology
Hofstra North Shore-LIJ School of
Medicine
New Hyde Park, NY
USA

Thomas O. Tailly
Division of Urology, Department of
Surgery
Ghent University Hospitals
Ghent
Belgium

Dominic A. Teichmann
Specialist Registrar in Urology
University Hospital of Wales and School
of Medicine
Cardiff University, Wales
UK

Andrew M. Todd
Department of Urology
The Ohio State University Wexner
Medical Center
Ohio
USA

Olivier Traxer
Professor of Urology
Department of Urology
Tenon University Hospital
Pierre & Marie Curie University
Paris, France

Graham Watson
Consultant Urologist and Chairman,
Medi Tech Trust
BMI The Esperance Hospital
Eastbourne
UK

Philip T. Zhao
The Smith Institute for Urology
Hofstra North Shore-LIJ School of
Medicine
New Hyde Park, NY
USA

Foreword

The Urology World has long awaited a book entirely devoted to ureteral stents.

Dr. Kulkarni has assembled an impressive selection of contributors to this book all of whom are experts in the field. Various types of stents are described and all aspects of stenting, including techniques of insertion and the complications that may ensue, are discussed.

It is now a relatively simple matter to insert a ureteral stent either to overcome an obstruction or to prevent it. Indeed, too frequently, ureteral stents are inserted with no thought given to the problems that may arise when they are subsequently removed (see chapter 20).

For example, patients with bilateral ureteral obstruction caused by a malignancy are invariably stented without discussing with the patient and/or family the alternative of non-intervention. In many instances, a fairly rapid demise from uraemia may in fact be preferable to stenting a patient and extending a life of poor quality and severe pain.

My single message to the readers of this book is that the possible consequences of stenting should always be considered before embarking on this form of therapy.

I congratulate Dr. Kulkarni for this major contribution to the urologic literature. This book will certainly be appreciated by its readers and will be invaluable in the treatment of their patients.

Professor Arthur Smith
The Arthur Smith Institute of Urology
Long Island
New Hyde Park
New York

Preface

Ureteric stenting is one of the most common urological procedures. The idea of writing a book on the subject seemed like stating the obvious. But when I thought about the subject, it lent itself as a little challenge. The changes in designs, materials and the evolution of technical alternatives over the past decades alone have been so extensive that a compilation felt worthwhile.

Many enthusiasts have done sterling work on different aspects of stents. These contributions have been published and are well recognised. However, not many have reached the operating theatres of the practicing urologist nor have these advances passed on to the patients who would benefit from these modifications. Making the urological community aware of these seemed like a good idea.

Original research on the physiology of the ureter to the new biodegradable materials has enriched our knowledge and has provided a platform to consider alternatives. The quantification of stent related morbidity and the cost benefits have also been brought to our attention in the new cost-conscious world in which clinical practice is critically evaluated.

This treatise of a wide spectrum of chapters written by some of the well-recognised authorities in the world will provide a valuable source of scientific and practical information to all those involved in managing ureteric obstruction. Aimed at all levels of urologists and radiologists, this book will hopefully offer some technical as well as conceptual hints. I anticipate, it will also generate enthusiasm so necessary to keep innovation at the forefront of this field.

I am most grateful to all the authors for their efforts and the time. Special thanks to Prof Arthur Smith, whose advice from the very concept to the selection of topics has been of enormous value.

I would like to thank my wife Meena for putting up with me during this work!

Ravi Kulkarni MS FRCS
Consultant Urological Surgeon
Ashford and St Peter's Hospital NHS Foundation Trust
Chertsey, Surrey, UK

1

Anatomy of the Human Ureter

Ravi Kulkarni

Consultant Urological Surgeon, Ashford and St Peter's Hospitals NHS Foundation Trust, Chertsey, Surrey, UK

The ureter is a muscular tube, which connects the renal pelvis to the urinary bladder. Approximately 25 to 30 cm long, it has a diameter of about 3 mm. It has three natural constrictions. The first at the pelvi-ureteric junction, the second at the pelvic brim where it crosses the iliac vessels, and finally at the uretero-vesical junction (Figure 1.1). The narrowest part of the ureter is the intra-mural segment at the uretero-vesical junction [1].

The ureter traverses the retro-peritoneal space in a relatively straight line from the pelvi-ureteric junction to the urinary bladder. Lying in front of the psoas major muscle, its course can be traced along the tips of the transverse processes of the lumbar vertebrae [2].

Its posterior relations in the abdomen are the psoas major muscle and the genito-femoral nerve. The right ureter is covered anteriorly by the second part of the duodenum, right colic vessel, the terminal part of the ileum, and small bowel mesentery. The anterior relations of the left ureter are the left colic vessels, the sigmoid colon, and its mesentery. The gonadal vessels cross both the ureters anteriorly (Figure 1.2) in an oblique manner [3–6].

The ureter enters the pelvis at the bifurcation of the common iliac artery. The segment of the ureter below the pelvic brim is approximately of the same length as the abdominal part. It traverses postero-laterally, in front of the sciatic foramen and then turns antero-medially. In its initial course, it lies in front of the internal iliac artery, especially its anterior division and the internal iliac vein – an important relationship for the pelvic surgeon [6, 7]. It crosses in front of the obliterated umbilical artery, obturator nerve and finally the inferior vesical artery (Figure 1.2).

The relations with the adjacent organs from this part vary in both the sexes and are of clinical significance.

In the male, it is crossed by the vas deferens from the lateral to the medial side. The ureter then turns infero-medially into the bladder base just above the seminal vesicles.

In a female, the ureter passes behind the ovary and its plexus of veins – an important relation that makes it vulnerable to trauma during the ligation of these veins (Figure 1.2). It lies in the areolar tissue beneath the broad ligament. It is then crossed by the uterine artery, which lies above and in front of the ureter and yet again renders the ureter to injury. The subsequent part of the ureter bears a close relationship to the cervix and the vaginal fornix. It lies between 1 and 4 cm from the cervix. The course in front of the

Ureteric Stenting, First Edition. Edited by Ravi Kulkarni.
© 2017 John Wiley & Sons Ltd. Published 2017 by John Wiley & Sons Ltd.

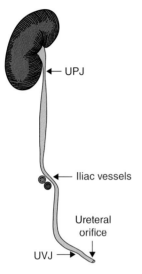

Figure 1.1 Anatomy of the ureter.

UPJ

Iliac vessels

Ureteral orifice

UVJ

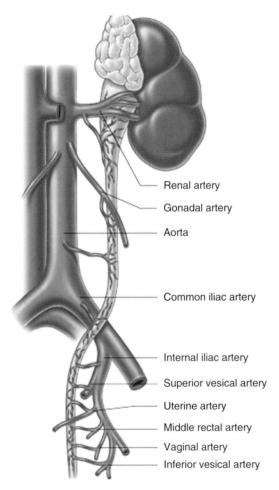

Figure 1.2 Blood supply of the ureter.

Renal artery

Gonadal artery

Aorta

Common iliac artery

Internal iliac artery

Superior vesical artery

Uterine artery

Middle rectal artery

Vaginal artery

Inferior vesical artery

lateral vaginal fornix can be variable. The ureter may cross the midline and therefore, a variable part may lie in front of the vagina [8–10].

The intra-mural part of the ureter is oblique and is surrounded by the detrusor muscle fibres. Both these features result in the closure of the lumen and are responsible for prevention of reflux of urine during voiding. The two ureteric orifices are approximately 5 cm apart when the bladder is full. This distance is reduced when the bladder is empty.

1.1 Structure

The ureter does not have a serosal lining. It has three layers: the outermost, fibrous and areolar tissue, the middle, muscular, and innermost, the urothelial. The fibrous coat is thin and indistinct (Figure 1.3).

The smooth muscle fibers that provide the peristaltic activity are divided in circular and longitudinal segments. The inner, circular bundles are mainly responsible for the forward propulsion of urine. The longitudinal coat is less distinct in its proximal part. Additional longitudinal fibers are seen in the distal part of the ureter. The muscle coat of the ureter is rarely arranged in two specific layers.

The inner, urothelial lining is of transitional epithelium. It is four to five cell layers thick in the main part of the ureter but is much thinner in its proximal part where it is two to three cell layers (Figure 1.3). It has very little sub-mucosa. Mostly folded longitudinally, it merges with the urothelium of the bladder at the distal end.

1.2 Blood Supply

The ureter draws its blood supply in a segmental fashion (Figure 1.2). There is a good anastomosis between the arterial branches arising from renal artery, abdominal aorta, gonadal vessels, common iliac, internal iliac, superior and inferior vesical arteries. Ureter also has branches arising from the uterine artery in females. Despite the extensive

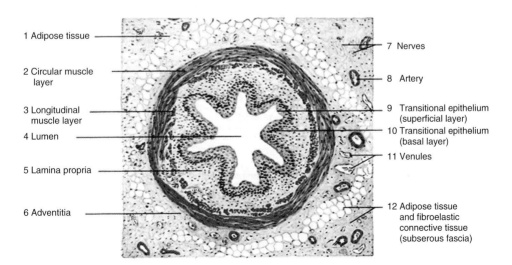

1 Adipose tissue

2 Circular muscle layer

3 Longitudinal muscle layer

4 Lumen

5 Lamina propria

6 Adventitia

7 Nerves

8 Artery

9 Transitional epithelium (superficial layer)

10 Transitional epithelium (basal layer)

11 Venules

12 Adipose tissue and fibroelastic connective tissue (subserous fascia)

Figure 1.3 Histology of the ureter.

internal anastomoses, the blood supply of the distal 2–3 cm of the ureter is unpredictable [9]. This makes this segment vulnerable to ischemia if dissected excessively.

The venous drainage of the ureter follows the arteries and ultimately leads into the inferior vena cava.

Lymphatic drainage of the ureter is also segmental. The internal, communicating plexus of lymphatics within the walls of the ureter drain into the regional lymph nodes. The lymphatics from the proximal part of the ureter drain into the para-aortic lymph nodes near the origin of the renal artery. The distal abdominal segment drains in the para-aortic as well as common iliac lymph nodes. The lymphatics from the pelvic segment of the ureter drain into the internal and subsequently into the common iliac lymph nodes [10–12].

1.3   Nerves

The autonomic nerve supply of the ureter arises from the lumbar and sacral plexuses. The proximal part of the ureter derives the nerve supply from the lower thoracic and the lumbar plexus whereas the distal and pelvic part from the sacral. Pain fibers to the ureter predominantly arise from L1 and L2 segments, which explain the referred pain to the relevant dermatome. The nerve fibers are sparse in the proximal part but plentiful in the distal segment. Ureteric peristalsis is largely independent of its innervation. A downward wave, initiated in the collecting system, much like the sino-atrial node in the heart, is believed to be responsible for the forward propulsion of urine towards the bladder. A paralysis of this intrinsic neuro-muscular activity can occur due to an obstructive or inflammatory process.

1.4   Embryology

Ureteric buds develop and grow in a cephalad fashion from the embryonic bladder. The superior ends of these buds are capped with the meta-nephros, which develops in to the adult kidney (Figures 1.4 and 1.5). The proximal extension of the ureteric bud develops into the renal pelvis, calyces and the collecting tubules. Meta-nephros, which develops from the mesoderm, forms up to 1000,000 nephrons, which join the collecting tubules to form the final functional units of the adult kidney. Once the meta-nephros and the developing collecting system have reached its lumbar destination, it gains attachment to the adrenals. Medial rotation of the embryonic kidney results in alteration of relationship of both kidneys to the neighbouring organs.

The separation and proximal growth of the ureteric buds has an important bearing on the ureteric and renal anomalies. The lack of separation of the meta-nephros will lead to the development of a horseshoe kidney (Figure 1.6). Similarly, any deviation in the normal development of the bud will lead to duplex or fused ectopia.

1.5   Congenital Variations

1.5.1   Reto-caval ureter

The right ureter may cross behind the inferior vena cava (retro-caval ureter). The incidence is reported to be 1 in 1500 patients. More common in males than in

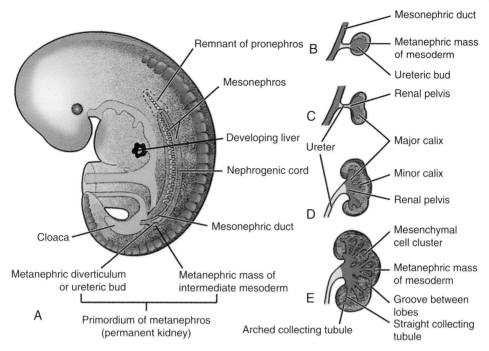

Figure 1.4 Ureter embryology, part one.

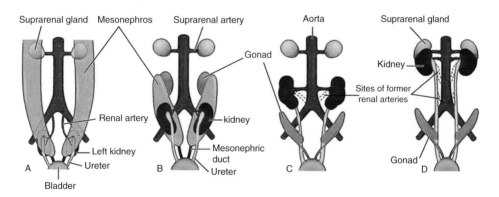

Figure 1.5 Ureter embryology, part two.

females, this congenital variation is considered an anomaly of the development of the vena cava rather than the ureter. So, the term pre-ureteral cava is more appropriate (Figure 1.7).

1.5.2 Duplex

Duplication of the ureteric bud may result in a variety of anomalies. This may be in the form of two separate systems on both sides or a duplex ureter at variable levels which get fused anywhere from the PUJ to the ureteric orifice. The location of the ureteric

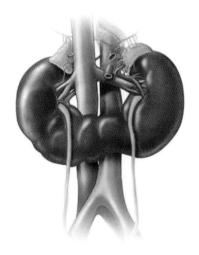

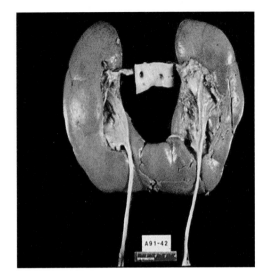

Figure 1.6 Horse-shoe kidney.

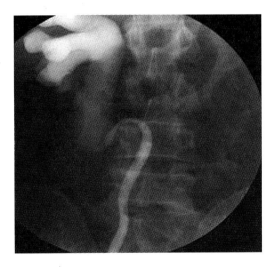

Figure 1.7 Retro-caval ureter.

orifices of a duplex system is governed by what is known as the Weigert-Meyer law, which states that the ureteric orifice of the upper moiety is more medial and caudal where as that of the lower segment is more cranial and lateral (Figure 1.8). The upper moiety is usually small and its ureter is more likely to suffer with obstruction or an ureterocoele. The lower moiety is more prone to reflux.

1.5.3 PUJ Obstruction

A functional narrowing of the uretero-pelvic junction results from muscular hypoplasia or a neuro-muscular abnormality. A lack of the progression of the peristaltic wave at this location results in functional obstruction. Progressive dilatation of the renal pelvis

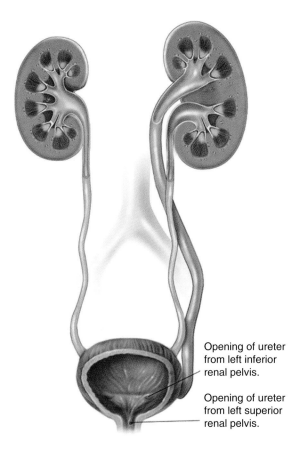

Opening of ureter
from left inferior
renal pelvis.

Opening of ureter
from left superior
renal pelvis.

Figure 1.8 Duplex ureter.

follows and causes stasis. These two features lead to complications such a formation of calculi, infection, pain, and a progressive loss of renal parenchyma if corrective surgery is delayed.

Other variations include a high attachment of the ureter to the pelvis, a long segment of atresia and segmentation of the renal pelvis. Associated with a PUJ obstruction, the renal artery or its branches may cross the ureter, potentially leading to obstruction. The role of crossing vessels near the pelvic-ureteric junction and their influence on obstruction to the upper tract is often difficult to assess. Whether they lead to the dilatation of the renal pelvis or the latter appears obstructed due to the over-hang is often debatable.

1.5.4 Ectopic Ureteric Orifice

This rare form of anomaly is often seen with the upper moiety of a duplex system. In a fully developed single renal unit, the ureter may drain in the posterior urethra, seminal vesicle, or the vas deferens. In a female, the orifice may be in the urethra, vagina, or the perineum, and presents with incontinence.

1.5.5 Ureterocoeles

Usually seen in the upper moiety of a duplex system or an ectopic ureter, these are due to the failure of canalization of the ureteric bud.

1.5.6 Mega-Ureter

A grossly dilated ureter with a narrow uretero-vesical junction is the typical appearance of this condition. An a-peristaltic segment of the distal segment is the possible cause. There may be an associated reflux. This anomaly may be seen with other abnormalities such as prune belly and other syndromes.

1.5.7 Ureteric Diverticulae

This rare anomaly is due to the variation in the development of the ureteric bud.

1.6 Clinical Significance

The importance of anatomy of any organ cannot be over-emphasised to a surgeon.

Awareness of the normal anatomy and its variations can help the surgeon to avoid trauma during procedures that involve dissection of the ureter. Accidental tears, trans-section, ligation, heat damage caused by diathermy, ligasure, harmonic scalpel, or laser energy can be reduced by careful separation of the ureter. Such heat damage can be subtle and manifest much later when tissue necrosis develops following ischemia. The knowledge of the blood supply is important. Avoiding excessive mobilization can prevent the development of ischemic strictures following ureteric surgery. Although distensible, the diameter of the ureter should be respected. Insertion of wide-bore instruments invariably leads to tears and subsequent scarring. Increasing use of ureteroscopy and the use of devices such as lasers has led to a rise of iatrogenic ureteric trauma.

References

[1] Davies DV, Coupland RE. *Grey's anatomy, 34th ed*. Orient Longman, Harrow, Essex, UK, 1989, 1538–1540.

[2] McMinn RMH. *Last's Anatomy, Regional and Applied, 9th ed*. Churchill Livingstone, Elsevier, UK, 2013, 371.

[3] Schenkman NS. Standard anatomy and variants. In: Ureter Anatomy, (Gest TR, ed). Medscape, New York, US. 2013.

[4] Knipe H, Butler, I. Ureter. Available at: https://Radiopaedica.org/articles/ureter (accessed October 19, 2016).

[5] Butler P, Mitchell A, Healy JC. *Applied radiological anatomy, 2nd ed*. Cambridge University Press, 2012, 110–113.

[6] Ryan S, McNicholas M, Eustace S. *Anatomy for diagnostic imaging, 2e*. Saunders Ltd., 2004.

[7] Pal M. Urogynecology & pelvic reconstructive surgery. April 2016. Available at: http://www.teachMeanAtomy.info (accessed October 19, 2016).

[8] Schlossberg L, Zuidema GD. 1997. The John Hopkins Atlas of Human Functional Anatomy. Available at: http://www.radiopaedia.org/articles/ureter (accessed October 19, 2016).

[9] Uninary Systems. Ureter. Chapter 33. 2016. Available at: http://www.www.mananatomy.com/body-systems/urinary-system/ureter (accessed October 19, 2016).

[10] My KenHub. The Ureter. n.d. Available at: http://www.kenhub.com/en/library/anatomy/the-ureters (accessed October 19, 2016).

[11] Anatomy of the Ureter. 2015. Available at: http://www.emedicine.medscape.com/article/378075-overview (accessed October 19, 2016).

[12] Anatomy of the Ureter. December 2015. Available at: http://www.anatomyatlases.org/AnatomicVariants (accessed October 19, 2016).

2

Anatomic Variations of the Ureter

Piruz Motamedinia[1], David A. Leavitt[2], Philip T. Zhao[1], Zeph Okeke[1] and Arthur D. Smith[3]

[1] *The Smith Institute for Urology, Hofstra North Shore-LIJ School of Medicine, New Hyde Park, NY, USA*
[2] *The Smith Institute for Urology, Hofstra-North Shore-LIJ Health System, New Hyde Park, NY, USA*
[3] *Professor of Urology, The Smith Institute for Urology, Hofstra North Shore-LIJ School of Medicine, New Hyde Park, NY, USA*

A normal ureter is a narrow, tubular structure that carries urine between the renal pelvis and the bladder. Far from a passive tube, the ureter has three distinct muscular layers surrounding a specialized urothelium, which actively propels urine to the bladder. The ureter narrows at distinct points along its course including the ureteropelvic junction (UPJ), the ureteral segment over the iliac vessels/pelvic brim, and the ureterovesical junction (UVJ). These act as common points of obstruction for a passing stone. However, variations in normal anatomy result in a higher likelihood or even increased degree of obstruction, and present several challenges to stent placement.

2.1 Horseshoe Kidney

Horseshoe kidney (HSK) is the fusion of the right and left kidneys at their lower pole across the midline. The point of fusion is referred to as the isthmus and varies in quality from a thin, fibrous band to thicker, functional renal parenchyma. HSK occurs in about 1 in 400 to 666 individuals and is twice as common in men [1, 2]. The higher incidence of HSK seen in children can be explained by the co-occurring non-urologic comorbidities limiting their overall survival. Associated urologic abnormalities include UPJ obstruction (17%), vesicoureteral reflux (20–50%), and ureteral duplication (10%).

Normally, kidneys ascend to the upper retroperitoneum, just below the liver or spleen. They rest on the psoas muscles resulting in a line with the upper pole slightly more medial to the lower pole. With HSK, the isthmus is tethered by the inferior mesenteric artery limiting kidney ascent resulting in the lateral rotation of the upper poles with an anterior displacement of the renal pelvises [3].

The ureter has a high insertion into the renal pelvis in HSK with an increased incidence of ureteropelvic junction (UPJ) obstruction of about 13–35% [2]. Moreover, the ureter courses over the isthmus creating another point of obstruction and urinary stasis, raising the risk of nephrolithiasis and urinary tract infection (UTI) [4–6].

Management of stones offers several challenges in patients with HSK given their abnormal renal and ureteral anatomy. Shock wave lithotripsy (SWL) is an option;

however, the reliance on passive clearance results in poor stone free rates (31–70%) [7, 8]. Ureteroscopy is plausible and one series was able to demonstrate excellent stone-free rates in patients with stones ≤10 mm [9]. Larger stones up to 16 mm were more likely to have residual fragments or require multiple procedures.

PCNL offers the best outcomes regarding stone-free rates (75–100%) [7, 8, 10]; however, major complications including bleeding, sepsis and bowel injury are more common, albeit still rare. Given the lower position and abnormal rotation of HSK pre-operative cross-sectional imaging is paramount to accurately assess stone burden and also proximity of major blood vessels and organs including bowel and pleura. The anterio-medial rotation of the lower pole results in the upper poles being the most posterior region of the HSK and so the preferred point of access. Patients with HSK have a higher incidence of retrorenal colon (3–19%) and as such are at an increased risk of bowel perforation during percutaneous access [11, 12].

In other cases of renal ectopia with or without fusion are far less common than HSK [13]. Ureteral anomalies similar to HSK continue to occur and their course is dependent on the kidneys final position relative to the intended ipsilateral trigone.

2.2 Duplex Ureter

The incidence of upper tract duplication is 0.5 to 0.7% of the asymptomatic population and 1% to 10% of children with UTIs [14]. The most common variation is a partial duplication (70%) with a common ureter entering the bladder [15]. Complete duplications are more likely to have additional comorbidities including reflux, ureteral obstruction, or ureterocele. Ureteral duplication is difficult to appreciate on a non-contrast CT scan and contrast enhancement is suggested when suspicion is high [16]. The Weigert-Meyer rule dictates that in a completely duplicated system, the lower-pole moiety implants more laterally in the bladder with a shorter intramural segment more prone to reflux [17]. Conversely, the upper-pole moiety implants caudally and is more likely to be ectopic and obstructed.

Stent placement in a partially duplicated ureter can be challenging. If electing to only stent a single system, the surgeon should chose a stent with side holes throughout its entire length. If retrograde wire placement does not preferentially cannulate the desired moiety, an angled-tip catheter can direct a glidewire at the point of bifurcation. Alternatively, ureteroscopy with direct visualization of the desired ureter at its bifurcation may be required. If a retrograde approach is unsuccessful, percutaneous antegrade ureteral stent is preferred. Surgeons should consider stenting both moieties to prevent de novo compression and obstruction of the unstented moiety.

2.3 Megaureter

A normal ureteral diameter is between 3–5 mm. Dilation greater than 7 mm may be considered a megaureter [18]. Etiologies include primary or secondary (due to bladder outlet obstruction) reflux, or ureteral obstruction attributable to segmental narrowing or aperistalsis. Megaureters have been described as obstructing and refluxing; however, this combination is less common [19]. Aperistaltic dilation without obstruction is thought to be secondary to abnormal muscle fibers or collagen deposition [20].

Congenital megaureter is primarily a pediatric diagnosis, often diagnosed in utero given the near ubiquitous use of neonatal sonographic screening. For children who escape discovery or remain asymptomatic, about half spontaneously resolve without the need for intervention [21, 22]. Congenital megaureter diagnosis in adults is rare and proceeded by symptoms secondary to obstruction or infection. Ureteral stones, which developed due to urine stagnation in the dilated segment have been described in 36% of patients with symptomatic megaureter [23].

Megaureter management derived from the pediatric literature states a primary goal of renal preservation [19]. Surgical management includes excision of the obstructing segment, tapering to allow for a normal length to diameter ratio, and re-implantation. In adults with obstructed megaureter, treatment may be indicated in the setting of recurrent urinary infections, ureterolithiasis, pain, or renal deterioration. Near complete loss of renal function secondary to longstanding obstruction may warrant simple nephrectomy rather than a salvage procedure. Percutaneous decompression with interval functional assessment would help guide surgical planning in this regard. Surgical tapering and reimplantation have been described in adults with good success. A less invasive approach with ureteral meatotomy and stenting has also been described and useful for patients with ureteral calculi [23].

Non-orthotopic ureteral reimplantation and irregularities in the inner lumen following megaureter repair may make subsequent ureteral stenting and instrumentation difficult. Antegrade percutaneous intervention or stent placement should be considered in these cases.

2.4   Ectopic Ureter

An ectopic ureter is a ureter that does not implant in the trigone of the bladder [24]. Similar to ureteroceles, the exact mechanism that results in ureteral ectopia is unknown; however, it is thought to be related to abnormal ureterotrigonal development [25, 26]. As stated earlier, following the Weigert-Meyer rule, ectopic ureters in a duplex system are commonly associated with the upper pole moiety and likely to be obstructed especially when implanted proximal to the external sphincter above the pelvic floor [17].

Ectopic ureters usually implant in a Wolffian structure, which in males include the vas, seminal vesicles, or ejaculatory ducts [26]. In women, an ectopic ureter may have a wider range of implantation from the bladder neck to the vagina, rectum, and perineum [27]. A young girl presenting with signs of continuous incontinence or dribbling while still voiding spontaneously should raise suspicions of an ectopic ureter distal to the bladder neck and should be investigated accordingly.

2.5   Ureterocele

A ureterocele is defined as a cystic dilation of the terminal portion of the ureter. The exact embryologic mechanism by which ureteroceles form is unknown; however, abnormal ureterotrigonal development, a defect in common nephric duct apoptosis, and failure in rupture of the distal membrane at the ureteral orifice are likely contributing events [25, 26]. Not all ureteroceles are obstructive and the cystic appearance of the non-obstructive variety is likely a result of poor muscularization and ballooning of the distal ureter.

Ureteroceles may be classified into two subtypes: intravesical ureterocele inserts into the bladder and is confined within its lumen; extravesical ureterocele results from an ectopic insertion of the ureter, commonly into the bladder neck or urethra. A cecoureterocele combines an ectopic with an intraluminal orifice. The result is a prolapsing ureterocele that obstructs the bladder outlet. Ureterocele incidence ranges from 1 in 500 to 1 in 1200 individuals and is 6 times more likely to affect women [26, 28]. Approximately 80% are associated with a duplicated system and affect the upper pole moiety, and 10% are bilateral [26].

Antenatal sonography has rendered ureteroceles primarily a pediatric diagnosis. Children often have concomitant hydronephrosis or UTIs, and treatment aims to prevent infection, maximize renal function, and preserve continence. In symptomatic patients or in the setting of hydronephrosis, endoscopic puncture using a Bugbee electrode, or more recently, a laser is regarded as the treatment method of choice [29].

Adult ureteroceles are less commonly encountered and are likely to be intravesical and orthotopic [26]. Ureteral atony with stasis increases the risk of ureteral stone formation to 4–39% of patients [30]. With the increase risk of ureteral stones, holmium laser unroofing with ureteroscopy and laser lithotripsy has been described [31]. In our own experience, adult ureteroceles tend to be thick-walled and a simple puncture is inadequate. Rather, a longitudinal incision or complete resection especially in the setting of prolapsed and bladder neck obstruction is necessary.

Anatomic variations can result from abnormal kidney development and localization, or are dependent on the embryologic development of the ureter relative to the bladder. Deviations from the normal anatomic course of the ureter increase the risk of ureteral obstruction and dilation resulting in a higher incidence of urinary stasis, urolithiasis, and infection. Surgical intervention should be reserved for symptomatic individuals or for cases that will preserve renal function.

Prior to operating on a patient, cross-sectional imaging with contrast and delayed-phase urogram will help delineate variant vasculature, the ureteral course, and the relative location of adjacent organs that may be different from those with normal anatomy.

References

[1] Hobbs CA, Cleves MA, Simmons CJ. Genetic epidemiology and congenital malformations: from the chromosome to the crib. Archives of pediatrics & adolescent medicine. 2002;156(4):315–320.

[2] Weizer AZ, Silverstein AD, Auge BK, Delvecchio FC, Raj G, Albala DM, et al. Determining the incidence of horseshoe kidney from radiographic data at a single institution. The Journal of urology. 2003;170(5):1722–1726.

[3] Natsis K, Piagkou M, Skotsimara A, Protogerou V, Tsitouridis I, Skandalakis P. Horseshoe kidney: a review of anatomy and pathology. Surgical and radiologic anatomy: SRA. 2014;36(6):517–526.

[4] Glenn JF. Analysis of 51 patients with horseshoe kidney. The New England journal of medicine. 1959;261:684–687.

[5] Shapiro E, Bauer SB, Chow JS. Anomalies of the upper urinary tract. In: Wein AJ, Kavoussi LR, Novic AC, Partin AW, Peters CA, editors. Campbell's Urology. 10th ed. Philadelphia, PA: Elsevier Saunders; 2012.

[6] Yavuz S, Kiyak A, Sander S. Renal Outcome of Children With Horseshoe Kidney: A Single-center Experience. Urology. 2015;85(2):463–466.

[7] Viola D, Anagnostou T, Thompson TJ, Smith G, Moussa SA, Tolley DA. Sixteen years of experience with stone management in horseshoe kidneys. Urologia internationalis. 2007;78(3):214–218.

[8] Symons SJ, Ramachandran A, Kurien A, Baiysha R, Desai MR. Urolithiasis in the horseshoe kidney: a single-centre experience. Bju Int. 2008;102(11):1676–1680.

[9] Molimard B, Al-Qahtani S, Lakmichi A, Sejiny M, Gil-Diez de Medina S, Carpentier X, et al. Flexible ureterorenoscopy with holmium laser in horseshoe kidneys. Urology. 2010;76(6):1334–1337.

[10] Shokeir AA, El-Nahas AR, Shoma AM, Eraky I, El-Kenawy M, Mokhtar A, et al. Percutaneous nephrolithotomy in treatment of large stones within horseshoe kidneys. Urology. 2004;64(3):426–429.

[11] El-Nahas AR, Shokeir AA, El-Assmy AM, Shoma AM, Eraky I, El-Kenawy MR, et al. Colonic perforation during percutaneous nephrolithotomy: study of risk factors. Urology. 2006;67(5):937–941.

[12] Kachrilas S, Papatsoris A, Bach C, Kontos S, Faruquz Z, Goyal A, et al. Colon perforation during percutaneous renal surgery: a 10-year experience in a single endourology centre. Urological research. 2012;40(3):263–268.

[13] Glodny B, Petersen J, Hofmann KJ, Schenk C, Herwig R, Trieb T, et al. Kidney fusion anomalies revisited: clinical and radiological analysis of 209 cases of crossed fused ectopia and horseshoe kidney. Bju Int. 2009;103(2):224–235.

[14] Amis ES, Jr., Cronan JJ, Pfister RC. Lower moiety hydronephrosis in duplicated kidneys. Urology. 1985;26(1):82–88.

[15] Joseph DB, Bauer SB, Colodny AH, Mandell J, Lebowitz RL, Retik AB. Lower pole ureteropelvic junction obstruction and incomplete renal duplication. The Journal of urology. 1989;141(4):896–899.

[16] Eisner BH, Shaikh M, Uppot RN, Sahani DV, Dretler SP. Genitourinary imaging with noncontrast computerized tomography-are we missing duplex ureters? The Journal of urology. 2008;179(4):1445–1448.

[17] Meyer R. Normal and abnormal development of the ureter in the human embryo; a mechanistic consideration. The Anatomical record. 1946;96(4):355–371.

[18] Hellstrom M, Jodal U, Marild S, Wettergren B. Ureteral dilatation in children with febrile urinary tract infection or bacteriuria. AJR American journal of roentgenology. 1987;148(3):483–486.

[19] Carr MC, Casale P. Anomalies and Surgery of the Ureter in Children. In: Wein AJ, Kavoussi LR, Novic AC, Partin AW, Peters CA, editors. Campbell's Urology. 10th ed. Philadelphia, PA: Elsevier Saunders; 2012.

[20] Rosenblatt GS, Takesita K, Fuchs GJ. Urolithiasis in adults with congenital megaureter. Canadian Urological Association journal = Journal de l'Association des urologues du Canada. 2009;3(6):E77–E80.

[21] Domini M, Aquino A, Pappalepore N, Tursini S, Marino N, Strocchi F, et al. Conservative treatment of neonatal primary megaureter. European journal of pediatric surgery: official journal of Austrian Association of Pediatric Surgery [et al] = Zeitschrift fur Kinderchirurgie. 1999;9(6):396–399.

[22] Oliveira EA, Diniz JS, Rabelo EA, Silva JM, Pereira AK, Filgueiras MT, et al. Primary megaureter detected by prenatal ultrasonography: conservative management and prolonged follow-up. International urology and nephrology. 2000;32(1):13–18.

[23] Hemal AK, Ansari MS, Doddamani D, Gupta NP. Symptomatic and complicated adult and adolescent primary obstructive megaureter--indications for surgery: analysis, outcome, and follow-up. Urology. 2003;61(4):703–707; discussion 7.

[24] Glassberg KI, Braren V, Duckett JW, Jacobs EC, King LR, Lebowitz RL, et al. Suggested terminology for duplex systems, ectopic ureters and ureteroceles. The Journal of urology. 1984;132(6):1153–1154.

[25] Mendelsohn C. Using mouse models to understand normal and abnormal urogenital tract development. Organogenesis. 2009;5(1):306–314.

[26] Peters CA, Schlussel RN, Mendelsohn C. Ectopic Ureter, Ureterocele, and Ureteral Anomalies. In: Wein AJ, Kavoussi LR, Novic AC, Partin AW, Peters CA, editors. Campbell's Urology. 10th ed. Philadelphia, PA: Elsevier Saunders; 2012.

[27] Weight CJ, Chand D, Ross JH. Single system ectopic ureter to rectum subtending solitary kidney and bladder agenesis in newborn male. Urology. 2006;68(6):1344; e1-e3.

[28] Vijay MK, Vijay P, Dutta A, Gupta A, Tiwari P, Kumar S, et al. The safety and efficacy of endoscopic incision of orthotopic ureterocele in adult. Saudi journal of kidney diseases and transplantation : an official publication of the Saudi Center for Organ Transplantation, Saudi Arabia. 2011;22(6):1169–1174.

[29] Pagano MJ, van Batavia JP, Casale P. Laser ablation in the management of obstructive uropathy in neonates. Journal of endourology/Endourological Society. 2015;29(5):611–614.

[30] Nash AG, Knight M. Ureterocele calculi. British journal of urology. 1973;45(4):404–407.

[31] Shah HN, Sodha H, Khandkar AA, Kharodawala S, Hegde SS, Bansal M. Endoscopic management of adult orthotopic ureterocele and associated calculi with holmium laser: experience with 16 patients over 4 years and review of literature. Journal of endourology/Endourological Society. 2008;22(3):489–496.

3

The Pathophysiology of Upper Tract Obstruction

Alexander P. Jay[1] and David L. Nicol[2,3,4]

[1] *Clinical Fellow, The Royal Marsden NHS Foundation Trust, London, UK*
[2] *Chief of Surgery/Consultant Urologist, The Royal Marsden NHS Foundation Trust, London, UK*
[3] *Professor of Surgical Oncology, Institute of Cancer Research, UK*
[4] *Professor of Surgery, University of Queensland, Australia*

3.1   Introduction

Obstruction of the upper urinary tract is a common clinical problem in urological practice. Obstruction to drainage of urine at any point along the urinary tract is termed an
obstructive uropathy. This can lead to irreversible damage to the renal parenchyma with
functional impairment described as *obstructive nephropathy*. Several factors determine
how an obstructive uropathy will affect a kidney as well as the likelihood of this developing. These factors include characteristics of the obstruction – unilateral or bilateral,
partial or complete, as well as the duration of obstruction together with underlying
characteristics of the kidney (pre-morbid function and renal anatomy).

3.2   Aetiology

Upper urinary tract obstruction may relate to pathology affecting either the ureters
(supra-vesical) or lower urinary tract conditions that impair bladder emptying (vesical
or infra-vesical). The causes of upper tract urinary obstruction are shown in Table 3.1.
These can relate to intra-luminal or mural (either intra-mural or extra-mural) pathology. Intra-luminal causes are the most common and ureteric calculi comprise the
majority of cases in clinical practice. Intra-mural causes relate to conditions of the ureteric wall resulting in stricture formation from ischemia or urothelial malignancy or
functional obstruction due to impaired peristalsis exemplified by congenital uretero-
pelvic junction obstruction. Extra-mural obstruction compromises the ureteric lumen
and peristaltic activity by mechanical circumferential compression of the ureter.

Intra-luminal obstruction frequently results in acute obstruction, which may be high
grade, although partial chronic obstruction may also arise or subsequently evolve.

In contrast, mural causes (both intra and extra-mural) tend to present more insidi-
ously but can progress to complete or high-grade obstruction over time. Obstruction
primarily related to conditions arising from or within the ureter tends to be unilateral.

Ureteric Stenting, First Edition. Edited by Ravi Kulkarni.
© 2017 John Wiley & Sons Ltd. Published 2017 by John Wiley & Sons Ltd.

Table 3.1 Etiology of upper urinary tract obstruction.

Intra-luminal causes	Mural causes		Lower urinary tract causes	
	Intra-mural	Extra-mural	Vesical	Infra-vesical
Ureteric calculus	Upper tract transitional cell carcinoma	Retroperitoneal fibrosis • Idiopathic • Secondary causes	Neuropathic bladder dysfunction	Benign prostatic hyperplasia
Sloughed renal papilla	Benign strictures • Inflammatory • Iatrogenic	PUJ obstruction • Crossing lower pole vessel		Urethral stricture disease
Fungal ball • Spinal cord injury • Neuropathic bladder	PUJ obstruction • High uretero-pelvic take off • Aperistalic segment	Pelvic cancers • Prostate • Cervical • Colorectal • Bladder Malignant lymphadenopathy • Pelvic cancers • Lymphoma		

In contrast, extrinsic causes such as retroperitoneal fibrosis and non-ureteric malignancy, including lymphadenopathy, can result in either unilateral or bilateral obstruction. Infra-vesical obstruction typically relates to bladder outflow obstruction, both mechanical and neurological, and is typically associated with chronic urinary retention as well as bilateral ureteric involvement.

3.3 Presentation

Presentation of upper urinary tract obstruction is dependent on etiology, particularly whether it relates to an acute or chronic process. Acute and complete obstruction, for example, from a ureteric calculus, results in the characteristic renal colic symptomatology. Chronic partial obstruction from an uretero-pelvic obstruction may also result in flank pain during periods of diuresis with increased fluid intake or alcohol consumption. This, however, reflects intermittent high-grade acute obstruction invoking similar pathways. Bilateral upper urinary tract obstruction may present as a result of the primary pathology or with renal impairment. The latter may include biochemical evidence of renal failure as well as signs and symptoms of uremia. Lower urinary tract symptoms may also be the only clinical manifestation of an underlying presence of an obstructive uropathy. Nocturnal or dribbling incontinence is a classic sign of chronic urinary retention, which on investigation reveals unilateral or, more commonly, bilateral upper tract urinary obstruction. Upper urinary tract obstruction with associated infection may also present with bacteremia and without definitive drainage of the obstruction can rapidly progress to septicemia and multi-organ failure.

3.4 Diagnosis

Diagnosis of upper urinary tract obstruction can be made using both anatomical and functional imaging techniques. Anatomical imaging may demonstrate hydronephrosis, which together with other clinical features may indicate obstruction as the underlying cause. Functional imaging is a more definitive means of diagnosis related to dynamic evaluation of renal function and urine flow.

3.4.1 Anatomical Imaging

Anatomical imaging can essentially detect the presence of hydronephrosis. Further information may, however, be necessary to determine whether this relates to obstruction as hydronephrosis can be secondary to non-obstructive causes.

Ultrasound (US) is usually the first imaging modality employed for investigation of upper tract urinary obstruction. As it does not involve ionizing radiation, it is the investigation of choice to diagnose upper urinary tract obstruction during antenatal screening and also employed when investigating maternal upper urinary tract obstruction in pregnancy. Non-obstructive hydronephosis is common in pregnancy and can make a diagnosis of obstructive uropathy challenging in this setting. Although US is a useful initial investigation it may not define either the etiology or level of obstruction. Consequently when hydronephrosis is detected on US, clinical management usually requires additional imaging studies [1].

Computed tomography (CT) is the usual investigation of choice when hydronephrosis is detected on US. It is also frequently the initial radiological assessment for patients presenting with symptoms of acute ureteric obstruction, particularly when this relates to suspected urolithiasis. In the acute setting it can demonstrate the presence or absence of hydronephrosis, as well as other vital features required for clinical management. For example, it may detect the presence of a ureteric calculus, a soft tissue mass or contrast enhanced features of delayed or reduced perfusion of the kidney, as well as impaired clearance from the renal parenchyma as features associated with obstruction. Poor clearance from the collecting system provides further evidence of obstruction, although this may require re-imaging (including plain abdominal x-ray) 20 minutes or more after injection of contrast. Although rarely used magnetic resonance imaging can be used as an alternative to CT if contrast use is problematic, providing morphological and functional information [2].

Retrograde pyelography and antegrade pyelography are now rarely used as a means of diagnosing ureteric obstruction. They are a preliminary to ureteric stent or nephrostomy insertion and may be useful to define the level and nature of obstruction in the acute setting if obstruction is suspected clinically and contrast imaging contraindicated.

3.4.2 Functional Studies

Functional studies can be used to determine whether the hydronephrosis is due to an obstructive uropathy or whether the hydronephrosis is non-obstructive in nature. Nuclear medicine scans are non-invasive functional studies that utilize radiopharmaceuticals. Typically, Technetium-99m (99mTc) mercaptoacetyltriglycine (MAG$_3$) is used as it is renally excreted and can be combined with a diuretic challenge to optimize distension of a large dilated renal pelvis [3]. Another functional study to diagnosis obstruction is the largely historical Whitaker test [4]. It requires the presence of nephrostomy and urethral catheter, which limits its applicability. It is a form of invasive urodynamics of the upper urinary tract to determine the presence of obstructive uropathy by measuring the renal pelvic pressure as well as the flow rate of saline infused via the nephrostomy. High intra-pelvic pressure associated with a slow flow rate is indicative of obstruction.

3.5 Consequences of Obstruction

Ureteric obstruction results in a series of pathophysiological events that ultimately, if left untreated, lead on to obstructive nephropathy. The specific pathological changes that occur during upper tract obstruction depend on the nature of the obstruction and particularly whether this is acute or chronic in nature.

Obstruction results in changes affecting the collecting system and ureter (obstructive uropathy) and parenchyma (obstructive nephropathy).

3.5.1 Obstructive Uropathy

3.5.1.1 Acute

With acute obstruction, such as a ureteric calculus or inadvertent operative ligation, the obstruction is usually both high grade or complete and of rapid onset. Ureteral pressure rises quickly with ureteral smooth muscle spasm and stretching of mechanoreceptors proximal to the point of obstruction [5]. Distension of the ureter and renal pelvis results in spinothalamic pain fiber excitation and the perception of pain as the characteristic renal colic. These effects are potentiated by prostaglandins and other kinins, which is why non-steroidal anti-inflammatory drugs are very effective for renal colic [6, 7]. On occasion, very rapid onset of a high-grade obstruction may result in a forniceal rupture with disruption of the junction of the collecting system and renal parenchyma. This occurs because the muscle and elastic connective tissue in the ureteric wall are unable to accommodate the flow rapidly enough, and consequently, high pressures are transmitted directly to this point [8]. Forniceal rupture leads to extravasation of urine into the perinephric space – rapidly reducing collecting system pressure. Consequently US may not delineate the clinical scenario due to difficulties detecting extravasated urine. Contrast imaging, however, may demonstrate contrast within the perinephric space associated with minimal pelvicalyceal dilatation.

3.5.1.2 Chronic

Typically, chronic obstruction, associated with more insidious changes, results from mural or extra-mural obstruction with examples including strictures, malignancy, or other forms of extrinsic compression. Ureteral pressure initially increases slowly. The ureteric wall deforms, accommodating the slowly rising pressure, which results in hydroureter. These effects may be mediated by the stimulation of nitric oxide release [9]. As urine production continues, pressure further increases with proximal progression of dilatation and hydronephrosis. As dilatation of the renal pelvis progresses, the calyces also dilate becoming clubbed in appearance. This stretches the renal papillae and they eventually develop ischemia. With time the deformation of the ureter results in ureteric lengthening and tortuosity, which together with substantial pelvicalyceal dilatation are the typical features of chronic obstruction.

Without relief of the obstruction, irreversible changes in ureteral wall dynamics occur. Ureteral smooth muscle initially hypertrophies but with persisting obstruction ischemia occurs resulting in fibrotic connective-tissue deposition within the wall impairing compliance and contractility [10]. At this point, even with relief of obstruction, the ureteric wall does not return to its normal caliber. This explains persisting hydroureter and hydronephrosis following resolution of the obstruction. This is a common and sometimes challenging dilemma post pyeloplasty where hydronephrosis and sluggish drainage on functional imaging persist post treatment.

3.5.2 Obstructive Nephropathy

Ureteric obstruction may precipitate changes within the renal parenchyma, including inflammation, tubular atrophy, and interstitial fibrosis with nephron loss, and ultimately, irreversible damage. The mechanisms underlying this have been extrapolated from laboratory animal studies measuring renal blood flow, histological changes, and biochemical changes following iatrogenic obstruction.

With animal models, studies have employed unilateral and complete ureteric obstruction – with the key physiological events shown in Table 3.2. Figure 3.1 depicts the relationship of renal blood flow in afferent and efferent arterioles and renal tubular pressure during unilateral ureteric obstruction (UUO).

In clinical practice, obstruction of this nature is uncommon with partial obstruction, which is either acute or chronic in nature, which is a more common scenario.

Table 3.2 Key events in unilateral ureteric obstruction (UUO).

Obstructive event
- Resulting increase in intra-ureteral pressure
- Hydrostatic pressure is transmitted retrograde to the renal tubules
- Glomerular filtration rate (GFR) declines

Acute hyperemic response
- An increase in renal blood flow maintains GFR countering the increased hydrostatic pressure in Bowman's capsule
  - This is mediated by afferent arteriole vasodilation
- This hyperemic response lasts a few hours [15]

Chronic phase
- Renal tubule pressure continues to rise and with this GFR reduces
- Reduction in renal blood flow to non-filtering cortical glomeruli, this results in a global reduction in renal blood flow [17]
- This reduces GFR and mitigates the effects of the increasing tubular pressure
  - This mediated by the renin-angiotensin pathway and vasoconstriction of afferent arterioles [13]
- Some of the obstructed urine flows out of the collecting system via hilar lymphatics and back into circulation and eventually excreted by the other kidney
- Micro-ruptures of the collecting system occur as the tubular lining stretch and atrophy releasing some urine into the interstitium

Irreversible phase
- Under-perfusion and ischemia lead to interstitial fibrosis.
- The glomeruli, interstitium, and tubules are replaced with connective and scar tissue in response to the insult and the renal function is permanently lost
- The contra-lateral kidney undergoes compensatory hypertrophy

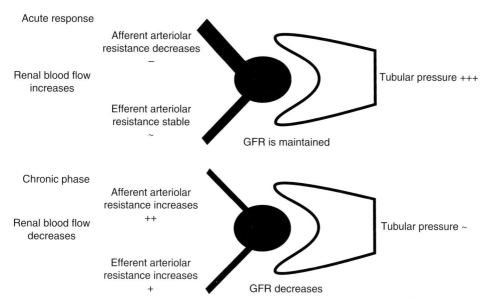

Figure 3.1 Renal blood flow, GFR and tubular pressure during UUO.

Acute obstruction, even if incomplete, will result in a rapid pressure rise within the ureter and collecting system, and thus, has some parallels with experimental models. Chronic obstruction, either unilateral or bilateral, is a gradual process, with intra-luminal and collecting system pressures rising slowly and often marginally.

Consequently, the pathophysiological changes defined experimentally may not entirely reflect those in many clinical scenarios. Nevertheless, as the histological changes seen in both are similar, the processes defined experimentally are likely to be valid explanations from a clinical perspective.

Obstruction of the kidney results in an initial rise in pressure proximal to the obstruction due to ongoing glomerular filtration at this point. This pressure rise is transmitted to renal tubular structures with several consequences [11]. Increased proximal tubular pressure reduces the hydraulic pressure gradient across the glomerular basement membrane reducing filtration. Mechanical stretching of tubular epithelium associated with tubular pressure rise activates the renin-angiotensin system with production of angiotensin II the active end product of this system [12, 13]. Other vasoactive compounds including endothelin-1 (ET-1) and inflammatory cytokines are also upregulated [14]. These include a number controlling cell cycle (e.g., caspases, intrinsic and extrinsic death pathway molecules, inhibitors of cyclin-dependent kinases p27 and p21, reactive oxygen species, and catalase), hypoxic response (HIF- α), epithelial-mesenchymal transformation (e.g., hepatocyte growth factor, bone morphogenic protein 7 m and nestin), and the upregulation of additional cytokines and growth factors (e.g., TGFβ-1, EGF, PDGF, VEGFm and TNF-α) as well as chemokines (MCP-1, osteopontin, IL-1, ICAM-1, VCAM-1, and selectins) [11, 14].

Nitric oxide (NO) production is also stimulated by tubular stretching [9]. As a vasodilatory cytokine, it is the likely mediator of the increase in renal blood flow that occurs in the very early phase of obstruction [15]. This effect is transient and subsequently overwhelmed by the release of angiotensin II and other vasoactive agents, which mediate intra-renal vasoconstriction, which reduces glomerular blood flow. This significantly reduces glomerular filtration, and thus, intra-tubular pressure over the course of several hours [16]. With persisting obstruction, renal vascular resistance remains elevated with ongoing tubular ischemia [17].

Inflammatory cells, and specifically macrophages, are recruited into the renal interstitium following obstruction – initially by activation of the renin-angiotensin system and subsequently by the influence of tubular-derived chemokines [14]. Additional recruitment of macrophages then occurs by autocrine mechanisms as several cytokines, chemokines, and their receptors are upregulated by the infiltrating inflammatory cells [18]. As a consequence, interstitial fibroblast numbers increase. These are derived through a combination of proliferation of existing interstitial fibroblasts, as well as cytokine-/chemokine-mediated renal homing of circulating bone marrow-derived fibroblasts, as well as transformation of tubular epithelial cells, endothelial cells, and pericytes into interstitial fibroblasts [19]. With activation these variously derived interstitial fibroblasts increase synthesis of extracellular matrix (ECM) proteins. In conjunction with this, fibrinolytic pathways are inhibited, enhancing the deposition of extracellular matrix protein (Figure 3.2).

The pathways outlined following obstruction with changes in intra-tubular pressure and secondary ischemia result in a cascade of inter-related pathological events comprising tubulo-interstitial inflammation, tubular cell death, and fibrosis.

3.5.2.1 Tubulo-Interstitial Inflammation

Cytokine release following the changes in intra-renal blood flow leads to inflammatory changes with interstitial infiltration by macrophages (Figure 3.3). This progressively increases after several hours after obstruction and may persist for several weeks. The mediators of this inflammatory response include Angiotensin II (AngII), tumor necrosis factor-alpha (TNFα), and nuclear transcription factor-kappaB (NF-κB).

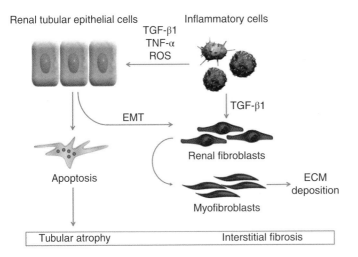

Figure 3.2 Renal cell types involved in the pathogenesis and progression of obstructive nephropathy. ECM: extracellular matrix; EMT: epithelial to mesenchymal transition; TGF- β1: transforming growth factor- β1; TNF-: tumor necrosis factor-; ROS: reactive oxygen species. *Source*: Lucarelli, et al., [18] http://www.hindawi.com/journals/bmri/2014/303298/. Used under CC-BY 3.0 https://creativecommons.org/licenses/by/3.0/.

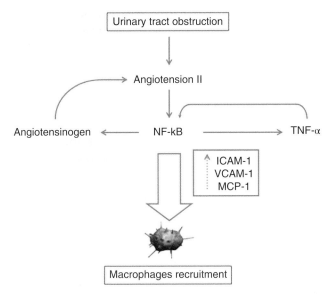

Figure 3.3 Autocrine-reinforcing loops amplifying angiotensin II (ANG II) and tumor necrosis factor- α (TNF- α) signaling. NF-kB: nuclear factor kappa-light-chain-enhancer of activated B cells; ICAM-1: intercellular adhesion molecule-1; MCP-1: monocyte chemotactic protein-1; VCAM-1: vascular cell adhesion molecule-1. *Source*: Lucarelli, et al., [18] http://www.hindawi.com/journals/bmri/2014/303298/. Used under CC-BY 3.0 https://creativecommons.org/licenses/by/3.0/.

A dramatic upregulation of adhesion molecules (ICAM-1 and VCAM-1) also occurs mediating macrophage adhesion and local proliferation. Macrophages themselves release cytokines and growth factors, which contribute to the ongoing cascade apoptosis and tubulo-interstitial fibrosis [14].

3.5.2.2 Tubular Cell Death

In contrast to severe direct vascular injury, tubular cell death following obstruction is felt, which is related to apoptosis. The initial trigger for this is the mechanical stretching of tubular epithelium, initiating an apoptotic-related cytokine expression as shown in Figure 3.4. This is an active energy-dependent form of cell death (cell suicide), which is triggered or accelerated by metabolic stress and inflammation. It is accelerated in tubular cells as interstitial inflammation compounds the metabolic stress of changes in blood flow and mechanical stretching. Tubular apoptosis begins within 24 hours of obstruction, whereas within interstitial cells, this commences several days later.

Factors contributing to apoptosis include AngII, TNF, and other inflammatory cytokines, as well as the oxidative stress and ATP depletion provoked by blood flow changes. Mechanical stretch on tubular epithelium may also provoke intracellular apoptotic pathways. Endogenous NO production, which is also activated, confers some protection from apoptosis and contributes to the reversibility of damage if obstruction is relieved before established interstitial damage has occurred [9, 20].

3.5.2.3 Tubulo-Interstitial Fibrosis

Progressive interstitial fibrosis is the ultimate cause of obstructive nephropathy. This is characterized by increased numbers of activated fibroblasts and diffuse accumulation of extra-cellular matrix (ECM) components, such as collagen, proteoglycans,

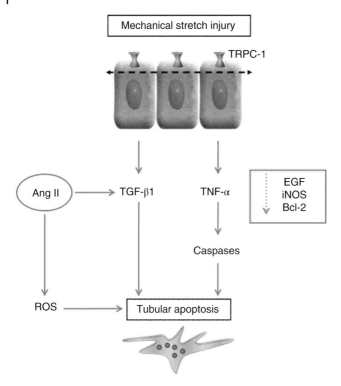

Figure 3.4 Pathogenesis of renal tubular apoptosis in obstructive nephropathy. Ang II: angiotensin II; EGF: epidermal growth factor; iNOS: inducible NO synthase; ROS: reactive oxygen species; TRPC-1: transient receptor potential cationic channel-1. *Source*: Lucarelli, et al., [18] http://www.hindawi.com/ journals/bmri/2014/303298/. Used under CC-BY 3.0 https://creativecommons.org/licenses/by/3.0/.

and fibronectin. The key events of fibroblast activation, epithelial-mesenchymal transition (EMT), and ECM accumulation begin to occur within several days of obstruction [19]. Fibroblast accumulation is clearly apparent after approximately 7 days of obstruction with evidence of deposition of active collagen and other components of ECM within 2 weeks.

3.6 Post-Obstructive Outcomes

Recovery of renal function depends primarily on the extent and the duration of the obstruction. With early intervention the sequence of events associated with ureteric obstruction may be truncated. Interventions can broadly be divided into initial drainage and then definitive options for management of the obstruction. Initial drainage of an upper tract obstruction is a temporizing measure to address an immediate clinical situation. This may be dictated by clinical emergency, including sepsis, acute renal failure, and also uncontrolled pain. It must also be considered in the absence of these problems as an urgent intervention to minimize irreversible parenchymal damage.

This is particularly the case with acute obstruction, and even more so if high grade or complete. In these scenarios the sudden and dramatic changes in pressure rapidly invoke the downstream events described above and irreversible parenchymal damage.

This contrasts with chronic, more incomplete obstruction. With this, the gradual distension of the collecting system buffers any dramatic or sudden pressure rise, which is far less threatening in terms of parenchymal consequences and damage in the short to intermediate term.

3.6.1 Parenchymal Damage and Functional Loss

The extent of tubular injury fundamentally underpins the degree of parenchymal and functional loss. If the tubular basement membranes remain intact at the time obstruction is relieved, which can be the case with acute ischemic injury related to pre-renal factors, acute high-grade obstruction of short duration and low pressure chronic obstruction epithelial recovery and repopulation will restore function. Once the inflammatory response, however, is sufficiently established tubular basement membranes become progressively disrupted as consequences of the inflammatory response and structural integrity were lost. Subsequent inflammation and fibrosis with ECM deposition result in both luminal obliteration and complete loss of glomerular function.

Animal studies have shown that in complete iatrogenic UUO in dogs there was full functional renal recovery at 2 weeks but no recovery of renal function beyond this time [21]. In humans, recovery of renal function after obstruction is more difficult to define. This relates to the individual variability of circumstances and response to obstruction. With complete obstruction, such as that seen with ureteric ligation, significant and irretrievable loss of function is likely to occur within days. Complete loss of function may occur within a relatively short time after this without relief of obstruction.

In clinical practice, complete obstruction is rare with an acute presentation. For example, in calculus disease, acute obstruction is generally only partial, even if high grade, and intermittent. Similarly with low pressure bilateral obstruction, significant recovery of renal function can occur even in the presence of significant renal dysfunction at the time of presentation [22]. Consequently, the extent and degree of permanent parenchymal damage represents a continuum from almost complete recovery to total loss of function. The latter is associated with diffuse parenchymal fibrosis with extensive tubular and interstitial fibrosis and loss of glomerular function. With lesser degrees of chronic damage, renal function may initially be adequate but impaired. This, however, may be associated with hyperfiltration injury, typically with a GFR of <30 ml/min, resulting in ongoing damage and progressive insidious ongoing damage over time, despite relief of obstruction [23]. Patients with GFR >30 ml/min following relief of obstruction, the presence of proteinuria and microalbuminemia are markers of risk for subsequent ongoing changes and decline in renal function [23].

3.6.2 Post Obstructive Diuresis

Post obstructive diuresis may occur following relief of bilateral ureteric obstruction or obstruction of a functionally solitary kidney [24, 25]. It does not occur in unilateral ureteric obstruction with a functional contralateral kidney. This is typically associated with relief of obstruction when tubular cell injury has been incomplete or sublethal and significant glomerular loss has not occurred. Providing tubular basement membranes are intact, epithelial cells will recover and repopulate allowing return of function. This scenario occurs in low-pressure bilateral partial chronic obstruction or acute high-grade obstruction of a solitary kidney (or both kidneys). Tubules remain intact populated by viable but functionally compromised tubular epithelium.

Post-obstructive diuresis comprises two components:

1. Physiological

If fluid retention has occurred a physiological diuresis can occur to excrete excess water and solutes. The latter includes urea, which may exert an osmotic diuretic effect [24]. Relief of obstruction usually leads to rapid restoration of glomerular filtration, which is reduced with obstruction. Consequently, the physiological diuresis related to fluid overload and an osmotic diuresis may be relatively short lived [26].

2. Pathological

Tubular epithelial injury results in impaired membrane fluxes of tubular cells. This specifically impacts on the counter current mechanisms within the Loop of Henle limiting fluid and electrolyte resorption from glomerular filtrate. Injury also reduces the sensitivity of tubular cells to antidiuretic hormone (ADH) [24, 26]. Increased serum osmolarity stimulates hypothalamic release of ADH, which normally stimulates fluid reabsorption by epithelial cells of the distal nephron and collecting ducts. Lack of response to ADH thus further disrupts the concentration of urine.

The pathological component of post obstructive diuresis thus persists for much longer than would be expected with a purely physiological diuresis. This results in ongoing fluid and electrolyte loss resulting in dehydration, hyponatremia and hypokalemia.

With time, tubular cell recovery and regeneration occurs although varies considerably in clinical practice [25]. In managing this, fluid and electrolyte balance is critical with the need for replacement ranging from days to weeks. This requires clinical skill, as recovery of tubular function occurs to ensure that replacement therapy does not prolong the process by potentiating a physiological diuresis.

3.7 Summary

Upper urinary tract obstruction occurs because of intra-luminal or mural (both intra-mural or extra-mural) ureteric pathology and some lower urinary tract conditions. The clinical presentation is dependent on the nature of the obstruction and the etiology. An obstructed kidney undergoes characteristic pathophysiological changes, which eventually result in obstructive nephropathy reflecting intra-renal ischemia, inflammation, and fibrosis. Timely diagnosis and subsequent drainage can prevent deterioration and promote recovery, allowing definitive management of the underlying pathological process.

References

[1] Iyasere O, Xu G, Harris K. Urinary tract obstruction. Br J Hosp Med (Lond). 2012;73(12):696–700.

[2] Emad-Eldin S, Abdelaziz O, El-Diasty TA. Diagnostic value of combined static-excretory MR Urography in children with hydronephrosis. J Adv Res. 2015;6(2):145–53.

[3] Taylor AT. Radionuclides in nephrourology, Part 2: pitfalls and diagnostic applications. J Nucl Med. 2014;55(5):786–98.

[4] Lupton EW, George NJ. The Whitaker test: 35 years on. BJU Int. 2010;105(1):94–100.

[5] Tillig B, Mutschke O, Rolle U, Gaunitz U, Asmussen G, Constantinou CE. Effects of artificial obstruction on the function of the upper urinary tract of Guinea pigs, rats and pigs. Eur J Pediatr Surg. 2004;14(5):303–15.

[6] Allen JT, Vaughan ED, Jr., Gillenwater JY. The effect of indomethacin on renal blood flow and uretral pressure in unilateral ureteral obstruction in a awake dogs. Invest Urol. 1978;15(4):324–7.

[7] Davenport K, Timoney AG, Keeley FX. Conventional and alternative methods for providing analgesia in renal colic. BJU Int. 2005;95(3):297–300.

[8] Gershman B, Kulkarni N, Sahani DV, Eisner BH. Causes of renal forniceal rupture. BJU Int. 2011;108(11):1909–11; discussion 12.

[9] Yoo KH, Thornhill BA, Forbes MS, Chevalier RL. Inducible nitric oxide synthase modulates hydronephrosis following partial or complete unilateral ureteral obstruction in the neonatal mouse. Am J Physiol Renal Physiol. 2010;298(1):F62–71.

[10] Dinlenc CZ, Liatsikos EN, Smith AD. Ureteral ischemia model: an explanation of ureteral dysfunction after chronic obstruction. J Endourol. 2002;16(1):47–50.

[11] Truong LD, Gaber L, Eknoyan G. Obstructive uropathy. Contrib Nephrol. 2011;169:311–26.

[12] Rohatgi R, Flores D. Intratubular hydrodynamic forces influence tubulointerstitial fibrosis in the kidney. Curr Opin Nephrol Hypertens. 2010;19(1):65–71.

[13] Frokiaer J, Djurhuus JC, Nielsen M, Pedersen EB. Renal hemodynamic response to ureteral obstruction during converting enzyme inhibition. Urol Res. 1996;24(4):217–27.

[14] Grande MT, Perez-Barriocanal F, Lopez-Novoa JM. Role of inflammation in tubulo-interstitial damage associated to obstructive nephropathy. J Inflamm (Lond). 2010;7:19.

[15] Moody TE, Vaughn ED, Jr., Gillenwater JY. Relationship between renal blood flow and ureteral pressure during 18 hours of total unilateral uretheral occlusion. Implications for changing sites of increased renal resistance. Invest Urol. 1975;13(3):246–51.

[16] Gaudio KM, Siegel NJ, Hayslett JP, Kashgarian M. Renal perfusion and intratubular pressure during ureteral occlusion in the rat. Am J Physiol. 1980;238(3):F205–9.

[17] Harris RH, Yarger WE. Renal function after release of unilateral ureteral obstruction in rats. Am J Physiol. 1974;227(4):806–15.

[18] Lucarelli G, Mancini V, Galleggiante V, Rutigliano M, Vavallo A, Battaglia M, et al. Emerging urinary markers of renal injury in obstructive nephropathy. Biomed Res Int. 2014;2014:303–298.

[19] Chevalier RL, Forbes MS, Thornhill BA. Ureteral obstruction as a model of renal interstitial fibrosis and obstructive nephropathy. Kidney Int. 2009;75(11):1145–52.

[20] Felsen D, Schulsinger D, Gross SS, Kim FY, Marion D, Vaughan ED, Jr. Renal hemodynamic and ureteral pressure changes in response to ureteral obstruction: the role of nitric oxide. J Urol. 2003;169(1):373–6.

[21] Vaughan ED, Jr., Shenasky JH, 2nd, Gillenwater JY. Mechanism of acute hemodynamic response to ureteral occlusion. Invest Urol. 1971;9(2):109–18.

[22] Organ M, Norman RW. Acute reversible kidney injury secondary to bilateral ureteric obstruction. Can Urol Assoc J. 2011;5(6):392–6.

[23] Cachat F, Combescure C, Chehade H, Zeier G, Mosig D, Meyrat B, et al. Microalbuminuria and hyperfiltration in subjects with nephro-urological disorders. Nephrol Dial Transplant. 2013;28(2):386–91.

[24] Harris RH, Yarger WE. The pathogenesis of post-obstructive diuresis. The role of circulating natriuretic and diuretic factors, including urea. J Clin Invest. 1975;56(4):880–7.

[25] Hamdi A, Hajage D, Van Glabeke E, Belenfant X, Vincent F, Gonzalez F, et al. Severe post-renal acute kidney injury, post-obstructive diuresis and renal recovery. BJU Int. 2012;110(11 Pt C):E1027-34.

[26] Gulmi FA, Matthews GJ, Marion D, von Lutterotti N, Vaughan ED. Volume expansion enhances the recovery of renal function and prolongs the diuresis and natriuresis after release of bilateral ureteral obstruction: a possible role for atrial natriuretic peptide. J Urol. 1995;153(4):1276–83.

4

Physiology of the Human Ureter

Robin Cole

Consultant Urological Surgeon, Ashford and St Peter's Hospitals NHS Foundation Trust, Chertsey, Surrey, UK

4.1   Historical Introduction

> *"Where observation is concerned, chance favours only the prepared mind."*
> —*Louis Pasteur (1822–1895)*
> From the address given on the inauguration of the Faculty of Science, University of Lille, December 7, 1854

Despite the considerable advances in the treatment of urinary tract stone disease, there remains a paucity of knowledge regarding the physiology of human ureteric smooth muscle. Such an understanding may allow for the development of mechanisms that may modify ureteric contractility to enhance the passage of ureteric stones. The mechanism by which the pain of ureteric colic is generated is often misunderstood and assumptions are passed down through the literature without clear scientific evidence, although the author demonstrated the effectiveness of non-steroidal drugs in the treatment of ureteric colic over a quarter of a century ago [1]. The driving force at that time to expand knowledge of the physiology of the upper urinary tract was the advent of extracorporeal shockwave lithotripsy as a means of fragmenting human kidney stones in vivo where the ultimate success of treatment was governed by the safe passage of stone fragments from the upper urinary tract [2]. The fundamental principle in managing acute ureteric obstruction caused by stones or stone fragments relates to the balance between the likelihood of spontaneous stone passage and the development of complications such as continuing pain, loss of renal function, and the development of infection within an obstructed system.

A complete understanding of the whole upper urinary tract is vital if pharmacological manipulation is to be developed for clinical benefit. Any treatment modality, which can increase the likelihood of stone passage is important for several reasons. Ureteric colic is a very common urological emergency and readmission rates are high for patients treated conservatively. The cost implications are obvious. The pain of ureteric colic is intense, unpredictable, and the ensuing complications can be profound and serious with the need for emergency intervention. There is undoubtedly a fear factor of ureteric colic among stone formers, which leads some to carry diclofenac suppositories and

Ureteric Stenting, First Edition. Edited by Ravi Kulkarni.

other analgesics for emergencies. While these sufferers understand the importance of fluid intake and avoidance of dehydration, there is a pharmaceutical vacuum when it comes to medication, which might promote the spontaneous passage of stones. Furthermore, stone disease itself is most prevalent in the working population. Travel can also become an issue in this group of patients. In addition, there is a belief that stone disease is becoming encountered more in the elderly population. This may be a consequence of improved imaging where non-contrast CT is the modality of choice for stone diagnosis. Furthermore, the widespread and sometimes over-enthusiastic use of modern imaging often reveals the presence of multiple asymptomatic abnormalities including urinary tract stone disease. This creeping universal change in investigative practice has now reached epidemic proportions and represents a significant and previously unrecognized addition to the cost of delivering healthcare.

There has been some evidence that by relaxing ureteric smooth muscle by alpha 1 receptor blockade or calcium channel pump inhibitors the likelihood of spontaneous stone passage is increased and the need for interventional procedures reduced. This treatment has been termed *medical expulsive therapy* and has become the adopted recommended standard of care for some patients with ureteric stones where conservative management is thought to be the initial treatment of choice. However, a recent multi-center, randomized, placebo-controlled trial has shown that tamsulosin and nifedipine are ineffective at decreasing the need for further intervention to achieve stone clearance within 4 weeks for patients with ureteric colic treated conservatively [3]. This high-quality study has cast doubt on the present concept of medical expulsive therapy generated by previously relatively small, single-center, low- to moderate-quality trials and variability in trial design with differing inclusion criteria and outcome measurement. However, the authors of this publication did acknowledge that the study may have been underpowered to detect a statistical difference between the clinical outcome of patients in the treatment arms and placebo group for larger stones (>5 mm) [4]. It must also be accepted that studies of this type are very difficult to construct and interpret simply because of the heterogeneous nature of urinary stones and the functional variability in the anatomy and physiology of the upper urinary tract. In the late 1980s, attempts were made to understand the optimal conditions, which would enhance the passage of stone fragments following extra-corporeal shockwave lithotripsy (ESWL) but these studies failed to come to fruition for those very reasons (Cole, R.S., unpublished observations).

New and alternative avenues of pharmacological manipulation of the ureter need to be explored particularly as human ureteric smooth muscle is relatively inert and largely outside the control of the autonomic nervous system. The first and fundamental question will revolve the nature of physiological change best suited to medical expulsive therapy. There has been an acceptance that smooth muscle relaxation is needed to increase the likelihood of stone passage, but the alternative, achieved by increasing the intensity of ureteric peristalsis, needs to be considered and the concept of a ureteric inotrope needs to be explored [5].

In this chapter the author will endeavour to explore what is known about the physiological properties of human ureteric smooth muscle, and relating these to ureteric colic, provide an arena that may lead to the discovery of promising new drugs that could be useful in relieving the pain of ureteric colic, increasing the likelihood spontaneous stone passage and facilitating the successful outcome of ureteroscopy as well as acting as an adjuvant for extracorporeal shockwave lithotripsy. The use of invasive ureteric stenting has played a pivotal role in all these aspects of stone management.

4.2   The Pain and Myths of Ureteric Colic

While those who have experienced ureteric colic describe it as the worst possible pain of all, its character is not that of a true colic as described by patients with small bowel colic secondary to bowel obstruction. Small bowel colic gives rise to cramping rhythmic and intermittent spasms of pain lasting a few minutes. It comes in peaks and depressions and the pain disappears completely during a trough. The pain of ureteric colic tends to build in a continuous manner to reach an agonizing and constant crescendo when there maybe an exacerbation of pain but importantly it never disappears.

In a very recent publication, ureteric colic was defined as an episodic severe abdominal pain from "sustained contraction of ureteric muscle" as a kidney stone passes down the ureter into the bladder [3]. This definition was referenced from a review article, which did not cite any scientific references for the statement [6]. The pain of ureteric colic has nothing to do with spasmodic contractions of ureteric smooth muscle, but relates specifically to ureteric obstruction with the rate of change of tension in the walls of the renal pelvis as the specific pain-provoking factor.

In 1954, Risholm postulated that the pain of ureteric colic resulted from acute upper urinary tract obstruction leading to distension and an increase of tension in the walls of the ureter and renal pelvis. Pain identical to ureteric colic could be evoked by inflating an obstructing balloon catheter within the ureter of conscious patients. Local distension of the ureter by a non-obstructing balloon (analogous to a doughnut) evoked discomfort of minor importance [7]. This hypothesis has subsequently been supported by a number of investigators. Kiil considered that the onset of pain was related to the rate of rise of pressure rise within the upper urinary tract [8]. In an elegant radiological study, Bretland demonstrated that the pain of ureteric colic occurred only in the presence of ureteric obstruction and subsided when the obstructing element, usually a stone, was removed [9]. Michaelson measured intra-pelvic pressure by means of percutaneous needle puncture and noted in two patients with ureteric colic that severe flank pain was simultaneously associated with highly elevated pelvic pressures [10]. It is commonly observed by those carrying out radiological studies via nephrostomy tubes in conscious patients that the rate of contrast instillation is the critical determinant in precipitating loin pain. Rapid infusion elicits pain, whereas a larger volume infused slowly give rise only to a mild awareness.

The current guidelines from the British Association of Urological recommend oral or parenteral diclofenac as the analgesic of choice for the treatment of patients with acute ureteric colic. It has been known historically for many years that non-steroidal anti-inflammatory drugs (NSAIDs) are effective in the treatment of ureteric colic [11–13]. Clinical studies have reported adequate pain relief in 80–90% of patients. Indeed, in a study from 1984, prophylactic indomethacin given for 7 days following an attack of ureteric colic reduced the frequency of recurrent attacks of colic and the total duration of recurrent pain without influencing stone passage [14]. A further study showed indomethacin to be effective in the prophylactic treatment of ureteric colic following extracorporeal shockwave lithotripsy [1]. Animal studies have clearly demonstrated that following acute unilateral ureteric obstruction, there is an initial increase in renal blood flow lasting 1–2 hours associated with a marked elevation in ipsilateral ureteric pressure [15]. It has been suggested that this initial hyperaemic response is mediated by prostaglandins as prior administration with indomethacin eliminates the response and the rise in ureteric pressure is less and slower than in untreated animals [16, 17].

The actions of increased synthesis and release of local prostaglandins, diuresis, and local afferent vasodilatation aggravates the already rising pressure in the renal pelvis, and therefore, the rate of change of tension in the walls of the real pelvis, which is considered to be the important pain-provoking factor. Hence it is suggested that the NSAIDs provide pain relief by blocking the normal physiological response to ureteric obstruction.

However, although this proposed mechanism of pain relief by the prostaglandin synthetase inhibitors can be neatly accommodated in the likely sequence of events giving rise to ureteric colic, the physiological consequences of widespread prostaglandin synthesis inhibition are complicated and other factors may be important in influencing the tension changes in the renal pelvis. Ureteric stones vary hugely in appearance, chemical, and crystalline composition with variable stone fragility. The vast majority are far from smooth "glass marbles," being rough and spiculated with scalloped edges [18]. Stone passage through the ureter causes significant inflammatory reactions of the urothelium and lamina propria, and this is an important factor aggravating spontaneous stone passage. The difficulties of maneuvering a ureteroscope past an impacted stone with a dense distal inflammatory stricture can make the procedure hazardous and unpredictable. The NSAIDs may act to reduce the inflammatory response and therefore may contribute to the lowering of renal pelvic pressure with a reduction in pain. The intrinsic hysteresis loops generated by the visco-elastic properties of the upper urinary tract are such that a very small seepage of urine past an obstructing stone results in a rapid and profound fall in intra-pelvic pressure. A similar analogy is observed in patients suffering the pain of acute urinary retention when catheter drainage of the first few milliliters of urine results in an immediate relief of pain.

In addition, in vitro studies of human ureteric smooth muscle have provided convincing evidence that both endogenous and exogenesis prostaglandin can profoundly influence the contractility of human ureteric smooth muscle [19]. Whilst the extrapolation of in vitro finding to a clinical situation can only be speculative, evidence is presented to suggest that prostaglandin synthetase inhibitors have a direct effect upon ureteric function and this in itself would have beneficial effects in terms of pain relief because of relaxation and the intrinsic nature of hysteresis loops of tension and pressure generated by ureteric smooth muscle.

4.3   Anatomical and Functional Studies

The essential function of the ureter is to transport urine from the kidney to the bladder. This is accomplished, under normal conditions, by peristaltic waves resulting from coordinated contractions of the various components of the ureteric musculature. Electrical activity, in the form of action potentials, originating in the primary pacemaker located in the proximal portion of the collecting system precede and initiate the peristaltic contraction and are propagated in an antegrade direction from cell to cell via low resistance electrical pathways allowing the ureter to behave as a functional syncitium. The normal ureter consists essentially of three layers: transitional cell urothelium with its supporting lamina propria, a muscle coat, and an outer adventitial layer of connective tissue. The muscle coat is 750 to 800 um thick and composed of bundles of tightly packed smooth muscle cells separated by large amounts of collagen and elastic fibrils. These bundles are not arranged in distinct layers, as in the gut, but form a complex interwoven and interconnected meshwork. The individual smooth muscle cells make up the primary functioning anatomical unit of the ureter. These cells are spindle shaped 250 to 400 um in length and 5–7 um in diameter. Within the cytoplasm of these cells can be seen longitudinally orientated myofilaments consisting of the contractile proteins, actin and myosin, which constitute the basic machinery responsible for cellular contraction [20]. Electron-dense bodies beneath the plasma membrane anchor the myofilaments. Flask shaped infoldings of the plasma membrane, the caveolae, increase the surface area of the cell and associated with the infolding are sacs of sarcoplasmic reticulum, which may play a role in controlling calcium movements within the cell.

The individual smooth muscle cells become intimately related to each other at specialised junctions [21]. These areas of close approach may serve as low-resistance pathways allowing electrical activity to be conducted throughout the cellular syncitium. Other junctions may provide mechanical linkage between the cells: peg and socket junctions and intermediate junctions [22]. The role of the autonomic nervous system in ureteric peristalsis has been a matter of controversy for over 100 years. Englemann [23] proposed that ureteric peristalsis was myogenic in origin on the basis that autonomic ganglia were absent from smooth muscle several animal species. In the human ureter ganglia have been identified but only in the adventitia in association with Waldeyer's sheath [24]. Nevertheless, there is substantial evidence to support Englemann's original hypothesis of myogenic conduction. Firstly, the action potentials associated with ureteric peristalsis and the rate of propagation is not compatible with nerve fibre conduction [25]. Secondly, although there is a rich, irregular network of nerve fibers in the adventitia, the "Grundplexus of Engelmann," the number of fibers and distribution of terminal axons in the muscle layer is inadequate and only rarely are terminal axons containing synaptic vesicles seen to run between the muscle bundles and lie in close proximity to the smooth muscle cells. Electron microscopy studies have demonstrated the very occasional ureteric muscle synapse. It seems therefore that only a very small proportion of ureteric muscle cells are innervated by autonomic nerves and even at these regions morphological specialisation of the post-synaptic membrane has not been demonstrated. Lastly, ureteric peristalsis persists after renal transplantation [26], denervation [27], reversal of a segment in situ [28], and in vitro isolated segments [29].

A further network of nerve fibers can be identified extending from the inner surface of the muscle layer toward the base of the urothelium in the lamina propria. These nerve terminals are probably afferent or sensory endings [21]. Some workers, using in vitro physiological techniques have provided evidence for the presence of excitatory alpha-adrenergic and inhibitory beta-adrenergic receptors in ureteric muscle [30, 31], and to lesser extent cholinergic receptors [32]. The functional significance of these receptors is unclear and controversial.

While the autonomic nervous system would seem relatively unimportant in ureteric contraction it provides the fundamental control of normal physiological contraction in the bladder.

4.4   Ureteric Transport Mechanisms

It has long been considered that the prime stimulus to ureteric contraction is the content of urine in its lumen, the empty ureter lies quiescent [33].

Under normal conditions regular, coordinated contractions of ureteric smooth muscle are responsible for the transport of urine from the kidney to the bladder. As the renal pelvis fills with urine, the intra-pelvic pressure rises and urine is extruded into the upper ureter, where it is formed into a bolus. The bolus, lying within a passive non-contracting segment of ureter, is propelled toward the bladder by the ureteric peristaltic wave [34]. Efficient propulsion of the bolus is dependent upon the ability of the ureter to completely coapt its wall. The resting intra-ureteric pressure is approximately 0–5 cm water with superimposed pressure waves of 20–80 cm water occurring during each ureteric contraction. At normal flows the peristaltic waves occur two to six times per minute [35].

Bozler [36] was the first to demonstrate using electrically placed surface electrodes, that under normal conditions, each ureteric contraction was preceded by an electrical event, the action potential. An action potential describes a discrete electrical event consisting of a regenerative depolarisation and repolarization occurring across the membrane of an electrically excitable cell. This event may occur spontaneously or as a result of an external stimulus, such as stretch, applied electrical stimulation, receptor activation by neurotransmitters or drugs, or an adjacent action potential spreading from an already excited cell. The initiation of an action potential is an all or none phenomenon and once generated can be propagated allowing synchronised electrical excitation to occur between electrical cellular connections. Other tissue factors will influence the speed and magnitude of these events but the sequence results in a synchronised contraction of the ureteric musculature. In the ureter, under normal physiological conditions, the pacemaker cells within the minor calyces trigger the generation of the spreading action potential by spontaneous slow depolarization that ultimately reaches a critical level, the threshold potential. Hence the peristaltic contraction waves originates in the most proximal part of the upper urinary tract, probably at one of the several spontaneously active calyceal pacemaker sites and are transmitted to the renal pelvis and ureter. However, at normal flow rates, the frequency exceeds that of the ureter. The pelvi-ureteric region appears to act as a "gating mechanism" with the transmission of the peristaltic waves beyond the pelvi-ureteric junction dependent upon the volume of urine present within the renal pelvis. As the urine flow increases, more pacemaker contractions become transmitted to the ureter and at high flow rates there is an exact correlation. As the flow rate of urine from the kidney increases, the number of peristaltic waves increase, followed by increases in the volume of the bolus. At high flow rates the boluses coalesce, the ureteric walls do not coapt, thus the transporting mechanism is dependent upon the hydrostatic pressure produced by urine production within the kidney.

The effect of obstruction upon ureteric physiology is complex and dependent upon several factors including the degree and duration of the obstruction, the rate of urine formation, and the presence of infection. An initial rise in intra-luminal pressure with an increase in ureteric dimensions is dependent upon the balance between the continued production of urine by the kidney and the degree of obstruction. It may be accompanied by a transient increase in the amplitude and frequency of peristaltic waves, although this phase is short lived [37]. As a result of changes in the ureteric dimensions the intra-luminal pressure falls. This and the inability of the ureteric walls to coapt as the ureteric diameter increases, further impairs the already failing transport mechanism and the likelihood of overcoming or actively extruding the obstructing element. The dynamic coordinated muscular properties of the ureter have been transformed into those of a static drainpipe. Furthermore, these changes may interfere with the activity of the pacemaker sites housed within the renal calyces and responsible for the coordination ureteric peristalsis [38]. The presence of infection will potentiate the deleterious effects of obstruction [39].

Relief of the obstruction or the diversion of urine by the insertion of a percutaneous nephrostomy tube allows the ureter to regain its normal dimensions and coapt its lumen with the restoration of effective ureteric contractility and peristalsis. There is some evidence from animal studies that after two weeks of ureteric obstruction there is smooth muscle hypertrophy and an increase in muscle contractility [40, 41]. This experimental observation may form part of the explanation for the passage of ureteric steinstrasse or ureteric stones following the placement of a nephrostomy tube. However, although the presence of a nephrostomy tube imposes a further set of changes to upper urinary tract physiology, which may result in dis-coordinated ureteric peristalsis because of interference with pacemaker sites, the placement of an intra-ureteric stent will effectively paralyse ureteric function until it is removed.

The presence of a percutaneous nephrostomy tube gives direct access to the upper urinary tract and this may provide a portal of entry for drugs, which may enhance ureteric contractility with the aim to expel the obstructing stone.

4.5 Physiological and Pharmacological Properties of Human Ureteric Muscle

There is considerable diversity in cellular functional organisation between various smooth muscle types and within different species. There is a need to investigate each type of smooth muscle as a separate entity and to avoid extrapolation of experimental data between both smooth muscle type and animal species. Fundamentally, it is not possible to use an animal model to make an attempt to understand the physiology of human ureteric smooth muscle.

The majority of workers have focused their efforts on isolating agents that would bring about relaxation and inhibition of ureteric peristalsis because they considered hyperperistalsis and "ureteric spasm" to be the initiating factors in the pain of ureteric colic. There are a considerable number of misconceptions held about the etiology of ureteric colic and the mechanisms of pain production. There appears to be no factual evidence to support the concept that either hyperperistalsis or spasm contribute to the pain of ureteric colic.

The number of scientific publications relating to the physiology of the human ureter over the last 20 years are relatively few and far between when compared to the pharmacological interest in bladder function and in particular, the drive by the pharmacological companies to provide effective medication for the overactive bladder. The mechanism of action of prostaglandins and prostaglandin synthetase inhibitors in the treatment of ureteric colic has already been mentioned. However, apart from these substances and the rather surprising action of carbon dioxide, human ureteric muscle appears relatively inert, particularly when compared to detrusor muscle.

In a comprehensive series of in vitro experiments using the technique of microsuperfusion, designed to ensure good tissue viability, the author was able to define the basic contractile properties of human ureteric muscle [19]. The tension produced during a phasic contraction, initiated by electrical field stimulation of an isolated muscle preparation, superfused with a physiological solution, and prevented from shortening (isometric contraction) was used as the index of contractility. Under certain conditions, such as raising the concentration of potassium in the superfusate, changes in the resting tension were observed. These contractions were termed tonic responses. Using this model, the effect of various agents added to the superfusate was investigated.

A summary of the effects of various agents upon human ureteric smooth muscle contractility is summarised in Table 4.1 below.

Table 4.1 Ureteric response to electrical stimulation. The effects of various agents upon the contractile response of human ureteric smooth muscle to electrical field stimulation.

No effect	Some effect	Significant effect
Tetrodotoxin 8×10^{-4} g/l	$[Ca^{2+}]_o$ 0.45–15 mM	Indomethacin $10^{-5} - 10^{-4}$ M
Atropine 1 μM	Noradrenaline 1–100 μM	Diclofenac $10^{-5}-5 \times 10^{-5}$ M
Phentolamine 30 μM		$PGF_{2\,alpha}$ $10^{-8} - 10^{-5}$ M
Propranolol 1 μM		PGE_2 $10^{-8} - 10^{-5}$ M
Acetylcholine 1–100 μM		$[K^+]_o$ 8–128 mM
Carbachol 5 μM		CO_2 5–30%
Isoprenaline 0.1–100 mM		
Glucagon 0.1–10mM		
Metaclopramide 0.1–10mM		
$[HCO_3^-]_o$ 6–48 mM		

Tetrodotoxin, a potent neurotoxin from the ovaries of the Japanese Puffer fish, Fugu, inhibits the generation of action potentials in nerve fibers, but not in smooth muscle, by selectively blocking an increase in sodium conductance. The insensitivity of the preparation to tetrodotoxin under any condition of stimulation, and the lack of effect of atropine, phentolamine, and propranolol suggests that the contractions elicited by electrical field stimulation are due to a direct effect upon the muscle and independent of the sparse autonomic nervous network that is embedded within it. This conclusion is of fundamental importance. The lack of effect of acetylcholine, carbachol, and isoprenaline provides further evidence that cholinergic and beta adrenergic receptors have no role in modulating ureteric contractility in human ureter in vitro. Noradrenaline produced a response that could be blocked by phentolamine (although phentolamine alone had no effect), suggesting it was mediated by alpha receptors. However, the high concentrations required might make the response of dubious physiological significance. It emerges that the local nervous networks, although present in the wall of the human ureter, are relatively unimportant in the control of ureteric contractility. This is in contrast to the situation, which exists in human detrusor muscle.

4.6 The Effect of Metoclopramide and Glucagon

Metoclopramide has been described as having a significant dose-dependent effect upon rat, canine, and human ureter [42]. This has not been confirmed in these studies and suggests that the clinical observation of vigorous ureteric peristalsis following administration of metoclopramide to four patients [43] was not due to a direct action upon ureteric smooth muscle.

Similarly, glucagon had been found to cause complete inhibition of canine ureteric peristalsis in vivo [44]. Further studies confirmed this finding [45]. However, the same authors were unable to demonstrate any significant effect upon ureteric peristalsis in man [46]. Our studies agree with the latter findings. These responses highlight the difficulty in extrapolating data between different species. It is of interest that the antispasmodic buscopan is still prescribed for the treatment of ureteric colic in some accident and emergency departments.

4.7 The Effect of Prostaglandin Synthetase Inhibitors

Both indomethacin and diclofenac sodium, two chemically different prostaglandin synthetase inhibitors, were shown to abolish almost completely the contractile response of human ureteric smooth muscle to electrical field stimulation (Figure 4.1). Contractile activity, in the presence of the inhibitors, could be restored by prostaglandin E2 or F2 alpha, or by increasing the external potassium concentration (Figure 4.2). Prostaglandins alone were shown to increase both the phasic and tonic component of the electrically stimulated contractions. Prostaglandins are not stored and their production is dependent upon a continual supply of substrate. In sheep, electron microscopy of the ureter has demonstrated the presence of large numbers of lipophilic granules in the vicinity of the smooth muscle cells, which could serve as prostaglandin precursors [47]. It is evident that the human ureter has the capacity to produce substantial quantities of prostaglandins, which in

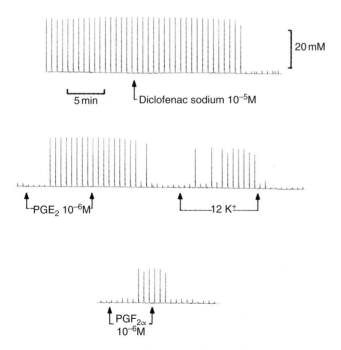

Figure 4.1 Top panel: the effect of diclofenac sodium (10-5 M) upon the contractile response of human ureteric muscle to electrical field stimulation. **Bottom Panels:** the restoration of contractile activity in the presence of diclofenac sodium (10-5 M) by prostaglandin E2 (10-6 M), increasing external potassium concentration to 12 mM or prostaglandin F2 alpha (10-6 M).

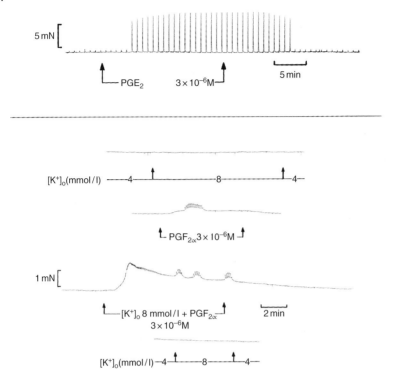

Figure 4.2 The actions of prostaglandin E2 and F2 alpha upon the contractile response of human ureteric smooth muscle. The upper trace demonstrates the increase in phasic contraction to electrical field stimulation. The bottom tracings illustrate tonic contractions with episodes of spontaneous activity induced by prostaglandin F2 alpha and the augmentation in isometric force initiated by simultaneously increasing the external concentration of potassium. The preparation is not receiving electrical stimulation.

in vitro have a profound effect upon contractility. Furthermore, cystoscopic biopsies of human bladder urothelium have been shown to produce substantial amounts of prostaglandin and other related substances in vitro and it has been postulated that these may have a role in modulating the tone and contractility of bladder muscle [48]. This study suggests that the administration synthetase inhibitors to patients could have a direct effect on ureteric function and possibility contribute to the pain-relieving qualities that these agents possess in ureteric colic. In addition, using an electrophysiological approach with intracellular microelectrodes, it was possible to measure the resting membrane potential (RMP) from a single human ureteric smooth muscle cell [19]. This had not been previously been reported in the literature. The value of the resting membrane potential is determined by the permeability and distribution of various ions across the cell membrane. For a single permeable ion distributing across the membrane, the RMP can be predicted by the Nernst equation. Furthermore, by inserting a microelectrode into a single ureteric smooth muscle cell within a ureteric strip, a simultaneous measurement of membrane potential and isometric tension could be recorded when the cell membrane was exposed to a superfusate containing a raised concentration of potassium or prostaglandin F2 alpha. During these experiments, the muscle preparations were not electrically stimulated as the microelectrode could easily be dislodged. The resting membrane potential was recorded as −55 mV and this is similar to that measured in animal preparations [49–51]. This value is very different from the potassium equilibrium potential for this tissue as predicted by the Nernst equation of approximately −93 mV, assuming an intracellular potassium concentration of 140 mM. This implies that the cellular membrane is not solely permeable to (K+), but there is a significant permeability to some other ion with an equilibrium potential positive compared to the recorded membrane potential. This is further substantiated by the fact that the magnitude of the depolarization observed by raising the external potassium from 4 to 48 mM was only 25 mV, whereas the Nernst prediction was 65 mV (Figure 4.3).

The depolarising action of raising the extracellular (K+) from 4 to 48 mM was demonstrated and prostaglandin F2 alpha (3x10−6 M) was shown to produce a small depolarization of the ureteric muscle cell membrane (Figure 4.4).

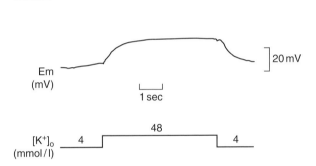

Figure 4.3 The effect of increasing the external potassium concentration from 4 to 48 mM upon the membrane potential, Em, of a single human ureteric muscle cell. The resting membrane potential was −61 mV in this experiment; the inside of the cell negative with respect to the outside.

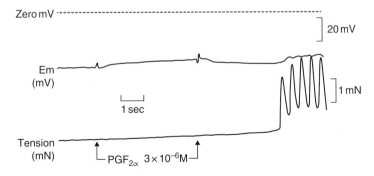

Figure 4.4 A simultaneous record of membrane potential, Em, of a single human ureteric muscle cell and isometric tension from the preparation showing the effect of prostaglandin F2 alpha (3 x 10-6 M). A small reversible depolarisation (7 mV) of the membrane is measured. There is a small rise in resting tension. Following return to the normal superfusate, this contracture persisted and culminated in spontaneous contraction with a further more marked increase in muscle tone.

4.8 The Effect of Acid-Base Changes Upon Ureteric Contractility

One of the most interesting areas of ureteric physiology relates to the contractile response to changes in acid-base balance [52]. In the early part of the last century, in vitro studies of animal ureteric function suggested that the pH of the muscle bath was an important factor in contractile activity. Indeed, Gruber [53], who introduced the concept of a ureteric pacemaker, demonstrated differing responses to changes in pH of the bathing solution of the upper and lower segments of the pig ureter.

The contractile response of human ureteric smooth muscle to changes in of extracellular pH is important for several reasons. Firstly, the pH of normal urine may vary between pH 4.5 and 8.0. Similarly, the partial pressure of carbon dioxide (PCO2) in urine fluctuates over a wide range. In general, the PCO2 seems to correlate best with urine pH, high levels occurring in alkaline diuresis and lower values (although still higher than plasma) following ingestion of ammonium chloride solution [54]. Furthermore, urine PCO2 varies inversely with urine flow in humans [55]. In certain groups of patients with a variety of renal tubular disorders, including renal tubular acidosis, Na-losing nephropathy, and adult Fanconi syndrome, urinary pCO2 was low, approximating to that of plasma [56]. Patients with chronic unilateral pyelonephritis affecting the tubular cells were noted to have a significantly lower pCO2 in urine from the diseased kidney [57].

Although the transitional cell urothelium of the urinary tract is considered to form a protective impermeable barrier, there is considerable evidence that CO2 can diffuse rapidly across cell membranes [58]. In addition, there is also evidence to suggest that urinary tract stone disease and infection may damage the protective nature of the urothelium, allowing the smooth muscle cells to be exposed to urine directly [59]. Experimental bacterial studies in dogs and primates in vivo have demonstrated that certain bacteria can have a profound effect on ureteric dynamics [60]. Similarly, in isolated animal and human ureters live pathogenic bacteria and *E. coli* endotoxin can produce cessation of muscle activity, which appears to be reversible and dose related [61]. The presence of urinary tract infection may in itself lead to considerable changes in urinary pH, via the urease splitting properties of certain strains of pathogenic bacteria, in particular Proteus, Pseudomonas, Klebsiella, and some strains of Staphylococcus. Infection has been used to explain the non-obstructive dilatation of the upper urinary tract associated with acute pyelonephritis and the ureteric dilatation observed below infective staghorn calculi [62]. In summary, therefore, wide fluctuations in urinary pH and carbon dioxide (pCO2) occur in both normal physiological circumstances and in a variety of pathological conditions, in particular, obstruction and infection. These changes may have a profound effect on ureteric muscle, and therefore, ureteric function.

One of the most interesting observations to emerge from these in vitro studies was the increased isometric phasic tension, which develops in response to an intracellular acidosis [52]. Reducing the superfusate pH from 7.8 to 6.8 by incrementally raising the pCO2 increased the contractions elicited by single electrical stimuli. Similar alteration of the superfusate pH by adjusting the bicarbonate (HCO3−) at constant calcium (Ca2+) and sodium (Na+) was without significant effect. Adjustment of both superfusate pCO2 and (HCO3−) so as to maintain constant pH produced an alteration to the contractile force that was quantitatively similar to that produced by changing the pCO2 alone. These observations suggest that modulation of contractile force maybe mediated by changes of intracellular pH and that the permeability of the muscle membrane to hydrogen (H+) and (HCO3–) is very low. The increase of force in the presence of an acidosis was a highly significant and unusual finding.

It is envisaged that a cyclical fluctuation in intracellular Ca2+ is responsible for the contraction relaxation cycle in human smooth muscle. The source of the activator Ca2+ is likely to vary between different types of smooth muscle. Extracellular Ca2+ may enter the cell through potential dependent and/or receptor-operated channels. Intracellular sources of Ca2+ are believed to be stored within the sarcoplasmic reticulum. In human ureteric muscle cells, the membrane potential appears to have a profound influence on muscle contractility, and although extracellular Ca2+ is necessary for contractile activity, it appears that intracellular sources are responsible for contractile activation. In detrusor muscle, transmembrane fluxes from extracellular sources appear to be responsible for detrusor muscle contractions. Fry *et al.* [63] reported in human and animal detrusor muscle that intracellular acidosis increased force as in the experiments reported here, but extracellular acidosis depressed force, unlike the situation here where there was no effect. The reason for the diverse response to extracellular acidosis may be related to the dependence of detrusor muscle contraction on extracellular Ca2+, but the relative independence of extracellular Ca2+ for ureteric muscle contraction. In addition, human detrusor muscle is also very sensitive to changes in the extracellular environment, such as alteration in extracellular Ca2+ and the presence of calcium channel blockers; the human ureter is relatively inert to these changes. In addition, the effect of intracellular and extracellular pH on the production of factors from the endothelial cells, known to have powerful effects on ureteric contractility within the smooth muscle syncitium, might also provide modulatory function.

It had been assumed that the classical association between acidosis, either extracellular or intracellular, and decreased cardiac contractility was also applicable to smooth muscle (Figure 4.5). However, a diversity of response exists between different types of smooth

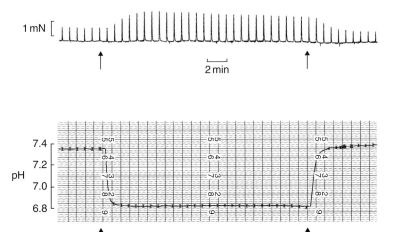

Figure 4.5 The response to extracellular acidosis by increasing superfusate pCO2. Upper trace, isometric force; lower trace, superfusate pH. The arrows mark the intervention. CO2 content of the equilibrating gas mixture was raised from 5–30%. Temperature 36 degrees C.

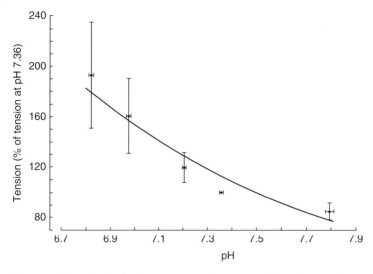

Figure 4.6 The relationship between superfusate pH and steady state phasic tension in isolated human ureteric muscle. Tension is expressed as a percentage of that measured in control solution, pH 7.36. Superfusate pH was altered by varying pCO2. Error bars represent SD of an observation, n = 13 pH 7.8; n = 24 pH 7.2; n = 20 pH 7.0; n = 17 pH 6.8. Temperature 36 degree C.

muscle. This is best exemplified by vascular smooth muscle. The main regulator of cerebral blood flow is the direct action of pCO2 on intracellular pH of vascular smooth muscle cells (Figure 4.6). Here a fall of intracellular pH leads to a vasodilatation and an increased blood flow. Similarly, relaxation of the ductus arteriosus in vitro occurs when the intracellular pH is lowered. In contrast, the pulmonary artery constricts in response to hypoxia and acidosis.

In the future the clear identification of the source of the activator calcium and the control mechanism, which govern its magnitude and distribution, may provide a basis for modulating contractile activity.

4.9 The Effects of Stents Upon Ureteric Function

The fundamental purpose of a ureteric stent is to allow drainage from an obstructed kidney. The German Surgeon, Gustav Simon, Professor at Heidelberg, who performed the first successful nephrectomy on August 2, 1869, is credited to be first to stent a ureter during an open bladder operation. Yoaquin Albarann created the first ureteric stent in 1900, and at that time, these were made from fabric and coated with a lacquer varnish. It was Gibbons in 1976 [64], who introduced the concept of a ureteric stent in clinical practice. The stent was radio-opaque and non-reactive and it provided considerable improvement in morbidity over a supravesical urinary diversion, particularly in the face of malignant obstruction. The obstruction could be corrected at the time of diagnosis and it was reversible as the stent could be removed. Since that time, stents have evolved from straight tubes prone to migration into a "double J configuration" to prevent migration either upward or downward [65]. If a silicone JJ stent is placed correctly at the time of insertion, spontaneous migration does not occur.

The indications for ureteric stenting further expanded in the 1980s following the introduction of extracorporeal shockwave lithotripsy (ESWL). Ureteric stents were inserted prior to ESWL in an attempt to reduce the likelihood of ureteric obstruction particularly when treating large stones of more than 1.5 cm were being treated. In this situation the presence of a ureteric stent would act as a "sieve," preventing any large stone fragments from entering the ureter and causing ureteric obstruction. Subsequent treatments to these fragments in the kidney would be feasible. Ureteric stents undoubtedly cause a partial ureteric obstruction and effectively paralyze the normal peristaltic transporting mechanism creating a drainpipe effect, and their presence also causes ureteric dilatation. This becomes advantageous when the stent is removed, as it facilitates the spontaneous passage of stone fragments or indeed obstructing steinstrasse. Furthermore, the emergency insertion of a ureteric stent as a means of safely treating acute ureteric obstruction caused by an impacted ureteric stone will make the subsequent definitive ureteroscopy both an easier and safer procedure.

Stents undoubtedly have a role in treating acutely obstructed and infected kidneys, but in the authors' experience, they do not effectively drain pus, and careful evaluation in this situation is needed to decide whether the insertion of a percutaneous nephrostomy tube would be a safer alternative. In some circumstances where ureteric drainage is considered appropriate, an 8–10Fr ureteric catheter is better suited to draining infected material from below, as it allows radiological access to the upper tract to establish that the system is indeed draining and for flushing.

Ureteric stents can generate significant inflammation, which can extend through the full thickness of the ureteric wall creating a very thickened, rigid, and woody structure, making any subsequent surgery very difficult. The best example here is the stenting of a pelvi-ureteric junction obstruction prior to reconstructive surgery, which is then sought with difficulty.

The etiology of ureteric obstruction in retroperitoneal fibrosis, whether benign or malignant, maybe more obscure than a simple physical obstruction. Infiltration into the wall of the ureter by either an inflammatory obstruction or a malignancy may disrupt normal ureteric peristalsis. In benign retroperitoneal disease, stent insertion is relatively straightforward as the ureter does not appear to have narrowed and even ureteroscopy can be relatively easy. It is as though the ureter has been paralyzed. However, stenting does seem to improve drainage and renal function. Ultimately, with malignant infiltration the progressive infiltration and fibrotic constricting nature of the process leads to an impassable stricture.

In general terms, ureteric stents achieve the purpose that they were designed to do, namely urinary drainage. However, the problem with stents is that they come with morbidity in terms of pain, irritative bladder symptoms, encrustation, obstruction, and haematuria. Some patients find them intolerable. Much effort has been made to improve stent design to reduce these side effects or to avoid their routine use, in particular after ureteroscopy. In stone disease, the use of a stent is often a short-lived maneuver, whereas definitive treatment is planned and executed. Ureteric stenting to treat malignant strictures imposes another set of conditions where periodic stent changes become necessary every three to six months with the prospect of blocking, because of the inability to counteract the external pressure caused by progressive malignant infiltration. Infection can become a significant problem, particularly fungal infection. The uses of metallic stents in these circumstances represent significant progress but cost and stent migration become additional possible setbacks. Extra-anatomic stents can be useful in rare clinical situations [66].

References

[1] Cole RS, Palfrey ELH, Smith SE, Shuttleworth KED. Indomethacin as prophylaxis against ureteric colic following extracorporeal shockwave lithotripsy. Journal of Urology 1989;141:9–12.

[2] Chaussy CG, Brendel W, Schmiedt E. Extracorporeally induced destruction of kidney stones by shockwaves. Lancet 1980;2:1265

[3] Pickard P, Starr K, MacLennan G, Lam T, Thomas R, Burr J, McPherson G, McDonald A, Anson K, N'Dow J, Burgess N, Clark T, Kilonzo M, Gillies K, Shearer K, Boachie C, Cameron S, Norrie J, McClinton S. Medical expulsive therapy in adults with ureteric colic: a multicentre, randomised, placebo-controlled trial. www.thelancet.com 2015;386:341–349.

[4] Zargar-Shoshtari K, Sharma P, Zargar H. Experts summary. European Urology 2015;68:910–911.

[5] Cole RS, Fry CH. Can prostaglandins facilitate the passage of ureteric stone streets? In: Lingeman JE, Newman DM, (eds.), Shock Wave Lithotripsy. Plenum Press, New York and London, 1989.

[6] Bultitude M, Rees J. Management of renal colic. British Medical Journal 2012:345:e5499.

[7] Risholm L. Studies on renal colic and its treatment by posterior splanchnic block. Acta Chir Scand, 1954;184:1.

[8] Kiil F. The function of the ureter and renal pelvis. WB Saunders Co., Philadelphia, 1957.

[9] Bretland PM. Acute ureteric obstruction. A clinical and radiological study. London: Butterworths, 1972.

[10] Michaelson G. Percutaneous puncture of the renal pelvis, intrapelvic pressure and the concentrating capacity of the kidney in hydronephrosis. Acta. Med. Scand 1974;(suppl)559:1.

[11] Holmlund D, Sjodin J-G. Treatment of ureteral colic with intravenous indomethacin. Journal of Urology 1978;120:676–677.

[12] Sjodin J-G, Holmlund D. Indomethacin by intravenous infusion in ureteric colic. A multicentre study. Scand. J. Urol Nephrol. 1982;16:221.

[13] Flannigan GM, Clifford RCP, Carver RA, Yule AG, Madden NP, Towler JM. Indomethacin—an alternative to pethidine in ureteric colic. British Journal of Urology 1983;55:6.

[14] Grenabo L, Holmlund DEW. Indomethacin as prophylaxis against recurrent ureteral colic. Scand. J. Urol. Nephrol 1984;18:325.

[15] Moody TE, Vaughan ED, Gillenwater JY. Relationship between renal blood flow and ureteral pressure during 18 hours of total unilateral ureteral occlusion. Implications for changing sites of increased renal resistance. Invest. Urol. 1975;13:246.

[16] Allen JT, Vaughan ED, Gillenwater JY. The effect of indomethacin on renal blood flow and ureteral pressure in unilateral obstruction in awake dogs. Invest. Urol. 1978;15:324–328.

[17] Wahlberg J. (1983) The renal response to ureteral obstruction. Scand. J Urol. Nephrol. 1983;(supplement)73:1–30.

[18] Lloyd-Davies RW, Parkhouse H, Gow JD, Davies DR. Color Atlas of Urology, Mosby, 1994, pp 127–156.

[19] Cole RS, Fry CH, Shuttleworth KED. The action of prostaglandins on isolated human ureteric smooth muscle. British Journal of Urology 1988;61:19–26.

[20] Perry SV, Grand RJA. Mechanisms of contraction and the specialised protein components of smooth muscle. British Medical Bulletin 1979;35:219–226.

[21] Notley RG. Ureteral morphology: anatomic and clinical consideration. Urology 1968;XII:8–14.

[22] Gosling JA, Dixon JS, Humpherson JR. Functional anatomy of the urinary tract. Churchill Livingstone. Edinburgh, London, New York, pp 2.2–2.13, 1983.

[23] Englemann TW. Zur Physiologie des ureters. Pflugers Archiv fur die gesamte Physiologie 1869;2:243–293.

[24] Schulman CC. Electron microscopy of the human ureteric innervations. British Journal of Urology 1974;46:609–623.

[25] Prosser CL, Smith CE, Melton CE. Conduction of action potentials in the ureter of the rat. American Journal of Physiology 1955;181:651–660.

[26] O'Conor VJ, Dawson-Edwards P. (1959) Role of the ureter in renal transplantation. 1. Studies of denervated ureter with particular reference to ureteroureteral anastomosis. Journal of Urology 1959;82:566–572.

[27] Wharton LR. The innervations of the ureter with respect to denervation. Journal of Urology 1932;28:639–673.

[28] Melick WF, Naryka JJ, Schmidt JH. Experimental studies of ureteral peristaltic patterns on the pig. II Myogenic activity of the pig ureter. Journal of Urology 1961;86:46–50.

[29] Malin JM, Deane RF, Boyarsky S. Characterization of adrenergic receptors in human ureter. British Journal of Urology 1970;42:171–174.

[30] Malin J M, Boyarsky S, Labay P, Gerber C. In vitro isometric studies of ureteral smooth muscle. Journal of Urology 1968;99:396–398.

[31] Weiss RM, Bassett AL, Hoffman BF. Adrenergic innervations of the ureter, Investigative Urology 1978;16:123–127.

[32] Weiss RM. Ureteral pharmacology. In: Finkbeiner AE, Barbour GL, Bissada NK. Pharmacology of the urinary tract and the male reproductive system. Appleton-Century-Crofts, New York, pp 137–173, 1982.

[33] Lapides J. The physiology of the intact human ureter. Journal of Urology 1948;59:501–537.

[34] Griffiths DJ, Notschaelen C. The mechanics of urine transport in the upper urinary tract: 1. The dynamics of the isolated bolus. Neurourology and Urodynamics 1983:2:155–166.

[35] Ross JA, Edmond P, Kirkland IS. Behaviour of the human ureter in health and disease. Churchill Livingstone, Edinburgh and London, pp 24–27, 1972.

[36] Bozler E. The activity of the pacemaker previous to the discharge of a muscle impulse. American Journal Physiology 1942;136:543–560.

[37] Rose JG, Gillenwater JY. Effects of obstruction upon ureteral function. Urology 1978;12:139–145.

[38] Djurhuus JC, Constantinou CE. Chronic ureteric obstruction and its impact on the coordinating mechanism of peristatsis (pyeloureteric pacemaker system). Urological Research 1982;10:267–270.

[39] Rose JG, Gillenwater JY. Effects on obstruction upon ureteral function. Urology 1973;12:139–145.

[40] Hausman M, Biancani P, Weiss RM. Obstruction induced changes in longitudinal force-length relations of the rabbit ureter. Investigative Urology 1979;17:223–226.

[41] Biancani P, Hausman M, Weiss RM. Effects of obstruction on ureteral circumferenteral force-length relations. American Journal of Physiology 1982;243:F204–F210.

[42] Berman DJ, Firlit CF. Effect of metoclopramide on ureteral motility. Urology 1984;13:150–156.

[43] Schelin S. Observations on the effect of metoclopramide (primperan) on the human ureter. Scand. J. Urol. Nephrol. 1979;13:79–82.

[44] Boyarsky S, Labay P. Ureteral Dynamics. Baltimore: Williams and Wilkins, pp. 262–266, 1972.

[45] Stower MJ, Wright JW, Hardcastle JD. The action of glucagon and commonly used antispasmodics and analgesics on the canine ureter. British Journal of Surgery 1983;70:89–91.

[46] Stower MJ, Clark AG, Wright JW, Hardcastle JD. Effect of glucagon on ureteric peristalsis in man, pig, rabbit and rat. Journal of Urology 1984;131:822–824.

[47] Al-Ugaily L, Thulesius O, Angelo-Khattar M. New evidence for prostaglandin induced motility of the ureter. Scand. J. Urol. Nephrol., 1986;20:225–229.

[48] Jeremy JY, Tsang V, Mikhailidis DP, Rogers H, Morgan RJ, Dandona P. Eicosanoid synthesis by human urinary bladder mucosa: pathological implications. British Journal of Urology 1987;59:36–39.

[49] Kuriyama T, Osa T, Toida N. Membrane properties of the smooth muscle of guinea pig ureter. Journal of Physiology 1967;191:225–238.

[50] Wooster MJ. Effects of prostaglandin E_1 on dog ureter in vitro. Journal of Physiology 1970;213:51P–53P.

[51] Aickin CC, Brading AF, Burdyga ThV. Evidence for sodium-calcium exchange in the guinea-pig ureter. Journal of Physiology 1984;347:411–430.

[52] Cole RS, Fry CH, Shuttleworth KED. Effects of acid-base changes on human ureteric smooth muscle contractility. British Journal of Urology 1990;66:257–264.

[53] Gruber CM. The peristalsis and antiperistaltic movements in excised ureters as affected by drugs. Journal of Urology 1928;28:27–59.

[54] Hong SK, Boylan JW, Tannenberg AM, Rahn H. Total and partial gas tensions of human bladder urine. Journal of Applied Physiology 1960;15:115–120.

[55] Ryberg C. Some investigations on the carbon dioxide tension of the urine in man. Acta Physiol. Scand. 1948;15:123–139.

[56] Pak Poy RK, Wrong O. The urinary PCO_2 in renal disease. Clinical Science 1960;19:631–639.

[57] Koch B, Zborowski DT, Dossetor JB, Collins WE. Oxygen and carbon dioxide tension of urine. Investigative Urology 1972;9:514–517.

[58] Jacobs MH. The production of intracellular acidity by neutral and alkaline solutions containing carbon dioxide. American Journal of Physiology 1920;53:457–463.

[59] Fussell EW, Roberts JA. Chronic pyelonephritis. Electron microscopic study. III The ureter. Investigative Urology 1979;17:108–119.

[60] Grana L, Donnellan WL, Swenson O. Effects of gram negative bacteria on ureteral structure and function. Journal of Urology 1968;99:539–550.

[61] King WW, Cox CE. Bacterial inhibition of ureteral smooth muscle contractility. 1. The effect of common urinary pathogens and endotoxin in an in vitro system. Journal of Urology 1972;108:700–705.

[62] Kass EJ, Silver TM, Konnak JW, Thornbury JR, Wolfman MG. The urographic findings in acute pyelonephritis: non-obstructive hydronephrosis. Journal of Urology 1976;116:544–546.

[63] Fry CH, Liston TG, Cole RS. The effects of pH on urinary tract smooth muscle function. Frontiers in Smooth Muscle Research, pp 717–723. Alan R Liss, Inc, 1990.

[64] Gibbons RP, Correa RJ Jr, Cummings KB, Mason JT. Experience with indwelling ureteral stent catheters. Journal of Urology 1976;115(1):22–26.

[65] Finney RP. Experience with new Double J ureteral catheter stent. Journal of Urology 1978;120:678–681.

[66] Minhas S, Irving HC, Lloyd SN, Eardley I, Browning AJ, Joyce AD. Extra-anatomic stents in ureteric obstruction: experience and complications. BJU International. 1999;84(7):762–764.

5

Etiology of Ureteric Obstruction

Philip T. Zhao[1], David A. Leavitt[2], Piruz Motamedinia[1], Zeph Okeke[1] and Arthur D. Smith[3]

[1] The Smith Institute for Urology, Hofstra-North Shore-LIJ School of Medicine, New Hyde Park, NY, USA
[2] The Smith Institute for Urology, Hofstra-North Shore-LIJ Health System, New Hyde Park, NY, USA
[3] Professor of Urology, The Smith Institute for Urology, Hofstra North Shore-LIJ School of Medicine, New Hyde Park, NY, USA

Ureteric obstruction is one of the most common urologic problems and can have a variety of intrinsic and extrinsic causes. The obstructive process itself can be further divided based on duration (acute versus chronic), severity (partial versus complete), totality (bilateral vs. unilateral), and the presence of complicating factors such as infection [1]. The variations in the etiology of obstruction presents different challenges to the urologist and understanding these perspectives plays an important role in the treatment of ureteric obstruction and their outcomes.

5.1 Congenital Causes

5.1.1 Ureterocele and Ureterovesical Reflux

Ureterocele is a cystic dilatation of the ureter that is commonly observed in females and children. It primarily affects the upper moiety of complete pyeloureteric duplication. Ureteroceles are divided into intravesical, completely contained inside the bladder, and extravesical when part of the cyst extends to the urethra or bladder neck. Most ureteroceles are diagnosed in utero and febrile urinary tract infection (UTI) is the most common postnatal presentation. It is necessary to evaluate for vesicoureteric reflux (VUR) once an ureterocele has been diagnosed. VUR in the lower pole is observed in 50% of cases and in the contralateral kidney in 25% [2]. Simple endoscopic puncture of the ureterocele can be an effective therapy for infected or obstructing ureteroceles. The reoperation rate after endoscopic treatment varies from 48 to 100% [3]. It is 15 to 20% after upper pole partial nephrectomy if VUR was absent before the operation, but can be as high as 50-100% when VUR was present [4]. Thus, endoscopic incision is appropriate when dealing with a completely intravesical ureterocele while upper pole partial nephrectomy is the elective treatment for an ectopic ureterocele without VUR.

5.1.2   Ureteric Valve

Congenital ureteric valves are a rare cause of ureteric obstruction in children, with less than 100 cases reported in the literature [5]. The ureteric valves can be managed by ipsilateral ureteroureterostomy, ureteropyelostomy, or longitudinal ureterotomy with excision of valve leaflets and reconstruction is curative.

5.1.3   Ectopic and Retrocaval Kidney

Ureteropelvic junction (UPJ) obstruction are frequently associated with other congenital anomalies of the kidney, including fusion abnormalities, malrotation, renal ectopia, and duplicated systems [6]. Often these anatomic variants can create mass effect and extrinsic pressure on the ureter causing an obstructed system. Treatment is dependent on the anatomic location and extent of the anomaly.

5.1.4   Prune Belly Syndrome

Prune belly syndrome is a rare genetic group of birth defects that involves poor development of abdominal muscles, cryptorchidism, and urinary tract abnormalities and effects 1 in 40,000 births [7]. Children present with megaureters, retention, UTI, and VUR. The ureteric system is obstructed in about 25% of all cases leading to renal failure due to persistent pyelonephritis or obstruction [8].

5.2   Metabolic Causes

5.2.1   Ureterolithiasis

Urolithiasis represents a major clinical and economic burden and one of the primary intrinsic causes of ureteric obstruction. Epidemiological data suggests the prevalence of stone disease has increased, with a rise in lifetime prevalence between 7 and 13%, for women and men, respectively [9, 10]. This rising prevalence is multi-factorial but can be attributed to poor dietary habits, decreased fluid intake, increasing levels of obesity, and metabolic syndrome [11, 12].

   The impact of obstruction on renal function is influenced by its extent or degree, the duration of obstruction, the baseline condition of the kidneys, and the presence of other mitigating factors [13]. Unilateral ureteric calculi typically present with renal colic, without any change in the overall measured renal function in a healthy individual. However, a small number of patients presenting with ureterolithiasis do have abnormal renal function tests and little is known about the factors that aggravate renal impairment in partial obstruction. Prolonged (>2 months) ureteric calculi impaction was associated with a rate of approximately 24% incidence of ureteric strictures at 7 months [14].

   In complete ureteric obstruction, interstitial inflammation, tubular cell injury, and ultimately fibrosis are present [15]. The duration of obstruction plays an important role in determining the degree of renal impairment and recoverability of function. Significant irreversible loss of functional renal parenchyma can occur if the obstruction persists for more than six weeks [16]. Short-term obstructions were also found to affect renal function. Although renal impairment was significantly associated with obstruction, it does not relate with the extent of the actual obstruction.

5.3 Neoplastic Causes

5.3.1 Primary Carcinoma of the Ureter

Urothelial cell carcinoma (UCC) is the fifth most common cancer worldwide, after prostate, breast, lung, and colorectal cancer [17]. Among UCC, upper tract urothelial carcinoma (UTUC) is rare and accounts for 5 to 10% of all urothelial carcinomas with an annual incidence of 2 per 100,000 inhabitants in the United States [18]. UTUC is more common in men than women by a factor of two and the mean age at diagnosis is 65 years old. It is located twice more often in the renal pelvis than in the ureter and in about 20% of the cases, concomitant urothelial carcinoma of the bladder is present. UTUC tends to recur in the bladder and progress through the lymphatic and vascular systems to distant organs.

UTUC remain largely clinically silent in the initial stage and its principal symptoms are gross hematuria or microhematuria, followed by ureteric obstruction causing flank pain and lumbar mass. UTUC in the ureter portends a worse prognosis than at other locations because the cancer can spread more rapidly due to the thin muscle layer of the ureter. Hydroureteronephrosis is often encountered but the degree of obstruction does not indicate the tumor grade or stage [19].

5.3.2 Non-Urologic Malignancies

Malignant ureteric obstruction is often the result of non-urologic malignancies including but not limited to ovarian, cervical, colorectal, breast cancer, and lymphoma [20, 21]. There can be extrinsic mass compression of the tumor bulk or buildup of micrometastatic disease within the wall of the ureter from these malignancies. Direct infiltration is most often caused by carcinomas of the bladder, prostate, cervix, ovary, endometrium, rectum, and sigmoid colon and they usually involve the distal ureter. Overall survival of patients diagnosed with malignant obstruction is consistently poor. Several studies have found mean and median survival to be between 6 and 8 months, and as low as 1.7 months for the highest-risk patients [22, 23]. Similarly, projected survival after the development of ureteric obstruction is approximately 50% or less within a year, and less than 15% in the highest risk patients [23].

5.4 Inflammatory Causes

5.4.1 Stricture

A ureteric stricture is a urological event defined as a narrowing of the ureter causing a functional obstruction. It can lead to renal failure if left untreated. Benign ureteric strictures can develop due to congenital or secondary causes after open or endoscopic surgical procedures, stones, trauma, radiotherapy, endometriosis, infections, abdominal aortic aneurysm, retroperitoneal fibrosis, or idiopathically [24]. Excluding the congenital ureteric strictures (discussed above), more than 70% of strictures are benign or iatrogenic [25]. This also includes strictures that resulted from renal transplantation and urinary diversion (ureteroenteric strictures). An additional 20% of ureteric strictures are characterized as idiopathic.

Incidence of iatrogenic ureteric injuries fluctuates between 0.3% and 1.5% [26]. In general, pelvic surgery accounts for more than 80% of all iatrogenic ureteric injuries, of which 73% are of gynecologic origin, 14% percent were general surgical procedures, and another 14% were urological [27, 28]. Endoscopic approaches exhibit the highest incidence of benign ureteric strictures (58%). Retroperitoneal and pelvic lymph node dissections are most commonly responsible for ureteric injuries.

Specifically, ureteric injury in gynecologic surgery ranges between 0.5 and 1.5%. The ureter is more commonly injured during an abdominal hysterectomy (2.2%), whereas in laparoscopic and vaginal hysterectomy, rates are 1.3 and 0.03%, respectively [29, 30]. Risk factors for ureteric injury during gynecological procedures are pelvic malignancy, extent of the operation, prior radiation, endometriosis, and congenital anomalies of the urinary tract.

Ureteric injury from ureteroscopy is rare with the incidence of ureteric strictures as 1% after ureteroscopy [31]. About a third of traumatic injuries and the majority of operative injuries from urologic surgery occur in the distal ureter.

Malignant causes can originate from primary ureteric pathology or extrinsic compression of the ureter from adjacent tumors. Radiotherapy for pelvic malignancies may lead to a distal ureteric stricture due to ischemic fibrosis. Radiation-induced strictures have an incidence of approximately 2 to 3% with 0.15% added risk per year for 25 years or more post-radiation [32]. Most often when obstruction is found after radiation therapy, it is due to the underlying malignancy.

Ureteroenteric strictures after urinary diversion with the use of ileum range between 1.4 and 15%, whereas a refluxing anastomosis exhibits a lower incidence compared with the non-refluxing techniques. Strictures are more common in the left ureter compared with the right ureter due to the transposition of the ureter under the sigmoid colon, which requires additional dissection of the left ureter increasing chance of injury and ischemia [33].

Ureteric stricture is the most common urological complication after kidney transplantation. Stricture incidence ranges from 3 to 8% [34]. Regarding stricture location, 73%, 12%, and 15% occur at the distal, mid, and proximal ureter, respectively [35].

5.4.2 Endometriosis and Tuberculosis

Ureteric endometriosis accounts for approximately 1%, among all women with endometriosis [36]. Distal ureteric strictures and more specifically strictures of the ureterovesical junction are encountered in less than 10% of patients suffering from tuberculosis of the genitourinary tract [37].

5.5 Miscellaneous Causes

5.5.1 Retroperitoneal Fibrosis

Retroperitoneal fibrosis (RPF) is an inflammatory disease that involves the abdominal aorta, the iliac vessels, and the ureters. If it occurs around a single ureter, it can cause extrinsic ureteric obstruction, and if it occurs around both, it may lead to renal failure. Antinuclear antibodies are positive in as many as 60% of patients with idiopathic RPF. Rheumatoid factor, antibodies against smooth muscle, double-strand DNA, extractable nuclear antigen, and neutrophil cytoplasm are also sometimes positive. Autoimmune disorders, such as lupus erythematosis and Hashimoto's thyroiditis, are also associated with RPF, but the pathogenic mechanism by which RPF develops is not well known [38].

Treatment centers around ureterolysis. The main surgical objective is to release and separate the stenotic ureter from the surrounding fibrotic tissue, but if this is all that is done, a recurrence of the problem is likely in 60% of cases [39]. Surgical options of separating the ureter from the circumjacent tissue include intra-abdominal transposition, omental wrap, and ureteric overwrapping with artificial vessel graft.

5.5.2 Pregnancy

Renal colic is an infrequent but potentially troublesome development during pregnancy that can lead to hospitalization, invasive investigations, and treatment, and adverse effects on both the mother and her fetus. Physiological hydronephrosis is more pronounced on the right side because of a dextrorotation of the enlarged uterus and a dilated uterine vein compressing the right ureter causing extrinsic obstruction. [40, 41] In contrast, the left ureter is protected by the sigmoid colon. Although standard management algorithm for documented nephrolithiasis has emerged over the past decade, there remains some uncertainty on how to best differentiate nephrolithiasis from physiological hydronephrosis of pregnancy.

Of the women presenting with colic, the majority sought attention during the second or third trimesters. Although there were a greater number of both colic and patients with stone in the third trimester, the trimester of presentation did not significantly alter the proportion of colic cases because of an actual stone. The progressive dilatation of the ureter during pregnancy can allow a greater number of previously asymptomatic renal calculi to migrate downward and cause pain when lodged at the pelvic brim.

5.6 Conclusion

The etiology of ureteric obstruction is multivariable and crosses a multidisciplinary spectrum. Great care and consideration should be made in regards to the cause of obstruction in its diagnosis and ultimate treatment. Surgical intervention should be tailored to each individual patient and address the root cause of obstruction. It is necessary to have adequate cross-sectional imaging with urogram to assess the level of blockage and renal scan to evaluate the degree of obstruction and function in order to formulate a treatment plan.

References

[1] Capelouto CC, Saltzman B. The pathophysiology of ureteric obstruction. J Endourol 1993;7(2):93–103.
[2] Caldamone AA, Snyder HM, Duckett JW. Ureteroceles in children: follow up of management with upper tract approach. J Urol 1984; 131:1130–1132.
[3] Merlini E, Lelli Chiesa P. Obstructive ureterocele-an ongoing challenge. World J Urol 2004;22(2):107–114.

[4] Husmann D, Strand B, Ewalt D, Clement M, Kramer S, Allen T. Management of ectopic ureterocele associated with renal duplication: a comparison of partial nephrectomy and endoscopic decompression. J Urol 1999; 162(4):1406–1409.

[5] Rabinowitz R, Kingston TE, Wesselhoeft C, Caldamone AA. Ureteric valves in children. Urology 1998; 51(5A Suppl):7–11.

[6] Das S, Amar AD. Ureteropelvic junction obstruction with associated renal anomalies. J Urol 1984;131(5):872–874.

[7] Baird PA, MacDonald EC. An epidemiologic study of congenital malformations of the anterior abdominal wall in more than half a million consecutive live births. Am J Hum Genet 1981; 33(3):470–478.

[8] Reinberg Y, Manivel JC, Pettinato G, Gonzalez R. Development of renal failure in children with the prune belly syndrome. J Urol 1991;145(5):1017–1019.

[9] Turney BW, Reynard JM, Noble JG, Keoghane SR. Trends in urological stone disease. BJU Int 2012;109:1082–1087.

[10] Wright AE, Rukin NJ, Somani BK. Ureteroscopy and stones: Current status and future expectations. World J Nephrol 2014; 3(4):243–248.

[11] Zaninotto P, Head J, Stamatakis E, Wardle H, Mindell J. Trends in obesity among adults in England from 1993 to 2004 by age and social class and projections of prevalence to 2012. J Epidemiol Community Health 2009; 63:140–146.

[12] Taylor EN, Stampfer MJ, Curhan GC. Obesity, weight gain, and the risk of kidney stones. JAMA 2005; 293:455–462.

[13] Al-Ani A, Al-Jalham K, Ibrahim T, Majzoub A, Al-Rayashi M, Hayati A, Mubarak W, Al-Rayahi J, Khairy AT. Factors determining renal impairment in unilateral ureteric colic secondary to calcular disease: a prospective study. Int Urol Nephrol 2015; 47(7):1085–1090.

[14] WW Roberts, JA Cadeddu, S Micali, et al. Ureteric stricture formation after removal of impacted calculi. J Urol 1998; 159:723–726.

[15] Ucero Alvaro C, Benito-Martin Alberto, Izquierdo Maria C, Sanchez-Nin˜o MD, Sanz AB. Unilateral ureteric obstruction: beyond obstruction. Int Urol Nephrol 2014; 46:765–776.

[16] Klahr S. Pathophysiology of obstructive nephropathy. Kidney Int 1983; 23:414–426.

[17] Siegel R, Ma J, Zou Z, et al. Cancer statistics. CA Cancer J Clin 2014; 64(1):9–29.

[18] Raman JD, Messer J, Sielatycki JA, et al. Incidence and survival of patients with carcinoma of the ureter and renal pelvis in the USA, 1973-2005. BJU Int 2011; 107(7):1059–1064.

[19] Williams SK, Denton KJ, Minervini A, et al. Correlation of upper-tract cytology, retrograde pyelography, ureteroscopic appearance, and ureteroscopic biopsy with histologic examination of upper-tract transitional cell carcinoma. J Endourol 2008; 22(1):71–76.

[20] Ganatra AM, Loughlin KR. The management of malignant ureteric obstruction treated with ureteric stents. J Urol 2005; 174:2125–2128.

[21] Chung SY, Stein RJ, Landsittel D et al. 15-year experience with the management of extrinsic ureteric obstruction with indwelling ureteric stents. J Urol 2004; 172:592–595.

[22] Wong LM, Cleeve LK, Milner AD, Pitman AG. Malignant ureteric obstruction: outcomes after intervention. Have things changed? J Urol 2007; 178:178–183.

[23] Izumi K, Mizokami A, Maeda Y, Koh E, Namiki M. Current outcome of patients with ureteric stents for the management of malignant ureteric obstruction. J Urol 2011; 185:556–561.

[24] Smith's Textbook of Endourology, 2nd ed., London: BC Decker, 2007, 285–290.

[25] JS Wolf Jr., OM Elashry, RV Clayman. Long-term results of endoureterotomy for benign ureteric and ureteroenteric strictures. J Urol 1997; 158:759–764.

[26] Parpala-Sparman T, Paananen I, Santala M, et al. Increasing numbers of ureteric injuries after the introduction of laparoscopic surgery. Scand J Urol Nephrol 2008; 42:422–427.

[27] Liapis A, Bakas P, Giannopoulos V, et al. Ureteric injuries during gynecological surgery. Int Urogynecol J Pelvic Floor Dysfunct 2001; 12:391–393.

[28] Dobrowolski Z, Kusionowicz J, Drewniak T, et al. Renal and ureteric trauma: Diagnosis and management in Poland. BJU Int 2002; 89:748–751.

[29] Vakili B, Chesson RR, Kyle BL, et al. The incidence of urinary tract injury during hysterectomy: A prospective analysis based on universal cystoscopy. Am J Obstet Gynecol 2005;192:1599–1604.

[30] Mathevet P, Valencia P, Cousin C, et al. Operative injuries during vaginal hysterectomy. Eur J Obstet Gynecol Reprod Biol 2001; 97:71–75.

[31] Geavlete P, Georgescu D, Niţa G, et al. Complications of 2735 retrograde semirigid ureteroscopy procedures: A single-center experience. J Endourol 2006; 20:179–185.

[32] Lau KO, Hia TN, Cheng C, et al. Outcome of obstructive uropathy after pelvic irradiation in patients with carcinoma of the uterine cervix. Ann Acad Med Singapore 1998;27:631–635.

[33] Ghoneim MA, Osman Y. Uretero-intestinal anastomosis in low-pressure reservoirs: Refluxing or antirefluxing? BJU Int 2007;100:1229–1233.

[34] Zavos G, Pappas P, Karatzas T, et al. Urological complications: Analysis and management of 1525 consecutive renal transplantations. Transplant Proc 2008; 40:1386–1390.

[35] Jaskowski A, Jones RM, Murie JA, et al. Urological complications in 600 consecutive renal transplants. Br J Surg 1987;74:922–925.

[36] Donnez J, Brosens I. Definition of ureteric endometriosis? Fertil Steril 1997; 68:178–180.

[37] Goel A, Dalela D. Options in the management of tuberculous ureteric stricture. Indian J Urol 2008; 24:376–381.

[38] Vaglio A, Corradi D, Manenti L et al. Evidence of autoimmunity in chronic periaortitis: a prospective study. Am J Med 2003; 114:454–462.

[39] Wagenknecht LV, Hardy JC. Value of various treatments for retroperitoneal fibrosis. Eur Urol 1981; 7:193–200.

[40] Biyani C, Joyce A. Urolithiasis in pregnancy. BJU Int 2002; 89:811–823.

[41] Lewis DF, Robichaux AG, Jaekle RK, et al. Urolithiasis in pregnancy. J Reprod Med 2003; 48:28–32.

6

The Role of the Interventional Radiologist in Managing Ureteric Obstruction

Stephen Perrio[1] and Alex Chapman[2]

[1] Ashford and St Peter's Hospitals NHS Foundation Trust, Chertsey, Surrey, UK
[2] Consultant Radiologist, Ashford and St Peter's Hospitals NHS Foundation Trust, Chertsey, Surrey, UK

6.1 Introduction

Upper urinary tract obstruction is a common clinical problem encountered by the urologists in day-to-day practice. It may be secondary to a benign or malignant pathology. In both cases, relief of the obstructed kidney is the first consideration. This may be achieved in the short term by a percutaneous nephrostomy or more definitively with ureteric stenting.

The first ureteric stents were placed during open operations on the bladder as early as the 1800s, but with the advent of cystoscopy in the early twentieth century, endoscopic stent placement became an established procedure for the management of ureteric obstruction. The first dedicated self-retaining ureteric stent was described by Zimskind in 1967 [1]. Shortly after, the first cases of percutaneous antegrade ureteric stenting were reported in 1978-1979 [2, 3]. More recently with advances in interventional radiology, antegrade percutaneous ureteric stent insertion has been increasingly utilized in the management of ureteric obstructions not amenable to primary endoscopic treatment.

The place of antegrade ureteric stenting in the management of ureteric obstruction is not clearly defined. In this chapter, we will review the evidence for antegrade stenting in the management of both malignant and benign ureteric obstruction with comparison to retrograde stenting. An overview of the procedure of antegrade stent placement and requisite patient preparation is described.

6.2 Indications for Antegrade Stenting

Ureteric obstruction is a common clinical scenario and may occur due to a wide variety of etiologies such as compressive pelvic malignancy, retroperitoneal fibrosis, and obstructing stone disease. Pragmatically, the causes of ureteric obstruction may be considered in terms of benign or malignant obstruction, the commonest cause of benign obstruction being obstructive stone disease and the most common cause of malignant obstruction being advanced pelvic malignant disease.

Ureteric Stenting, First Edition. Edited by Ravi Kulkarni.
© 2017 John Wiley & Sons Ltd. Published 2017 by John Wiley & Sons Ltd.

In the case of compressive pelvic malignant disease causing ureteric obstruction, retrograde stenting has been shown to have a poor success rate. Danilovic *et al.* showed a retrograde stent success rate of 52% for obstruction secondary to extrinsic compression. In these patients, the failure of retrograde stenting was due to non-identification of the ureteric orifice in 77% [4]. Antegrade stenting has been demonstrated to offer significantly improved success rates in this situation based on the available literature. A study by Chitale *et al.* demonstrated a 21% primary success rate with retrograde stenting of obstruction secondary to malignant pelvic disease compared with a 98% success rate with a two-stage antegrade approach [5]. The most frequent reason for failure of retrograde stenting was an inability to cannulate the ureteric orifice or failure to negotiate the lower segment of the ureter in 89% of cases. Subsequently, Uthappa and Cowan showed an initial success rate via the retrograde approach of 50% in cases of malignant pelvic obstruction from a number of primary tumor types. The commonest cause of failure was documented as tumor involving the bladder base. Those patients who failed the retrograde approach progressed to antegrade stenting with a 98% success rate [6]. Therefore, the antegrade placement of a ureteric stent is suggested as the first-line approach in those patients with pelvic ureteric obstruction or extensive bladder involvement with a involvement of the ureteric orifices by malignancy confirmed on imaging.

The place of antegrade stent insertion for benign obstruction is less well established with no comparative studies available. Retrograde stent insertion has been demonstrated as a successful approach with a success rate of over 90% in the treatment of benign ureteric obstruction [4]. In a large group of patients reported by Venyo *et al.*, the success rate of antegrade stenting was 87% (105/121) including 30 patients with obstruction secondary to stone disease, 13 benign strictures of varied cause, 3 with retroperitoneal fibrosis, 2 patients with benign prostatic hypertrophy, and one each of compressive fibroids, endometriosis, compressive abdominal aortic aneurysm and a pelvi-ureteric obstruction following laparoscopic pyeloplasty [7].

Given the high success rate of retrograde stent insertion, it seems appropriate that antegrade stenting be considered only as a second-line intervention when retrograde stenting is unsuccessful and decompression with percutaneous nephrostomy is required. There is then a high success rate with the antegrade approach.

6.3   Patient Preparation for Antegrade Stent Insertion

6.3.1   Pre-Procedure

Prior to an antegrade stent insertion, the patient should be reviewed by the clinical team to ensure suitability for the procedure. This must include a review of anticoagulant therapy to minimize the risk of bleeding complications. The Society of Interventional Radiology (SIR) consensus document suggests an INR of less than 1.5 is advisable prior to procedure similarly a platelet count of $> 50 \times 10^9$/L is suggested. Coumadin (Warfarin) should be stopped for 5 days or reversed with vitamin K or FFP and a repeat INR performed pre-procedure. Patients on unfractionated heparin should have this stopped for 3 hours and fractionated heparin should be withheld for 24 hours. Similarly anti-platelet therapy with clopidogrel or aspirin should be withheld for 5 days [8].

An assessment of the patient's respiratory status and ability to lie prone is advised with a low threshold for anaesthetic review if there is any concern. The prone position of the patient during stent insertion will exacerbate any pre-existing respiratory or ventilatory deficiencies and will also limit monitoring during the procedure. Any concern should be raised with the clinician performing the procedure early to allow adequate discussion or preparation [8].

A major risk of antegrade stent insertion is that of infection, hence prophylactic antibiotic therapy is suggested with the routine administration of 500 mg of oral ciprofloxacin 1 hour prior to the procedure having been shown to be safe and cost effective [9], although consultation with local antimicrobial guidelines is advised. Any pre-procedural or intra-procedural medications including antibiotics should be prescribed prior to the procedure to ensure timely dosing.

6.3.2 Contra-Indications

Contra-indications to antegrade ureteric stenting largely relate to the major risk of bleeding inherent in percutaneous renal puncture. The Society of Interventional Radiologists lists un-correctable severe coagulopathy and terminal illness/imminent death as relative contra-indications [10] to percutaneous nephrostomy.

Although a definitive list of relative contra-indications to antegrade ureteric stenting has not been agreed, and will vary by department, suggested contra-indications include:

- Uncorrected coagulopathy (INR >1.5; Platelets <50 x 10^9/L)
- Anaphylactoid contrast allergy
- Recent antiplatelet therapy
- Inability to lie prone without respiratory support [8]

6.3.3 Procedure

Antegrade ureteric stenting is usually performed in the interventional radiology suite by a consultant interventional radiologist and is largely well tolerated with local anesthesia and light conscious sedation only.

With the patient lying in the prone position, the dilated pelvicalyceal system is identified with ultrasound and a suitable site for puncture of an upper or mid pole calyx marked. This is often preferable to a lower pole puncture if antegrade stenting is planned, as it offers a more favorable tracking by reducing tortuosity. The skin is then cleaned and the area draped in preparation for calyceal puncture. Constant monitoring of the patient's pulse, heart rate, and cyclical blood pressure measurements are required throughout the procedure with regular relay to the operator to ensure patient safety.

Local anesthetic is injected to the skin and infiltrated to the level of the renal cortex under ultrasound guidance using a 22G spinal needle. If the patient experiences discomfort or distress, light sedation is achieved with a combination of opioid analgesic (fentanyl) and a benzodiazepine (midazolam).

This needle is exchanged for a micropuncture set with which the definitive calyceal puncture is made under direct ultrasound visualisation. Once urine is aspirated, dilute contrast is injected to confirm calyceal position with fluoroscopy. This should be done prior to the insertion of a guidewire and sheath to ensure a secure and satisfactory position.

A hydrophilic wire is then advanced down the ureter into the bladder. A vascular catheter commonly a Cobra or biliary manipulation catheter is used to provide stability and facilitate bridging of any stenosis and entry into the bladder. When the position in the bladder is confirmed with contrast fluoroscopically, a peel-away sheath may be inserted over a support wire to lie in the mid ureter place; this supports the insertion and positioning of the stent. It is sometimes necessary to pre-dilate a malignant or benign stenosis to allow the stent to be inserted; in the author's experience a 5 mm balloon is usually sufficient for this purpose. A double J stent is then advanced over a stiff wire to sit with the distal loop in the bladder.

Once safe position in the bladder is confirmed, the proximal loop is formed in the renal pelvis and contrast is instilled to ensure patency. A covering nephrostomy drain may then be inserted if required.

6.3.4 Complications

The complications of antegrade stent placement may be considered in terms of those relating to percutaneous renal puncture, which are indistinguishable to the risks of percutaneous nephrostomy and are unique to the antegrade approach, and those relating to stent placement. The latter are similar to a retrograde stenting as they are related to the stent itself, which are ubiquitous irrespective of the route of placement. The majority of complications are the former and may be further considered as systemic or local and minor or major, dependent on requirement for further treatment [10].

The major systemic complication is that of sepsis, usually secondary to *E. coli*, Klebsiella, and Proteus species. This results from bacterial translocation from renal pelvis to systemic circulation due to increased pressure in an infected system during puncture, contrast injection, and wire manipulation [11].

The reported rate of post nephrostomy insertion fever has been reported at between 21 [12] and 100% [13]. The rate of sepsis, however, is relatively small and has been reported in 1-3% of all patients post percutaneous nephrostomy, increasing to 7-9% in patients with pre-existing pyonephrosis in one review [10]. The SIR suggest a threshold rate of 4% and 10% respectively for these complications [10]. Lower rates of septicemia were demonstrated in the UK Nephrostomy Audit of 3263 procedures with a reported rate of 0.9%. However, sepsis was the cause of death in all four cases recorded, totalling 0.1% of all nephrostomy insertions [14]. To reduce this risk, over distension of the collecting system should be avoided during contrast injection. Evidence also suggests that the routine administration of 500 mg of oral ciprofloxacin 1 hour prior to nephrostomy insertion significantly reduces complications and is cost effective [9]. It stands to reason that a similar protocol for antegrade stenting would be effective but local microbiology protocols should be consulted.

Bleeding is the major local complication of percutaneous renal puncture and may occur from parenchymal or, if a high approach is taken, intercostal vessels. Venous bleeding is normally self-limiting but may be ameliorated by upsizing the catheter to cause tamponade. Rarely, venous bleeding may require transfusion [11]. In fact, some degree of venous bleeding is reported in up to 95% of cases but is a minor complication that rarely requires intervention [10].

Arterial bleeding may be more significant. It arises either from branches of the renal artery or inter-costal vessels if a high approach is taken. Depending on the severity, this may require transfusion, embolization, and rarely, open surgical management. The risk of bleeding correlates directly with the size of tract, and as such, a smaller sheath will carry a lower bleeding risk. The long-term complications of arterial injury include arterio-venous fistula formation, peri-renal/retroperitoneal hematoma, and pseudo-aneurysms. Although these are rare, they may be significant and should be considered in a patient who deteriorates following intervention [11]. The overall rate of bleeding complications requiring transfusion or other intervention is reported at 1 to 4% [10]. The UK Nephrostomy Audit included 3262 nephrostomy insertions and recorded an overall bleeding complication rate of 2% [14].

Less common local complications of percutaneous renal puncture include pleural complications of pneumothorax, hydrothorax, or hemothorax with reported rates of 0.06 [14] and 0.2% [15]. Urinoma formation following percutaneous puncture is a further recognized local complication with a reported rate of 0.1% [14]. Complications relating to trans-colonic puncture are uncommon but have been reported [16].

Local complications related to stent insertion are similar to those with a retrograde approach and include bladder irritation, pain, hematuria, infections, stent displacement, and blockage. These complications are not specific to antegrade stenting and are discussed in detail elsewhere.

The current overall complication rate for antegrade stenting is reported at 2-6% [17] for major complications and the complication rate of percutaneous nephrostomy in the UK Nephrostomy Audit was 6.3% with 4.1% requiring therapy [14]. These figures are comparable to the reported complication rate of retrograde stent insertion at 5.9% [18] and should not alter the decision of whether antegrade or retrograde stenting is most appropriate (Figures 6.1 and 6.2).

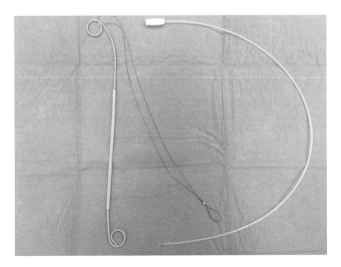

Figure 6.1 6 French 22cm Flexima Ureteric Stent System. Boston Scientific, MA, USA. The Glidex Hydrogel Coating on stent requires activation by soaking in sterile water or saline prior to use. This is inserted over a 0.038/0.035in guidewire. The suture at the proximal end enables retraction to facilitate optimal positioning; this must be removed once appropriate placement is achieved. The stent pusher has a radio-opaque distal marker.

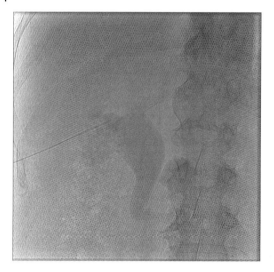

Figure 6.2 21-G introducer needle with stylet inserted into the mid pole calyx under ultrasound guidance. Satisfactory position confirmed with radiographic contrast. Midpole puncture may allow easier stent placement due to greater pushability particularly in the context of a distal ureteric stricture.

6.4   Stent Design

The ideal ureteric stent does not exist but has been well described as providing optimal flow dynamics, ease of insertion and removal, no complications, and being easily visible on imaging [19]. Modern stents are almost exclusively double J in design and formed of polymeric material. Polymeric stents provide a largely biologically inert stent and are usually coated with a variety of substances to provide a hydrophilic coating and reduce the formation of biofilms. Polymeric stents do, however, have limitations in terms of strength to resist radial force and acting as a nidus for infection formation [20]. In a bid to overcome these problems, there is ongoing research into the development of both metallic ureteric stents, to provide greater radial force, and biodegradable stents, to reduce complications of stent encrusting and infection [21]. At present, no biodegradable antegrade stents are used in clinical practice and these will not be considered further.

As discussed previously, antegrade stent insertion is most beneficial in the situation of external ureteric compression due to pelvic malignancy [5, 6] and as such the ability to withstand high radial force is especially desirable in stents placed via the antegrade route. Initial experience with metallic mesh stents was promising showing good patency rates in the treatment of malignant obstruction [22]. A more recent publication demonstrated a primary patency rate at 18 months of 54% but showed that placement of these stents did not result in adequate correction of renal failure to allow chemotherapy, the intended aim, in 21% of recipients [23]. Although all stents in this study were placed endourologically it is reasonable to suggest long-term patency and correction of renal function would be similar irrespective of the route of placement (Figures 6.3 and 6.4).

Experience with newer covered metallic stents placed via the antegrade approach has been more encouraging. Chung *et al.* [24] have shown favorable patency rates with

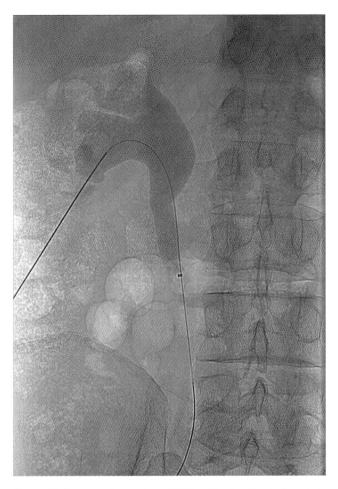

Figure 6.3 Lower pole puncture. 0.018in nitinol guidewire inserted to distal ureter and co-axial introducer, dilator and sheath inserted (tip of sheath has a radiographic marker lying in proximal ureter). The sheath accomodates both the 0.018in wire and a 0.035in standard wire, allowing the subsequent catheters and stents to be passed over the 0.035in wire, leaving the 0.018in wire in situ as a safety wire.

this new stent at 1 (100%), 3 (94.5%), 6 (74.7%), 9 (70.3%), 12 (65.3%), 18 (65.3%), and 24 months (65.3%) when compared to patency of double J stents (37.8% at 18 months) in the treatment of malignant ureteric obstruction. Although this was not a randomized study and the numbers small, initial results are promising and further large trials are required.

6.5 The One-Stage Antegrade Stent

Antegrade ureteric stenting has traditionally been performed as a two-stage procedure. Initially, a percutaneous nephrostomy tube is inserted acutely to relieve obstruction and after a delay the antegrade stent is inserted. Recent advances in interventional radiology

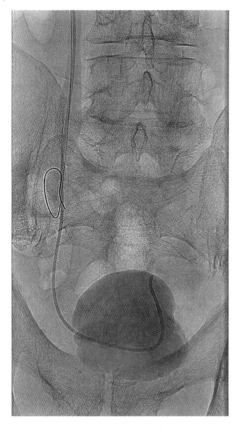

Figure 6.4 Catheter advanced into the bladder over a hydrophillic 0.035in wire and the approriate intravesical position confirmed with contrast.

have, however, allowed for more precise renal puncture, easier stent manipulation, and lower complication rates. These advances and increasing demand on interventional uro-radiologists has led to research in to the utility of a one-stage approach to antegrade ureteric stenting.

Current small studies have suggested that the use of a one-stage procedure in certain instances is both safe and cost effective. A one-stage procedure should not be considered if there is obstruction complicated by acute sepsis or untreated renal failure [25]. Other studies have, however, demonstrated a lower clinical success rate with a one-stage tubeless approach [17] and at present, the result of larger studies are awaited to inform day-to-day practice.

6.6 The Rendezvous Procedure

In patients with complex ureteric obstruction or where retrograde/antegrade stenting alone has failed, a combined procedure with both antegrade and retrograde access to the ureter can be used. This has become known as the rendezvous procedure and allows bidirectional traction to be applied across a stricture, as long as a wire can be passed across the lesion initially [26]. In patients with long length, mid ureteric, ischemic- or radiation-related strictures this approach has increased antegrade stent success from 78.6% to 88.09% in one series [27]. In these patients, the consensus opinion is that a decompressing nephrostomy via a mid or upper calyx should be performed initially and stent insertion only attempted as a two-stage procedure (Figures 6.5 and 6.6).

In the author's experience, the appropriate use of analgesia and sedation is vital to ensure the procedure is well tolerated. A semi-prone position is also often helpful for the patient's comfort. The use of a buddy wire, which can be introduced via the peel-away sheath, can aid stability in challenging anatomy and stenotic disease. Also, a staged approach to nephrostomy and stent insertion is frequently preferable in the emergent setting and while rarely an antegrade stent cannot be suitable advanced into a satisfactory position, this is mostly overcome with the use of a rendezvous technique.

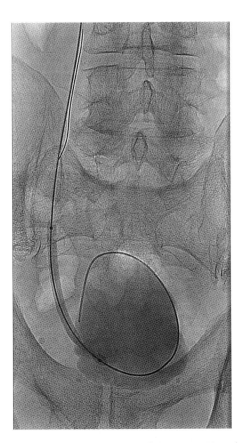

Figure 6.5 A stiff 0.035in guidewire is positioned within the bladder and 5mm balloon dilatation of the distal ureter sticture secondary to muscle invasive transitional cell carcinmoma is performed to enable stent placement. Waisting of the distal 1/3rd of the balloon is noted at the level of the vesicoureteric junction.

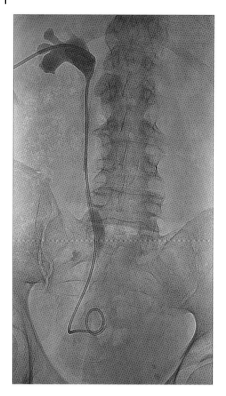

Figure 6.6 Following satisfactory stent placement, a covering nephrostomy tube is placed. This is then removed under flouroscopic guidance following a nephrostogram, as is the authors' normal practice.

6.7 Summary

Current evidence suggests that antegrade ureteric stenting has a similar safety profile to retrograde stenting and is more effective as a method for managing ureteric obstruction resulting from pelvic malignancy. As such, antegrade stenting is considered the optimal initial approach in this patient group. The place of antegrade stenting in benign ureteric obstruction is uncertain and no large studies exist. The limited case numbers available suggest that antegrade stenting is a reasonable second-line treatment if the retrograde approach fails.

In complex situations where retrograde or antegrade stenting alone are unlikely to succeed, a rendezvous procedure is an effective and established approach requiring close cooperation of both interventionalist and urologist.

Ongoing research in to a one-stage approach to antegrade ureteric stenting is required, but the available evidence suggests this is a cost-effective and safe approach in malignant ureteric obstruction without concomitant sepsis or renal failure.

The use of antegrade metallic stents has in the past shown varied results but newer covered metallic stents are a promising area of ongoing research for the treatment of malignant ureteric obstruction. Biodegradable antegrade stents are still under investigation but to date are not in regular clinical use.

Best treatment of ureteric obstruction requires close collaboration between both urologists and interventional radiologists. Robust guidelines governing optimal approach for stenting, pre-intervention optimization, and appropriate antibiotic prophylaxis should be encouraged and agreed on locally in the absence of national guidelines.

References

[1] Zimskind PD, Fetter TR, Willierson JL. 'Clinical use of longterm indwelling silicone rubber ureteral splints inserted cystoscopically.' Journal of Urology, 1967; 97:840–844.

[2] Smith AD, Lange PH, Miller RP *et al.* 'Introduction of the Gibbons ureteral stent facilitated by antecedent percutaneous nephrostomy.' Journal of Urology, 1978; 120(5):543–544.

[3] Mazer MJ, LeVeen RF, Call JE *et al.* 'Permanent percutaneous antegrade ureteral stent placement without transurethral assistance.' Urology 1979; 14(4):413–419.

[4] Danilovic A, Antonopoulus IM, Mesquite JL *et al.* 'Likelihood of retrograde double J stenting according to ureteral obstructing pathology' International Brazilian Journal of Urology, 2005;31(5):431–436.

[5] Chitale SV, Scott-Barrett S, Ho ETS *et al.* 'The management of ureteric obstruction secondary to malignant pelvic disease.' Clinical radiology, 2002; 57:1118–1121.

[6] Uthappa, M.C. Cowan NC. 'Retrograde or antegrade double-pigtail stent placement for malignant ureteric obstruction.' Clinical radiology, 2005; 60:608–612.

[7] Venyo AK, Hanley T, Barrett M *et al.* 'Ante-grade ureteric stenting, retrospective experience in managing 89 patients: indications, complications and outcome.' Journal of biomedical graphics and computing, 2014; 4(3):47–56.

[8] Dagli M, Ramachandri P. 'Percutaneous nephrostomy: technical aspects and indications.' Seminars in interventional radiology, 2011; 28(4):424–437.

[9] Sutcliffe JA, Briggs JH, Little MW *et al.* 'Antibiotics in interventional radiology.' Clinical Radiology, 2015; 70:223–234.

[10] Ramchandani P, Cardella JF, Grassi CJ *et al.* 'Society of Interventional Radiology Standards of Practice Committee. Quality improvement guidelines for percutaneous nephrostomy.' Journal of Vascular Interventional Radiology, 2003; 14(9 Pt 2):S277–S281.

[11] Hausegger KA, Portugaller HR. 'Percutaneous nephrostomy and antegrade ureteral stenting: technique – indications – complications.' European Radiology, 2006; 16:2016–2030.

[12] Cochran ST, Barbaric ZL, Lee JJ *et al.* 'Percutaneous nephrostomy tube placement: an outpatient procedure?' Radiology, 1991; 179(3):843–847.

[13] Lee WJ, Patel U, Patel S *et al.* 'Emergency percutaneous nephrostomy: results and complications.' Journal of Vascular Interventional Radiology, 1994;5(1):135–139.

[14] Chalmers N, Jones K, Drinkwter K *et al.* 'The UK nephrostomy audit. Can a voluntary registry produce robust performance data?' Clinical Radiology, 2008; 3:888–894.

[15] Farrell TA, Hicks ME. 'A review of radiologically guided percutaneous nephrostomies in 303 patients.' Journal of Vascular Interventional Radiology, 1997; 8:769–774.

[16] Wah TM, Weston MJ, Irving HC. 'Percutaneous nephrostomy insertion: outcome data from a propspective multi-operator study at a UK training centre.' Clinical Radiology, 2004; 59:255–261.

[17] Patel U and Abubacker Z. 'Ureteral stent placement without postprocedural nephrostomy tube: experience in 41 patients.' Radiology, 2004; 230:435–442.

[18] Geavlete P, Georgescu D, NiţĂ G *et al*. 'Complications of 2735 retrograde semirigid ureteroscopy procedures: A single center experience.' Journal of Endourology, 2006; 20(3):179–185.

[19] Al-Aown A, Kyriazis I, Kallidonis P *et al*. 'Ureteral stents: new ideas, new designs.' Therapeutic Advances in Urology, 2010; 2(2):85–92.

[20] Venkatesan N, Shroff S, Jayachandran K *et al*. 'Polymers as ureteral stents.' Journal of Endourology, 2010; 24(2):191–198.

[21] Chew BH and Denstedt JD. 'Technology insight: Novel ureteral stent materials and designs.' Nature Clinical Practical Urology, 2004; 1(1):44–48.

[22] Lugmayr H, Pauer W. 'Self-expanding metal stents for palliative treatment of malignant ureteral obstruction.' American Journal of Roentgenology, 1992; 159(5):1091–1094.

[23] Lang EK, Winer AG, Abbey-Mensah G *et al*. 'Long-term results of metallic stents for malignant ureteral obstruction in advanced cervical carcinoma.' Journal of Endourology, 2013; 27(5):646–651.

[24] Chung HH, Kim MD, Won JY *et al*. 'Multicenter Experience of the Newly Designed Covered Metallic Ureteral Stent for Malignant Ureteral Occlusion: Comparison with Double J Stent Insertion.' CardioVascular and Interventional Radiology, 2014; 37(2):463–470.

[25] Chitale S, Raja V, Hussain N *et al*. 'One-stage tubeless antegrade ureteric stenting: a safe and cost-effective option?' Annals of the Royal College of Surgeons of England, 2010; 92(3):218–224.

[26] Watson JM, Dawkins GPC, Whitfield HN *et al*. 'The rendezvous procedure to cross complicated ureteric strictures.' British Journal of Urology, 2002; 89:317–319.

[27] Macrì A, Magnoa C, Certob A *et al*. 'Combined antegrade and retrograde ureteral stenting: the rendezvous technique'. Clinical Radiology, 2005; 60:257–260.

7

Emergency Management of Ureteric Obstruction

Steeve Doizi[1] and Margaret S. Pearle[2]

[1] Research Fellow, Endourology and Stone Disease, Department of Urology, University of Texas Southwestern
Medical Center, Dallas, Texas, USA
[2] Professor of Urology and Internal Medicine, University of Texas Southwestern Medical Center, Dallas, Texas, USA

7.1 Introduction

The prevalence of urolithiasis has increased over the past three decades and now affects approximately 9% of the American adult population, with comparable increases in prevalence in other developed countries [1–10]. Accordingly, complications associated with stone disease have increased over time as well. Obstructive pyelonephritis, the occurrence of urinary infection proximal to a site of ureteral obstruction, is considered a urologic emergency that requires prompt drainage of the kidney to prevent life-threatening sepsis. According to data obtained from the Nationwide Inpatient Sample, hospital discharges associated with a diagnosis of renal or ureteral calculi and urinary tract infection/pyelonephritis increased by 96% between 1999 and 2009. Taking into account the increase in population, this represents a 12% increase in incidence per 100,000 U.S. adults [11]. Interestingly, despite a higher prevalence of nephrolithiasis in men than women, women were more than twice as likely to have infected urolithiasis than men (22.3 per 100,000 versus 10.2 per 100,000, respectively).

There are no randomized trials comparing surgical decompression with conservative management in patients with obstructive pyelonephritis. Only one older retrospective trial evaluated the outcome of 14 febrile patients with ureteral calculi in whom conservative therapy with fluid and antibiotics was initiated [12]. All patients became a-pyrexial and 11 patients required no further intervention. However, concern for pyonephrosis, the most feared and extreme form of obstructive pyelonephritis, which carries a high mortality rate and risk of renal loss, leads most practitioners to recommend prompt drainage of the collecting system in the setting of obstruction and infection. Indeed, data from the Nationwide Inpatient Sample from 2007 to 2009 revealed a higher mortality rate in patients with ureteral calculi and sepsis treated conservatively than with surgical decompression (19.2% versus 8.8%, respectively, $p < 0.001$) [13]. Furthermore, this disparity in mortality rates is likely an underestimate because of selection bias, by which only less sick patients were likely selected for conservative management.

Ureteric Stenting, First Edition. Edited by Ravi Kulkarni.
© 2017 John Wiley & Sons Ltd. Published 2017 by John Wiley & Sons Ltd.

7.2 Identifying Patients with Obstructive Pyelonephritis

The precise criteria needed to identify patients with obstructive pyelonephritis are not known. Elevated white blood count, fever, and bacteriuria are generally accepted indicators of pyelonephritis, although the exact cut-points defining abnormal parameters are not well-established. Markers of systemic inflammatory response syndrome (SIRS, defined as two or more of the following: temperature >38 °C or <36 °C; heart rate >90 beats/minute; respiratory rate >20 or partial pressure $CO_2 < 32$ mm Hg; white count >12,000/mm^3 or <4000/mm^3 or >10% immature neutrophil) provides a more objective means of identifying those at risk of sepsis who should undergo prompt upper tract drainage in the setting of obstruction. Yoshimura and associates retrospectively identified 53 patients who underwent 59 emergency drainage procedures and found that among those who underwent drainage for obstruction due to calculi, multivariate analysis revealed that patient age (≥75 years versus ≤74, OR 2.1, 95% CI 1.1-4.0); gender (female versus male, OR 1.8, 95% CI 1.0-3.2) and performance status (≤70% versus ≥80%, OR 2.9, 95% CI 1.5-5.6) were independent risk factors for sepsis [14].

7.3 Outcomes by Drainage Modality

Effective drainage of the collecting system can be accomplished by either retrograde stent placement or percutaneous nephrostomy (PN), both of which are generally readily available at most institutions. However, the optimal choice of drainage in the setting of obstruction and infection is controversial (Table 7.1). Proponents of nephrostomy drainage favor avoiding manipulation of the ureter and stone for fear of urinary extravasation or sepsis and cite the larger caliber nephrostomy tube, ability to directly monitor drainage and placement under intravenous sedation as advantages. On the other hand, stent advocates cite the lower serious complication rate with stent placement, greater comfort for patients with an internal drainage tube, and the ability of all urologists to perform the procedure.

The success of the procedure has been investigated for both PN and retrograde stent placement, although most series have not looked at outcomes specifically in patients with ureteral obstruction in the setting of infection. Retrograde stent placement is exclusively performed by urologists, most often in the operating room under general anesthesia using fluorosocopic guidance. Yossepowitch and colleagues prospectively evaluated 92 patients with ureteral obstruction, 61 of whom had intrinsic obstruction (from ureteral stones in 52, ureteropelvic junction obstruction in 5 and ureteral stricture in 4) [15]. Stent placement was successful in 94% of the patients with intrinsic obstruction and in 73% of the patients with extrinsic obstruction. On univariate analysis, the cause of obstruction, location of obstruction, and degree of hydronephrosis predicted the likelihood of successful stent insertion.

Early complications of retrograde stent placement include sepsis, stent migration, and stent occlusion. The incidence of sepsis associated with stent placement in the absence of stone manipulation has not been well evaluated. Upward or downward stent

Table 7.1 Advantages and disadvantages of ureteral stent versus percutaneous nephrostomy for drainage of the obstructed kidney.

Ureteral Stent		Percutaneous Nephrostomy	
Advantages	Disadvantages	Advantages	Disadvantages
Urologist-driven	High incidence of patient symptoms	External access to monitor urine drainage	External tube and collection device
No external collection device	High failure rate for extrinsic obstruction	External access for irrigation/exchange in case of occlusion	Greater risk of bleeding
Low risk of injury	Unable to monitor unilateral drainage	Potential for larger drainage tube	Greater risk of injury to surrounding organs
Uncorrected coagulapathy not contraindication	No access to irrigate obstructed stent	Local anesthesia/IV sedation	Radiologist-driven
Less urgency for definitive management	Requires manipulation of obstructed ureter	Avoids manipulation of ureter	Uncorrected coagulopathy a contraindication
	Precludes radiographic study of obstructed kidney or ureter	No bladder symptoms	
		Access for antegrade nephrostogram to plan definitive treatment	

migration occurs in 3-10% of patients. Stent occlusion or failure increases with duration of stenting, but the likelihood of immediate stent failure in the setting of pyonephrosis or obstructive pyelonephritis has not been reported.

PN is most often performed by interventional radiologists in the interventional radiology suite under conscious sedation with local anesthesia, using sonographic and/or fluoroscopic guidance in the emergency setting. Successful PN has been reported in 92-100% of patients [16–21]. Lee and colleagues showed that initial technical success rates were unaffected by operator experience once the operator had performed at least 10 PN procedures/year [22].

Major complications of PN, including hemorrhage requiring transfusion, sepsis, pleural injury (pneumothorax, empyema, hydrothorax, or hemothorax), and adjacent organ injury, occur in 4-7% of patients [23–26]. The need for blood transfusion related to nephrostomy insertion is as high as 3.2% in some series [27]. Among 92 patients undergoing PN specifically for pyonephrosis, Ng and coworkers reported a mortality rate of 2% and an overall complication rate of 14% [28]. Likewise, Watson and colleagues reported a 9.2% incidence of serious complications among 315 patients who underwent nephrostomy drainage for pyonephrosis, including significant bleeding in 2.2%, infected urinoma in 2.2%, perinephric abscess in 0.6%, pneumothorax in 0.3%, and perinephric hematoma in 0.3% [29].

7.4   Comparative Effectiveness

Few studies have compared the efficacy of retrograde stent placement and PN for drainage of the obstructed, infected kidney. In the only randomized trial (RCT) comparing the efficacy of retrograde stent placement and PN for the management of patients with infection and ureteral obstruction due to stones, Pearle and colleagues enrolled 42 patients meeting selection criteria [ureteral stone with temperature >38 °C and/or white blood cell count (WBC) >17,000/mm^3] over a 2-year time period [30]. The primary outcome parameters were time to normalization of WBC and temperature. The two groups were comparable with regard to pre-operative patient and stone characteristics.

Among 21 patients randomized to PN, an 8Fr nephrostomy tube was placed in 90%, 10Fr in 5%, and 12Fr in 5% of patients. Among the 21 patients randomized to stent placement, a 7Fr double pigtail stent was placed in 81% of patients and 6Fr stent in 19%. A Foley catheter was placed for bladder drainage in 71.4% of patients in the stent group and in 33.3% in the PN group. Only one failure occurred, a PN patient, who was successfully salvaged with stent placement. Procedural and fluoroscopy time were significantly shorter in the stent group compared with the PN group by 16.5 minutes and 2.6 minutes, respectively (p < 0.05 for both). However, no significant differences were found between the 2 groups with regard to successful drainage (100% for stent placement versus 95% for PN), clinical normalization of index parameters (time to normalization of WBC and temperature 2.6 and 1.7 days, respectively, for the stent group and 2.3 and 2.0 days for PN group, respectively) and length of hospital stay after drainage (3.2 days for the stent group versus 4.5 days for the PCN group). Using a visual analog pain scale, only flank pain symptoms were perceived to be greater in the PN group compared to the stent group, and more PN patients required parenteral narcotics than stent patients (38% versus 4.8%). Cost was more than twofold higher for stent placement than PN ($2401 versus $1137, respectively), most likely due to the high cost of the operating room. Because of no difference in efficacy between the two modalities, the authors concluded that the choice of drainage should be left to the discretion of the treating physician, taking into account stone size and location, subsequent planned definitive treatment modality and availability of operative room time and interventional radiologists.

Another comparative RCT by Mokhmalji and coworkers in 40 patients with obstructive hydronephrosis due to stones compared stent placement (n = 20) with PN (n = 20), although in this trial only 65% of stent patients and 55% of PN patients showed signs of infection [31]. The primary outcome parameters in this trial included success of drainage, relief of accompanying symptoms, duration of tube drainage, and effect of diversion on quality of life. Both procedures were performed under local anesthesia or conscious sedation in all patients. All PN patients underwent successful drainage while stent placement failed in 20% of stent patients. Reasons for failure were enlarged prostate precluding access to the ureteral orifice and discomfort during stent insertion. The proportion of patients in whom the drainage tube was left indwelling longer than 4 weeks was greater for the stent group than the PN group (56% versus 20%, respectively, p = 0.043), although the indication for tube removal was not well defined. Antibiotic duration was marginally longer in the stent group compared to the PN group, but the difference did not reach statistical significance.

Subgroup analysis of patients with obstructive pyelonephritis revealed longer duration of intravenous antibiotics in the stent patients than the PN patients (6.6 days versus 4.3 days, respectively, p = NS), although the difference was not statistically significant. The endpoint for antibiotic treatment was not well defined. No significant difference was reported for pain relief or quality of life between the two groups. Because of a shorter duration of drainage and marginally shorter antibiotic duration, the authors favored PN over stent placement in patients with obstructive hydronephrosis due to stones.

Using the Nationwide Inpatient Sample (1999–2009), Sammon and associates identified 113,439 patients with infection and obstruction due to stones who underwent drainage of the kidney. Among this group, 87.7% of patients underwent stent placement and 12.3% of patients underwent PN. Using propensity-score matching for patient and hospital characteristics, patients undergoing nephrostomy tube placement had higher rates of sepsis (OR 1.63, 95% CI 1.52-1.74), severe sepsis (OR 2.28, 95% CI 2.06-2.52), prolonged length of stay (OR 3.18, 95% CI 3.01-3.32) and in-hospital mortality (OR 3.14, 95% CI 2.13-4.63) than those undergoing stent placement [11].

In a similar retrospective study of 130 patients with obstructing renal or ureteral calculi and SIRS who underwent drainage with a percutaneous nephrostomy or retrograde ureteral stent, Goldsmith and colleagues identified three treatment failures (two stent placement and one PN), each of which was successfully salvaged by the other drainage procedure [32]. The two groups were *not* comparable with regard to either stone size (larger for PN group versus stent group, 10 mm versus 7 mm, respectively, p = 0.031) or severity of illness (higher APACHE scores for PN versus stent, 15 versus 11, respectively p = 0.003). On univariable analysis, PN was associated with a significantly longer length of stay (7.6 versus 4.2 days, respectively p = 0.001) and higher likelihood of ICU admission (42% versus 20%, respectively, p = 0.006) than stent placement. On multivariable logistic regression analysis, after adjusting for age, APACHE score and Charlson Comorbidity Index score, PN was an independent risk factor for longer length of hospital stay (ß = 0.47, 95% CI 0.2-0.74, p = 0.001) and risk of ICU admission (OR 3.23, 95% CI 1.24-8.41, p = 0.016). However, in both of these studies, selection bias may have confounded the findings because of the possibility that sicker patients were more likely to be treated with nephrostomy drainage than stent placement because of perceived greater safety and efficacy of PN.

7.5 Quality of Life (QOL)

Few studies have evaluated patient preferences regarding the choice of drainage modality in the setting of ureteral obstruction. Joshi and colleagues used a validated health index (EuroQol EQ-5D) and intervention-specific questionnaire to assess pain, urinary symptoms and perceived daily problems at a mean of 12 days after PN and 28 days after stent drainage [33]. They found no difference in the mean EuroQol and analogue pain scores between the two groups. However, patients with stents experienced significantly more irritative urinary symptoms and trended toward having greater discomfort for a longer duration and requiring more analgesia than patients undergoing PN drainage. However, patients in the PN group required more help in the daily care of the nephrostomy tube than did stent patients.

7.6 Conclusions

Ureteral obstruction in the setting of urinary infection can have life-threatening consequences. Prompt drainage of the collection system under these circumstances is considered mandatory, even through in some cases infection may not subsequently be proven. The choice of drainage modality, percutaneous nephrostomy versus ureteral stent placement, has been debated, but no clear evidence demonstrates superiority of one modality over the other with regard to clinical parameters. Consequently, the choice of drainage modality is left to the discretion of the clinician and should take into account patient preference, availability of an operating room or interventional radiologist, the size and location of the stone, and the subsequent surgical plan for definitive treatment.

References

[1] Scales CD Jr, Smith AC, Hanley JM, Saigal CS. Urologic Diseases in America Project. Prevalence of kidney stones in the United States. Eur Urol. 2012; 62(1):160–165.

[2] Romero V, Akpinar H, Assimos DG. Kidney stones: a global picture of prevalence, incidence, and associated risk factors. Rev Urol. 2010;12(2-3):e86–e96.

[3] Trinchieri A, Coppi F, Montanari E, Del Nero A, Zanetti G, Pisani E. Increase in the prevalence of symptomatic upper urinary tract stones during the last ten years. Eur Urol. 2000;37(1):23–25.

[4] Amato M, Lusini ML, Nelli F. Epidemiology of nephrolithiasis today. Urol Int. 2004;72 Suppl 1:1–5.

[5] Serio A, Fraioli A. Epidemiology of nephrolithiasis. Nephron. 1999;81 Suppl 1:26–30.

[6] Daudon M, Traxer O, Lechevallier E, Saussine C. Épidémiologie des lithiases urinaires. Prog Urol. 2008;18(12):802–814.

[7] Hesse A, Brändle E, Wilbert D, Köhrmann KU, Alken P. Study on the prevalence and incidence of urolithiasis in Germany comparing the years 1979 vs. 2000. Eur Urol. 2003;44(6):709–713.

[8] Sánchez-Martín FM, Millán Rodríguez F, Esquena Fernández S, Segarra Tomás J, Rousaud Barón F, Martínez-Rodríguez R, Villavicencio Mavrich H. Incidence and prevalence of published studies about urolithiasis in Spain. A review. Actas Urol Esp. 2007;31(5):511–520.

[9] Akinci M, Esen T, Tellaloğlu S. Urinary stone disease in Turkey: an updated epidemiological study. Eur Urol. 1991;20(3):200–203.

[10] Pinduli I, Spivacow R, del Valle E, Vidal S, Negri AL, Previgliano H, Farías Edos R, Andrade JH, Negri GM, Boffi-Boggero HJ. Prevalence of urolithiasis in the autonomous city of Buenos Aires, Argentina. Urol Res. 2006;34(1):8–11.

[11] Sammon JD, Ghani KR, Karakiewicz PI, Bhojani N, Ravi P, Sun M, Sukumar S, Trinh VQ, Kowalczyk KJ, Kim SP, Peabody JO, Menon M, Trinh QD. Temporal trends, practice patterns, and treatment outcomes for infected upper urinary tract stones in the United States. Eur Urol. 2013; 64(1):85–92.

[12] Klein LA, Koyle M, Berg S. The emergency management of patients with ureteral calculi and fever. J Urol. 1983;129(5):938–940.

[13] Borofsky MS, Walter D, Shah O, Goldfarb DS, Mues AC, Makarov DV. Surgical decompression is associated with decreased mortality in patients with sepsis and ureteral calculi. J Urol. 2013;189(3):946–951.

[14] Yoshimura K, Utsunomiya N, Ichioka K, Ueda N, Matsui Y, Terai A. Emergency drainage for urosepsis associated with upper urinary tract calculi. J Urol. 2005;173(2):458–462.

[15] Yossepowitch O, Lifshitz DA, Dekel Y, Gross M, Keidar DM, Neuman M, Livne PM, Baniel J. Predicting the success of retrograde stenting for managing ureteral obstruction. J Urol. 2001;166(5):1746–1749.

[16] Lee WJ, Patel U, Patel S, Pillari GP. Emergency percutaneous nephrostomy: results and complications. J Vasc Interv Radiol. 1994;5(1):135–139.

[17] Farrell TA, Hicks ME. A review of radiologically guided percutaneous nephrostomies in 303 patients. J Vasc Interv Radiol. 1997;8(5):769–774.

[18] Sim LS, Tan BS, Yip SK, Ng CK, Lo RH, Yeong KY, Htoo MM, Cheng CW. Single centre review of radiologically-guided percutaneous nephrostomies: a report of 273 procedures. Ann Acad Med Singapore. 2002;31(1):76–80.

[19] Mahaffey KG, Bolton DM, Stoller ML. Urologist directed percutaneous nephrostomy tube placement. J Urol. 1994;152(6 Pt 1):1973–1976.

[20] von der Recke P, Nielsen MB, Pedersen JF. Complications of ultrasound-guided nephrostomy. A 5-year experience. Acta Radiol. 1994;35(5):452–454.

[21] Kehinde EO, Newland CJ, Terry TR, Watkin EM, Butt Z. Percutaneous nephrostomies. Br J Urol. 1993;71(6):664–666.

[22] Lee WJ, Mond DJ, Patel M, Pillari GP. Emergency percutaneous nephrostomy: technical success based on level of operator experience. J Vasc Interv Radiol. 1994;5(2):327–330.

[23] Lewis S, Patel U. Major complications after percutaneous nephrostomy-lessons from a department audit. Clin Radiol. 2004;59(2):171–179.

[24] Wah TM, Weston MJ, Irving HC. Percutaneous nephrostomy insertion: outcome data from a prospective multi-operator study at a UK training centre. Clin Radiol. 2004;59(3):255–261.

[25] Ramchandani P, Cardella JF, Grassi CJ, Roberts AC, Sacks D, Schwartzberg MS, Lewis CA; SCVIR Standards of Practice Committee. Quality improvement guidelines for percutaneous nephrostomy. J Vasc Interv Radiol. 2001;12(11):1247–1251.

[26] Hausegger KA, Portugaller HR. Percutaneous nephrostomy and antegrade ureteral stenting: technique-indications-complications. Eur Radiol. 2006;16(9):2016–2030.

[27] Mendez-Probst, CE, Ravzi, H, Denstedt, JD: Fundamentals of instrumentation and urinary tract drainage. In: Wein A, Kavoussi L, Novick A, Partin A, Peters C (eds) in *Campbell-Walsh Urology, Tenth Edition*. Philadelphia: Elsevier Saunders, pp 177–191.

[28] Ng CK, Yip SK, Sim LS, Tan BH, Wong MY, Tan BS, Htoo A. Outcome of percutaneous nephrostomy for the management of pyonephrosis. Asian J Surg. 2002;25(3):215–219.

[29] Watson RA, Esposito M, Richter F, Irwin RJ Jr, Lang EK. Percutaneous nephrostomy as adjunct management in advanced upper urinary tract infection. Urology. 1999;54(2):234–239.

[30] Pearle MS, Pierce HL, Miller GL, Summa JA, Mutz JM, Petty BA, Roehrborn CG, Kryger JV, Nakada SY. Optimal method of urgent decompression of the collecting system for obstruction and infection due to ureteral calculi. J Urol. 1998;160(4):1260–1264.

[31] Mokhmalji H, Braun PM, Martinez Portillo FJ, Siegsmund M, Alken P, Köhrmann KU. Percutaneous nephrostomy versus ureteral stents for diversion of hydronephrosis caused by stones: a prospective, randomized clinical trial. J Urol. 2001;165(4):1088–1092.

[32] Goldsmith ZG, Oredein-McCoy O, Gerber L, Bañez LL, Sopko DR, Miller MJ, Preminger GM, Lipkin ME. Emergent ureteric stent vs percutaneous nephrostomy for obstructive urolithiasis with sepsis: patterns of use and outcomes from a 15-year experience. BJU Int. 2013; 112(2):E122–E128.

[33] Joshi HB, Adams S, Obadeyi OO, Rao PN. Nephrostomy tube or 'JJ' ureteric stent in ureteric obstruction: assessment of patient perspectives using quality-of-life survey and utility analysis. Eur Urol. 2001;39(6):695–701.

8

The History and Evolution of Ureteral Stents

Husain Alenezi[1] and John D. Denstedt[2]

[1] *Endourology Fellow, Division of Urology, Department of Surgery, Schulich School of Medicine & Dentistry-Western University, London, Ontario, Canada*
[2] *Professor of Urology, Division of Urology, Department of Surgery, Schulich School of Medicine & Dentistry- Western University, London, Ontario, Canada*

8.1   Introduction

Ureteral stent use has become an integral fundamental part of contemporary urological practice. The indications for ureteral stent insertion encompass virtually any operative intervention involving the ureter and a variety of renal surgeries [1]. By allowing urine flow through both intra- and extra-luminal routes, ureteral stents provide a conduit for urinary drainage from the kidney to the bladder to relieve obstruction and associated pain or infection. Despite the apparent advantages of ureteral stents, their use can be associated with complications such as infection, migration, perforation and encrustation [2]. Additionally, nearly 80% of patients experience stent-related bothersome symptoms such as loin pain, hematuria and lower urinary tract symptoms [3]. Thus, there is significant interest in developing the "ultimate stent" leading to better drainage accompanied by ease of insertion and removal together with fewer associated symptoms and infections. Recent statistics showed a significant rise in the number of new stent-related patents in the last two decades with a peak of 62 new registrations in 2005 alone (Figure 8.1). Although the number of new registered technologies per year has declined since 2005, modifications of technologies may hold considerable promise to develop a better stent design in the future.

8.2   History and Evolution of Stent Nomenclature

The designation of the word "stent" to describe ureteral hollow drainage tubes in the urological literature was not uniformly applied until the 1970s, whereas earlier publications used varying terms such as tubes, splints, stints, catheters, and stents interchangeably [4]. The first appearance of the term "stent" in the literature originated from a new dental impression material described by an English dentist, Charles T. Stent, and subsequently manufactured by himself and his sons, Charles R. and Arthur H., at home [4]. Esser of Holland, a plastic surgeon in Vienna during the First World War, successfully utilized stents dental impression compound to stabilize skin grafts in plastic surgery

Ureteric Stenting, First Edition. Edited by Ravi Kulkarni.
© 2017 John Wiley & Sons Ltd. Published 2017 by John Wiley & Sons Ltd.

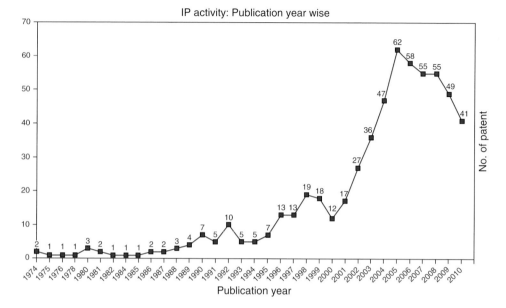

Figure 8.1 Patent activity for ureteral stents. *Source*: Reproduced with permission of Dolcera Corporation.

and subsequently in hypospadias repair [5]. Thus, two different descriptions were used to define "stent" in medical dictionaries. First, a stent is "a device that is used to maintain a bodily orifice or cavity during skin grafting, or to immobilize a skin graft following placement," and second, it is "a slender thread, rod, or catheter placed within the lumen of tubular structures, such as a blood vessel, to provide support during or after anastomosis" [6]. In 1972, Goodwin expressed his concerns on "a serious misuse of the language" by urologists in using the words splint, stent, and stint [7]. In his editorial comment, Goodwin concluded that when urologists place a tube in the ureter or urethra "it is not a splint. It may be a stent. It probably is never a stint" [7]. After that the term "stent" was adopted in the urological literature to describe intraluminal devices used to maintain the patency of a hollow structure [4].

8.3 Ancient History

Intubation of the urinary system using hollow tubes for drainage purposes dates back to ancient Egypt [8]. Bladder catheterization to relieve the pain associated with urinary retention was accomplished with different plant materials such as reeds, straws, and curled-up palm leaves [9]. Chinese history describes use of leaves of allium, which are thin and hollow, to drain the obstructed bladders after properly drying them [9]. But, difficulty in passing those fragile catheters and troubles with breaking inside the bladder was recognized and prompted the use of more rigid materials such as gold, copper, bronze, and tin [8, 9]. Further advancements in catheters were achieved by Galen (BC 131–210), who described the famous S-shaped metal catheter used in men and women, and by Avicenna, after demonstrating a more malleable catheter [9, 10]. In 1844, Goodyear described the revolutionary process of rubber vulcanization involved in shaping and forming rubber in any desired shape [8, 9]. This was shortly followed by the development of the Nelaton red rubber catheter by Auguste Nelaton of Paris, with improved flexibility leading to easier less traumatic insertion [8, 9]. The need for self-retaining catheters was realized and multiple mechanisms were developed with the most successful being the balloon self-retaining catheter (Foley catheter).

The development of ureteral catheters received only passing interest until the development of the cystoscope in the nineteenth century [9]. Gustav Simon, a German surgeon with many contributions to urology, was the first to probe the ureter using hollow tubes during an open cystostomy [9, 11]. While Alexander Brenner, a surgeon from Austria, initially reported endoscopic ureteral catheterization in a female patient around 1887, surgeons from John Hopkins were able to replicate the procedure in a female patient and shortly after were able to perform the first successful endoscopic ureteral catheterization in a male patient in 1893 [12]. Of course early stents were not specifically designed for ureteral catheterization, so they were radiolucent and lacked graduation marks [9]. Joaquin Albarran, renowned for his important innovations in urological instrumentation, designed the first manufactured models of stents intended for ureteral catheterization [9].

8.4 Recent History

The majority of advancements in ureteral stenting were accomplished during the twentieth century. In the 1940s, the development of plastics such as polyethylene and polyvinyl allowed for improved stents and catheters including enhanced rigidity and subsequently were easier to place while maintaining their flexibility. In 1949, J. P. Herdman from Oxford examined the feasibility of utilizing polyethylene tubes to bridge the gap in a cut ureter using an animal model [13]. Herdman found significant blockage of the tubes by urinary deposits (encrustations) with detrimental effects on the ipsilateral kidney after leaving the tubes indwelling for variable times [13]. W. S. Tulloch, a surgeon from Edinburgh, was able to successfully repair bilateral ureters with the aid of polyethylene tubes in a female patient who suffered from bilateral ureteric injury during hysterectomy [14]. Tulloch found the polyethylene tubes to be "as clean on removal as when first introduced" after nine indwelling days [14]. Later in the twentieth century, the incorporation of silicone elastomer in the catheter industry further improved the ease of stent placement with an added advantage of increased resistance to encrustation and infection [15], leading to the adoption of silicone catheters as the standard against which other materials were compared. In the 1960s, Blum examined the implantation of silicone catheters as ureteral prosthesis in dogs and found them functioning after several months with no evidence of encrustation, which encouraged Paul D. Zimskind in 1967 to place silicone tubes through the cystoscope as ureteral stents in human patients (Figure 8.2) [16]. Zimskind successfully treated 13 patients with malignant ureteral obstruction, ureterovaginal fistulas and ureteral strictures by leaving the silicone stents indwelling for up to 19 months [16]. In 1970, Marmar produced a silicone stent with a closed proximal tip, which facilitated cystoscopic placement of the stent over a guidewire [17], whereas Orikasa and colleagues from Japan further modified Marmar's insertion technique by introducing a hard polymer tube to act as a "pusher" [18]. The pusher held the ureteral stent in proper position during removal of the guidewire (Figure 8.3). Yet, the lack of self-retaining mechanisms lead to distal or proximal migration of the ureteral stents with subsequent discomfort and recurrent obstruction.

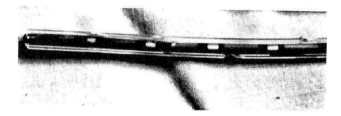

Figure 8.2 Silicone tube used by Zimskind as indwelling ureteral stents. Note the internal ureteral catheter used to support the silicon tube during cystoscopic insertion. *Source*: Zimskind *et al.*, 1967 [16]. Reproduced with permission of Elsevier.

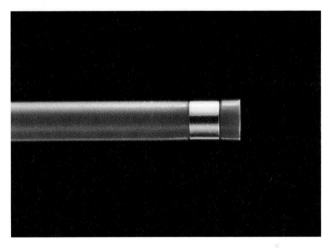

Figure 8.3 Stent pusher with radiopaque tip. Reproduced with permission of Cook Medical Incorporated, Bloomington, Indiana.

Thus, further modifications were focused on maintaining the proper position of the stent after cystoscopic placement, leading to the first stent that successfully prevented downward migration known as "Gibbons stent" (Figure 8.4) became commercially available in 1974 [19]. This silicone stent had multiple sharp barbs along its shaft to prevent distal migration and a distal flange intended to prevent proximal migration [19]. Despite providing adequate drainage and an effective mechanism to prevent distal migration, the barbs increased the diameter from 7Fr to 11Fr rendering insertion difficult in addition to failure to adequately prevent proximal migration. In 1978, Hepperlen *et al.* described a new polyethylene ureteral stent with a single proximal pigtail and a distal flange that effectively prevented distal migration accompanied by enhanced ease of insertion due to the smaller diameter (6Fr) [20]. The new placement technique demonstrated by Hepperlen *et al.* relied on the initial passage of a Teflon coated guidewire endoscopically to the renal pelvis prior to stent placement over the guidewire, which formed the basis for the modern technique in ureteral stenting [20]. Until 1978, there was still no effective mechanism to prevent proximal migration of ureteral stents, at which time Roy Finney reported his experience in using the new silicon double J ureteral stent [21]. The double J stent was suitable for placement by both open and endoscopic techniques. The J ends were formed in opposite directions (Figure 8.5), thus

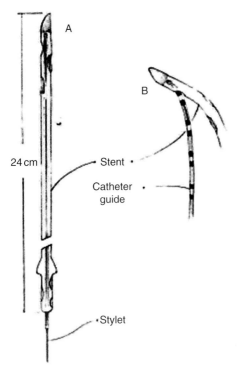

Figure 8.4 The original illustration of "Gibbon's stent." *Source*: Gibbons *et al.*, 1974 [19]. Reproduced with permission of Elsevier.

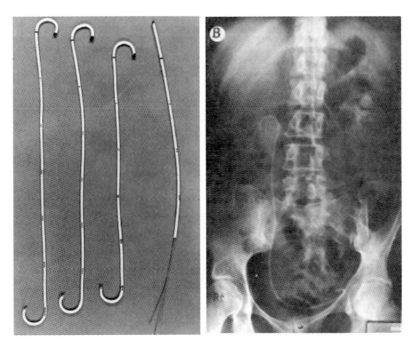

Figure 8.5 The original "Double J" used by Finney. Note the "J" ends that are straightened by a guidewire. *Source*: Finney *et al.*, 1978 [21]. Reproduced with permission of Elsevier.

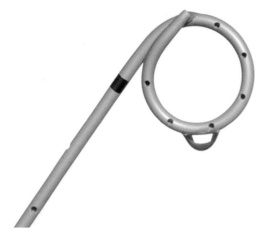

Figure 8.6 The pigtail retentive coil. *Source*: Reproduced with permission from Cook Medical Incorporated, Bloomington, Indiana.

the proximal J can hook into the renal pelvis, whereas the distal J curled in inside the bladder. In addition to effectively preventing proximal displacement of the stent, the distal J also reduced patient discomfort by elevating the distal tip from impinging on the sensitive bladder trigone [21]. Commercial production of the double J stent by Surgitek (Racine, WI, USA) began in 1978, and was an immediate success with wide acceptance by urologists worldwide. Since Surgitek held the patent for the original double J design of ureteral stents, most of the modern stents come with double pigtails (with full retentive coils) as the self-retaining mechanism (Figure 8.6).

8.5 Further Advances in Ureteral Stent Technology

Although it was a major revolution in the field of urology, the double J stent did not represent the ideal stent mainly due to its associated bothersome symptoms together with risks of related infections and stent encrustation. Thus, further research was warranted in an effort to produce the ideal stent with optimal physical characteristics such as a low friction coefficient for ease of insertion, easy to remove, has high biodurability and biocompatibility to withstand the harsh urinary environment without interfering with the host tissues, and highly radiopaque to facilitate easy recognition of the stent with imaging, while providing adequate drainage of the upper urinary tract [22]. In order to compare the impact of different stents on the patient's health related quality of life, stent specific questionnaires were developed notably the Ureteral Stent Symptom Questionnaire (USSQ) [23].

Various new technologies have been implemented in the stent industry to solve the associated problems. The use of new biomaterials and additional stent coatings represents one of the fast growing technologies focusing mainly on minimizing stent encrustation and biofilm formation along with easy atraumatic placement and less discomfort to the host [22, 24, 25]. Silicone and synthetic polymers such as polyethylene and polyurethane were originally used to fashion ureteral stents, however proprietary modifications of those materials were developed to overcome their shortcomings [22, 24, 25]. Examples of the new polymers include but not limited to C-Flex, Silitek, Percuflex, and

Sof-Flex. The addition of a stent coating, such as hydrogel, heparin, hyaluronic acid, and various other compounds, is a promising technology to improve stent design. Drug-eluting stents, a technology that has gained widespread interest in the medical field including urology, is encouraging and might play a major role in the stent industry in the future [25]. These advancements are elaborated on further in other chapters in this text.

Stent design is another variable amenable to modification and improvement [24]. The production of dual-durometer, mesh, and tail stents was meant to reduce patient's symptoms and discomfort, whereas other designs were manufactured to allow removal without the need for repeat cystoscopy. Examples include stents with distally attached suture and magnetic material-tipped stents [24]. Other design modifications serve particular purpose such as endopyelotomy stents, metallic stents, fistula stents, and nephrovesical subcutaneous urinary diversion stents.

Future advances in technology such as drug elution and tissue engineering may further improve stent design and mitigate or eliminate the current problems associated with ureteral stents.

References

[1] Chew BH, Knudsen BE, Denstedt JD. The use of stents in contemporary urology. Curr Opin Urol. 2004;14:111–115.

[2] Mohan-Pillai K, Keeley FX, Moussa S A., Smith G, Tolley D A. Endourological Management of Severely Encrusted Ureteral Stents. J Endourol. 1999;13(5):377–379.

[3] Joshi HB, Okeke A., Newns N, Keeley FX, Timoney A. G. Characterization of urinary symptoms in patients with ureteral stents. Urology. 2002;59(4):511–516.

[4] Bloom D A., Clayman R V., McDougal E. Stents and related terms: A brief history. Urology. 1999;54(4):767–771.

[5] Esser JF. Studies in Plastic Surgery of the Face: I. Use of Skin From the Neck To Replace Face Defects. II. Plastic Operations About the Mouth. III. the Epidermic Inlay. Ann Surg. 1917;65(3):297–315.

[6] Stent. Dictionary.com. *The American Heritage® Stedman's Medical Dictionary.* Houghton Mifflin Company. http://dictionary.reference.com/browse/stent [accessed June 10, 2015].

[7] Goodwin WE. Splint, Stent, Stint. Urol Dig. 1972;11:13–14.

[8] Nacey J, Delahunt B. The Evolution and Development of the Urinary Catheter. Aust NZ J Surg. 1993;63:815–819.

[9] Herman JR. Urology: A view through the retrospectroscope. 1973:35–36.

[10] Kardeh S, Choopani R, Mahmoudi Nezhad GS, Zargaran A. The Urinary Catheter and Its Significant Applications Described by Avicenna (980–1037 AD) in the Canon of Medicine. Urology. 2014;84(5):993–996.

[11] Moll F, Rathert P. The surgeon and his intention: Gustav Simon (1824–1876), his first planned nephrectomy and further contributions to urology. World J Urol. 1999;17(3):162–167.

[12] Arcadi J A. Dr. James Brown and catheterization of the male ureter: June 9, 1893. Urology. 1999;54(1):188–192.

[13] Herdman JP. Polythene tubing in the experimental surgery of the ureter. Br J Surg. 1949;37:105–106.

[14] Tulloch WS. Restoration of the continuity of the ureter by means of polythene tubing. Br J Urol. 1952;24:42–45.

[15] Blum J, Skemp C, Reiser M. SILICONE RUBBER URETERAL PROSTHESIS. J Urol. 1963;90:276–280.

[16] Zimskind PD, Fetter TR, Wilkerson JL. Clinical use of long-term indwelling silicone rubber ureteral splints inserted cystoscopically. J Urol. 1967;97:840–844.

[17] Marmar JL. The management of ureteral obstruction with silicone rubber splint catheters. J Urol. 1970;104(3):386–389.

[18] Orikasa S, Tsuji I, Siba T, Ohashi N. A new technique for transurethral insertion of a silicone rubber tube into an obstructed ureter. J Urol. 1973;110:184–187.

[19] Gibbons RP, Mason JT, Correa RJJ. Experience with indwelling silicone rubber ureteral catheters. J Urol. 1974;111:594–599.

[20] Hepperlen TW, Mardis HK, Kammandel H. Self-retained internal ureteral stents: a new approach. J Urol. 1978;119:731–734.

[21] Finney RP. Experience with new double J ureteral catheter stent. J Urol. 1978;120:678–681.

[22] Venkatesan N, Shroff S, Jayachandran K, Doble M. Polymers as ureteral stents. J Endourol. 2010;24(2):191–198.

[23] Joshi HB, Newns N, Stainthorpe A, MacDonagh RP, Keeley FX, Timoney A G. Ureteral stent symptom questionnaire: development and validation of a multidimensional quality of life measure. J Urol. 2003;169(3):1060–1064.

[24] Beiko DT, Knudsen BE, Denstedt JD. Advances in ureteral stent design. J Endourol. 2003;17(4):195–199.

[25] Mendez-Probst CE, Fernandez A, Denstedt JD. Current status of ureteral stent technologies: Comfort and antimicrobial resistance. Curr Urol Rep. 2010;11(2):67–70.

9

Ureteral Stent Materials: Past, Present, and Future

Andrew M. Todd[1] and Bodo E. Knudsen[2]

[1] Department of Urology, The Ohio State University Wexner Medical Center, Ohio, USA
[2] Interim Chair, Program Director, Associate Professor and Henry A. Wise II Professorship in Urology, Department of Urology, The Ohio State University Wexner Medical Center, USA

9.1 Introduction

Long have there existed different types of non-biological materials placed into the human genitourinary tract for instrumentation and drainage. The usage of materials within the urinary tract dates back to the third century B.C., where the Greek physiologist and anatomist, Erasistratus used metal tubing he coined as "catheter" for the treatment of urinary retention [1]. The first usage of instrumentation within the urinary tract is thought to date back to ancient Egypt, where papyrus and lead were reportedly used as urinary catheters [2]. The early Indian surgical text, *Sushruta Samhita*, which dates to approximately 1000 B.C. also described the use of catheters. It reported the use of gold, silver, iron, and wood smeared with a liquid butter, called "ghee," which was utilized for the drainage of the urinary tract and management of strictures [3]. The use of metals for urinary drainage continued into the early first few centuries A.D. Subsequently in the fourth century A.D., the Roman physician Oribasius, who served the Emperor Julian, described using treated paper for catheterization [5–7]. Not long thereafter, wool was used by the Byzantine physician Paul of Aegina within catheters in the seventh century [4].

Catheters made of soft or flexible materials were first described by Avicenna, the Saracen scientist and philosopher. In addition to rigid catheters of silver, gold, tin, and lead, he stated that the best catheters were those that were soft and made of stiffened sea animal skins adhered with cheese glue [8–10]. Despite this innovation, rigid catheters made from metal materials were still widely used until the 1700s. During that time period, leading Renaissance surgeon Fabricius of Acquapendente introduced a cloth catheter, impregnated with wax and molded over a silver sound. Additionally, Pickel of Wurtzburg developed silk woven catheters that were formed over probes. At the turn of the nineteenth century, natural rubber was beginning to be used by Michele Troia. These were limited by the disadvantage of becoming softer at body temperature. In the 1840s, Charles Goodyear developed vulcanized rubber catheters by treating natural rubber with lead. He received a patent in 1851, which promoted less-expensive development and more widespread use. The flexible red rubber catheter that is still used today has its roots from a particularly popular model of those catheters developed by Auguste Nélaton in 1860.

Ureteric Stenting, First Edition. Edited by Ravi Kulkarni.

Table 9.1 Biomaterials: Advantages and Disadvantages.

Material	Commercial Products	Advantages	Disadvantages
Silicone	Silitek	Greatest bicompatibility	Decreased drainage efficacy
		Decreased struvite and CaP stones	Increased CaCarb and CaOx stones
		High resistence to extrinsic compression	Higher bacterial adhesion
Modified Polyurethane	Tecoflex	Softens quickly - ease of insertion	Severe COM and UA stone encrustation
	Percuflex	Soft and smooth, enhanced physical properties	Very compressible
	Sof-Flex	Low frictional coefficient	Increased CaCarb and CaOx stones
	Inlay/Optima	66–79% less encrustation than competitors	
	C-Flex	Highly resistant to external force	Higher bacterial adhesion
Metal Alloys	Resonance	Very highly resistant to external compression	Encrustation difficult to detect
Biodegradable materials	TUDS	Almost all eliminated at 15 days	Small number breakage and retained fragments
	Uriprene	No reported retained fragments	4 weeks to completely dissolve

In the twentieth century the birth of numerous polymeric materials allowed for the development of many novel types of urethral catheters, stents, nephrostomy tubes, and other biomaterials used in the urinary tract (Table 9.1). Some of the materials developed included the continued use of latex rubber (polyisoprene), as well as polyethylene, polyvinylchloride, polyurethane, silicone, and a myriad of proprietary polymers [11].

Today there are a variety of materials that we still use with some iterations that trace their roots back to these original materials. They will be listed systematically in the ensuing sections, with the primary focus on ureteral stent materials. These include polyurethane, silicone, polyester, hydrogel/urethane/silicone blends, polyisobutylene, polystyrene, polyglycolic acid, polymethacralate, and metallic stents. Additionally, there are also some key issues that will be addressed at the end of the chapter that globally encompass some of the challenges and pitfalls associated with indwelling materials in the urinary tract.

A review of stent materials is not complete without a review of some of the challenges and complications that come part and parcel with indwelling ureteral stents. The complications that are associated with indwelling ureteral stents have impacted the choice and evolution of the materials used, which has driven the technological advances in their designs. These include, but are not limited to, irritative voiding symptoms, encrustation, bacterial colonization, pyuria, hematuria, urinary tract infections, migration, ureteral erosion, fistulization, and fracture. This has shaped the advances in materials that we will see, as we move chronologically through the different kinds of materials used. Rather than listing the ideal characteristics of indwelling ureteral stents, we will see how each material demonstrates pros and cons that can collectively add to the repository of "ideal characteristics of a stent."

9.2 Materials

9.2.1 Silicone and Silitek

Silicon was first introduced in the 1960s and is composed of alternating silicon and oxygen atoms. It is a biomaterial that is regarded as the "gold standard" in terms of its tissue compatibility due to its nontoxic and inert nature [12]. Despite having the greatest biocompatibility, it has been seen to have a lower drainage efficacy as compared to other materials [13]. Due to its uniform surface, there are fewer irregularities that provide footholds for bacteria and stones. In terms of encrustation, there is a decreased incidence of struvite and calcium phosphate hydroxyapatite stones compared to polyurethane-based materials. However, it is still prone to encrustation by calcium carbonate and calcium oxalate stones [14,15]. With regards to bacterial adherence and colonization, there is a higher proclivity of hydrophobic *Enterococcus faecalis* than *Escherichia coli*. Overall, there is a greater rate of bacterial adhesion with this material than with polyurethane. This fact, when coupled with the high coefficient of friction for silicone, has lead to pure silicone not being used as a stent. Coatings of lecithin, silver citrate, and liquid silicone have been found to decrease this and blending with polymers has become commonplace. An example of this is Silitek (ACMI/Olympus, Southborough, MA), a polyester copolymer that is firm and therefore resists extrinsic compression. However, it too has been shown to experience higher bacterial adhesion rates [16].

9.2.2 Polyurethane

Polyurethane is from a class of condensation polymers. It is versatile and inexpensive compared to many other stent materials. Sometimes known as the third-generation polymer to be used, it replaced polyethylene in the 1980s and gained wide usage. This was due to polyethylene's unstable nature in the urinary environment that made it subject to fracture. Polyurethane is chemically composed of a backbone of carbamate groups with urethane links. It is created from a reaction between polyol and diisocyanate. Polyurethane is prone to greater encrustation as compared to silicone, predominantly from calcium oxalate, struvite, and hydroxylapatite [14,17]. In terms of bacterial adherence, *E. faecalis* is seen more commonly, and *E. coli* less commonly, as compared to silicone. Expectedly, indwelling time for encrustation is significantly higher in recurrent stone formers, compared to patients without urolithiasis [17,18]. With regards to mechanical properties; fractures are most commonly noted at the drainage holes. Additionally, it has been concluded that urine flows primarily around these hollow stents, rather than through them [19].

Pure polyurethane poses a number of problems that have curtailed its modern-day usage. It is known to cause long-lasting changes to the urothelium, with urothelial ulceration and erosion being reported [20,21]. Encrustation and bacterial adhesion can also be problematic. This has been demonstrated to have an adverse effect on renal function. So despite its good mechanical properties, biocompatibility, and low occurrence of migration or fractures, pure polyurethane had numerous shortcomings that required modification prior to widespread acceptance. This has given rise to polymer blending (modification of the substrate) and special coatings.

9.2.3 Modified Polyurethanes and Proprietary Materials

Tecoflex is an aliphatic polyurethane with high radio-opacity. Its property of softening not long after insertion led to its use. However, it was found to severely encrust with calcium oxalate monohydrate, protein, and uric acid. An example of a stent that is constructed with tecoflex is the Quadra-Coil Multi-Length ureteral stent (Olympus), which is covered with a hydrophilic coating.

Other modified polyurethanes are Chronoflex and Hydrothane. Neither of these is currently in commercial production. Another experimental material from the late 1990s, Aquavene (Menlo Care, Menlo Park, CA, USA), is made from a mixture of a hydrophilic polymer and a urethane/silicone/polyvinyl chloride mixture. Gorman *et al.* described its ability to soften when hydrated while being firmer when dry. In a simulated 24-week urine flow study, it had superior resistance to encrustation and intraluminal blockage, but this study was performed in artificial urine from a reservoir in the lab, not in vivo [22]. Percuflex is a proprietary olefinic block copolymer (Boston Scientific, Natick, MA, USA) that softens and becomes flexible at room temperature [28]. It shows similar encrustation rates to polyurethane and similar bacterial adherence profiles with *Enterococcus spp.*, though it has improved physical characteristics [28].

There are a variety of other products utilizing this material from the manufacturer, some with hydrophilic coating, dual durometer, bladder loops, and softer bladder coils. The market for ureteral stents today has become quite saturated with mixtures of modified polyurethanes and "proprietary materials," which can include a variety of polymer mixtures that often remain proprietary to the manufacturer. Another modified polyurethane polymer used today is Sof-Flex® (Cook Medical, Bloomington, IN, USA). Advantages of this particular proprietary polymer include a low frictional surface, but it is prone to calcium carbonate and oxalate encrustation [28].

Another polymer utilized by Cook Medical in stent production is C-flex. This is a blend of styrene/ethylene/butylene/styrene block copolymers. Its advantage is being highly resistant to external compressive forces, but is efficient only in a protein free environment [23,24]. Therefore, it has been suggested that there is room for further modification, as urine contains proteins.

Another example of blending modified polyurethane with proprietary materials in actual stent composition is the mixture of Polytetrafluoroethylene (PTFE) and proprietary materials within the Inlay® and Inlay Optima® stents (Bard Medical, Covington, GA, USA). These have been compared head to head with several other non-disclosed stent materials and the manufacturer reports a 66–79% reduction in encrustation compared to competing products. These too have a proprietary coating to aid in placement and reduce salt accumulation, which is named "pHreeCoat." In vitro studies were performed by Whitfield *et al.* at University College of London, where atomic absorption spectrometry (AAS) showed less calcium urine salt accumulation than the four other competitors [39]. The Inlay Optima® stents were evaluated by Lee *et al.* in 2005 in a clinical trial. A total of 44 patients (73%) completed all USSQ validated stent symptom questionnaires. Urinary symptom scores were significantly lower for the Inlay stent on day 3 than for the Vertex ($P = 0.01$), Contour ($P = 0.05$), Endo-Sof ($P = 0.03$), and Classic ($P = 0.02$) stents. No significant differences were noted in pain and general symptom scores or narcotic use [35].

There are other polymer and polyester blends that have been studied, such as mixtures of polycaprolactone (PCL) and polyvinyl pyrrolidone (PVP), vinyl polymers like polymethylmethacrylate (PMMA). To our knowledge, none of these materials are currently being utilized in currently commercially available urinary stents, presumably secondary to their undesirable physical properties [36].

9.2.4 Metallic Stents

There are several types of metal stents including self-expandable polytetrafluoroethylene-covered nitinol stents, thermoexpandeable stents, and balloon-expandable nickel-titanium alloy stents. One of the primary challenges of metallic stents is the high rate of migration due to the inability of the coating material to properly anchor the stent. One metallic stent in commercial production is a nickel-cobalt-chromium-molybdenum alloy stent (Resonance, Cook Medical). It is magnetic resonance imaging (MRI)-compatible if specific parameters are followed for the imaging study (https://www.cookmedical.com/data/IFU_PDF/IFU0020-14.PDF), an important consideration for patient with malignant obstruction who may undergo surveillance imaging. Placing and changing these stents can be more difficult than that of polymer stents, but studies have shown that the extrinsic force needed to compress them is significantly greater than that of Silhouette®, Sof-Curl®, Percuflex®, and Polaris Ultra® stents [25]. This stent has been marketed to allow for indwell times of up to one year but must be monitored for evidence of encrustation. In a multicenter review, encrustation was difficult to visualize on plain film radiography due to the radio-density of the stents. Therefore, if encrustation is clinically suspected (recurrent UTIs, increased stent symptoms, worsening hydronephrosis), cystoscopy may be indicated to better assess the degree of encrustation on the distal coil. In the clinical study, several stents became encrusted and required surgical removal. Three of 76 stents required operative removal with either PCNL or cystolitholapaxy [37].

9.2.5 Coatings

In order to try and reduce the incidence of encrustation and bacterial adherence, a variety of compounds have been used. Each has inherent advantages and disadvantages. The first, hyaluronic acid, is a glycosaminoglycan and a natural inhibitor of growth, nucleation, and salt aggregation. This led to its inception as a coating for polyurethane through a plasma-activated surface modification. In vitro, it has demonstrated decreased bacterial cell adhesion and encrustation compared to silicone coating [26,27]. However, there are no clinical trials in vivo to validate efficacy and to date has not been used in clinical stent applications [28]. Another experimental coating is termed hydrogel. It is a hydrophilic polymer that allows for anchoring of water molecules to the stent surface. Hydrogel-coated stents have improved substrate material biocompatibility, hydrophilization, and lubrication [29]. Hydrogel-coated stents have been dipped into various antibiotic solutions and then have been shown to retain their antibacterial properties [30]. Other coatings used include sequential interpenetrating polymer networks (SIPNs), heparin, silver, polyvinylpyrrolidone (PVP), and diamond-like carbon (DLC). These have the goal of increased lubricity, decreased biofilm formation, and decreased encrustation. Clinical efficacies in vivo with most are either mixed or not reported to date [28].

9.2.6 Future Directions: Biodegradable Materials and Changes in Design

On the forefront of technology in ureteral stent design are biodegradable materials and polymers. The most notable of these are TUDS, PGA, and PLA. TUDS, or temporary ureteral drainage stents (Boston Scientific), are composed of a proprietary polymeric material. They were designed to allow for intervention-free drainage for approximately 48 hours after uncomplicated ureteroscopy, with no need for in-office removal. Lingeman *et al.* demonstrated in Phase II clinical trials that 89% of patients reported satisfaction with these, with an overall stent effectiveness rate of 78%. However, 3/80 patients required either ESWL or URS to remove retained materials, and the median time to complete stent elimination from the body was 15 days [34]. Concerns were raised secondary to the stent not fully dissolving in this small subset of patients and currently the stent is no longer available for clinical use.

Another biodegradable stent, Uriprene^{TM}, has been developed. Similar to absorbable suture, it is comprised of L-glycolic acid, polyethylene glycol, and barium sulfate. There are two layers: a hydrophobic outer mesh that dissolves rapidly, and an inner coil that takes longer to breakdown and provides structure. In a pig study, at 4 weeks 9/10 of these stents had completely dissolved as seen on IVP, and the last one had a few small pieces left in the bladder (<1.5 cm each) [38].

Still another biodegradable material is polyactic acid (PLA). PLA is an aliphatic polyester that has been tested in dogs to assess for changes in renal function during the biodegradation process. Similarly, polyglycolic acid (PGA) is a linear thermoplastic polymer of glycolic acid. Neither encrustation nor biofilm adherence was observed on the PGA stent, however poor mechanical properties have limited its propensity for usage. These stents have not been tested in humans and are not currently in commercial production [31].

9.2.7 Autologous and Engineered Tissue

In recent years, the use of small intestine in surgical replacement of ureteral segments has been investigated in pigs. As results were mixed, this is still purely investigational [32]. Tissue-engineered stents have also been investigated. Bovine shoulder chondrocytes fabricated over polyglycolic acid mesh scaffolding has been examined both in vitro and in vivo, and has been demonstrated to withstand high degrees of pressure [33]. This holds promise for the future stent designs.

In conclusion, ureteral stents have a rich history and have experienced many years of evolution and innovation. However, there remains significant morbidity associated with their use. Problems such as stent colic, encrustation, and bacterial adhesion remain despite the advances in stent materials and coatings. Currently, the most commonly used stents are composed of modified polyurethane blends. Metal stents have provided another option for patients who have extrinsic compression, although they are also not without their shortcomings. Biodegradable stents may provide an option in the future for patients requiring routine short-term stent placement, but concerns regarding incomplete breakdown remain. The ongoing development of new materials and coatings will likely lead to new product options in the coming decades.

References

[1] Mardis HK, Kroeger RM, Morton JJ, Donovan JM. Comparative evaluation of materials used for internal ureteral stents. J Endourol. 1993; 7:105.

[2] Galen C. Opera Omnia. Editionem Curavit C. G. Kuhn. Lipsiae: C. Cnobloch, vol. 14, p. 751, 1821–1833.

[3] Bitschay J, Brodny ML. A History of Urology in Egypt. New York: Riverside Press, p. 56, 1956.

[4] Das S. Shusruta of India, the pioneer in the treatment of urethral stricture. Surg Gynecol Obstet 1983; 157:581.

[5] Bloom DA, McGuire EJ, Lapides J. A brief history of urethral catheterization. J Urol 1994; 151:317.

[6] Celsus AC. De Medicina. Birmingham: Classics of Medicine Library, pp. 569–570, 1989.

[7] Denos E. From the Renaissance to the nineteenth century. In: The History of Urology. Edited by LJT Murphy. Springfield: Charles C. Thomas, ch. 4, pp. 70–72, 1972.

[8] Adams F. The Seven Books of Paulus Aegineta. London: Sydenham Society, 1846.

[9] Wershub LP. Urologic surgery from antiquity to the 20th century, part III. In: Urology: From Antiquity to the 20th century. St. Louis: Warren H. Greene, Inc., ch. 16, pp. 253–255, 1970.

[10] Marino RA, Mooppan UM, Kim H. History of urethral catheters and their balloons: drainage, anchorage, dilation, and hemostasis. J Endourol 1993;7:89.

[11] Beiko DT, Knudsen BE, Watterson JD, Cadieux PA, Reid G, Denstedt JD. J Urol. 2004; 171(6 Pt 1):2438–2444. Review.

[12] Denstedt JD, Wollin TA, Reid G. Biomaterials used in urology: Current issues of biocompatibility, infection, and encrustation. J Endourol 1998; 12:493.

[13] Hofmann R, Hartung R. Ureteral stents—materials and newforms. World J Urol 1989; 7:154–157.

[14] Tunney MM, Keane PF, Gorman SP. Assessment of urinary tract biomaterial encrustation using a modified Robbins device continuous flow model. J Biomed Mater Res 1997; 38:87–93.

[15] Reid G, Tieszer C, Denstedt J, Kingston D. Examination of bacterial and encrustation deposition on ureteral stents of differing surface properties, after indwelling in humans. Colloids and Surfaces B: Biointerfaces 1995; 5:171–179.

[16] Tunney MM, Keane PF, Gorman SP. Bacterial adherence to ureteralstent biomaterials. Eur J Pharmaceut Sci 1996; 4:177–177.

[17] Tunney MM, Keane PF, Gorman SP. Encrustation assessment using the Modified Robbins device. Eur J Pharmaceut Sci 1996;4:177–177.

[18] Robert M, Boularan AM, Sandid ME, Grasset D. Double-J ureteric stent encrustations: Clinical study on crystal formation on polyurethane stents. Urol Int 1997;58:100–104.

[19] Gorman SP, Jones DS, Bonner MC, *et al.* Mechanical performance of polyurethane ureteral stents in vitro and ex vivo. Biomaterials 1997; 18:1379–1383.

[20] Cormio L. Ureteric injuries: Clinical and experimental studies. Scan J Urol Nephrol 1995;171(suppl):1–66.

[21] Marx M, Bettmann MA, Bridge S, Brodsky G, Boxt LM, Richie JP. The effects of various indwelling ureteral catheter materials on the normal canine ureter. J Urol 1988; 139:180.

[22] Gorman SP, Tunney MM, Keane PF, *et al*. Characterization and assessment of a novel poly(ethylene oxide) = polyurethane composite hydrogel (Aquavene) as a ureteral stent biomaterial. J Biomed Mater Res 1998; 39:642–649.

[23] Hendlin K, Vedula K, Horn C, Monga M. In vitro evaluationof ureteral stent compression. Urology 2006; 67:679–682.

[24] Miyaoka R, Monga M. Ureteral stent discomfort: Etiology and management. Indian Journal of Urology: IJU: Journal of the Urological Society of India 2009;25(4):455–460. doi:10.4103/0970-1591.57910.

[25] Christman MS, L'Esperance JO, Choe CH, *et al*. Analysis of ureteral stent compression force and its role in malignant obstruction. J Urol 2009; 181:392–396.

[26] Kitamura T, Zerwekh JE, Pak CY. Partial biochemical and physicochemical characterization of organic macromolecules in urine from patients with renal stones and control subjects. Kidney Int 1982; 21:379–386.

[27] Robertson WG, Peacock M, Nordin B. Inhibitors of the growth and aggregation of calcium oxalate crystals in vitro. Clin Chim Acta 1973; 43:31–37.

[28] Venkatesan N, Shroff S, Jayachandran K, Doble M. Polymers as ureteral stents. J Endourol 2010;24(2):191–198. doi: 10.1089/end.2009.0516.

[29] Chew BH, Denstedt JD. Technology insight: novel ureteral stent materials and designs. Nat Clin Pract Urol 2004; 1:44–48.

[30] John T, Rajpurkar A, Smith G, Fairfax M, Triest J. Antibiotic pretreatment of hydrogel ureteral stent. J Endourol 2007; 21:1211–1216.

[31] Pe´tas A, Vuopio-Varkila J, Siitonen A, *et al*. Bacterial adherence to self-reinforced polyglycolic acid and self-reinforced polylactic acid 96 urological spiral stents in vitro. Biomaterials 1998; 19:677–681.

[32] Sofer M, Rowe E, Forder DM, Denstedt JD. Ureteral segmental replacement using multilayer porcine smallintestinal submucosa. J Endourol 2002; 16:27.

[33] Amiel GE, Yoo JJ, Kim B-S, Atala A. Tissue engineered stents created from chondrocytes. J Urol, 165: 2091, 2001.

[34] Lingeman JE, Preminger GM, Berger Y, *et al*. Use of a temporary ureteral drainage stent after uncomplicated ureteroscopy: Results from a phase II clinical trial. J Urol 2003; 169:1682–1688.

[35] Lee C, Kuskowski M, Premoli J, Skemp N, Monga M. Randomized Evaluation of Ureteral Stents Using Validated Symptom Questionnaire. Journal of Endourology 2005;19(8):990–993. doi:10.1089/end.2005.19.990.

[36] Jones DS, Djokic J, McCoy CP, Gorman SP. Poly(e-caprolactone) and poly(e-caprolactone)-polyvinylpyrrolidoneiodine blends as ureteral biomaterials: Characterisation of mechanical and surface properties, degradation and resistance to encrustation in vitro. Biomaterials 2002; 23:4449–4458.

[37] Modi AP, Ritch CR, Arend D, Walsh RM, Ordonez M, Landman J, Gupta M, Knudsen BE. Multicenter experience with metallic ureteral stents for malignant and chronic benign ureteral obstruction. J Endourol. 2010; 24(7):1189–1193. doi: 10.1089/end.2010.0121.

[38] Chew BH, Paterson RF, Clinkscales KW, Levine BS, Shalaby SW, Lange D. In vivo evaluation of the third generation biodegradable stent: a novel approach to avoiding the forgotten stent syndrome. J Urol. 2013;189(2):719–725. doi: 10.1016/j.juro.2012.08.202. Epub 2012 Oct 8.

[39] Choong SKS, Wood S, Whitfield HN. A model to quantify encrustation on ureteric stents, urethral catheters, and polymers intended for urologic use. BJU International 2000;86:414–421.

10

Physical Characteristics of Stents

Chad M. Gridley[1] and Bodo E. Knudsen[2]

[1] Department of Urology, The Ohio State University Wexner Medical Center, Ohio, USA
[2] Interim Chair, Program Director, Associate Professor and Henry A. Wise II Professorship in Urology, Department of Urology, The Ohio State University Wexner Medical Center, USA

10.1 Introduction

There may be no tool more versatile to the practicing urologist than that of the ureteral stent. The objects first placed within ureters bear little resemblance to the dedicated ureteral stents that now exist. As the physical characteristics of ureteral stents have evolved over the years, they have proven to be a vital component of the urologist's arsenal.

10.2 History

Bloom *et al.* defines a stent as "a cylindrical device to ensure patency of a lumen or anastomosis and usually to allow drainage," with the object deriving its name from Charles T. Stent, an English dentist of the mid-1800s [1]. Stents in their current form are very different from their original conception, however, and evolved through a long process that can be traced back to the early Egyptians [2]. It was the 1800s that had the first case reported of placement of a tube within the ureter by Gustav Simon, which was performed at the time of a cystotomy [3]. Joaquin Albarrano created the first tube specifically for the ureter in the early twentieth century [3]. It was then in the early 1950s, with the advancements in plastic technology, where polyethylene tubing was used in the repair of ureters and fistulas by Tulloch [4]. The year 1967 saw the creation of an open-ended silicone stent [5]. Modifications were made to this initial blueprint to help anchor the stent in place through flanges and barbs [6]. The stent continued to evolve until Finney reported in 1978 on the design of a stent still in use today, the double-J stent [7]. Many of the characteristics of the "ideal stent" as described by Finney still form the core of our present day ureteral stent: described as being made of soft flexible material that resists encrustation, radiopaque, uniform diameter without flanges to facilitate passage, passable in either direction during open or endoscopic surgery, and possessing means to prevent migration in either direction [7].

Ureteric Stenting, First Edition. Edited by Ravi Kulkarni.
© 2017 John Wiley & Sons Ltd. Published 2017 by John Wiley & Sons Ltd.

10.3 Standard

The double-J or "double-pigtail" is beneficial to the practicing urologist for several reasons. It can be used to provide drainage to an obstructed kidney due to renal calculus, uretero-pelvic junction obstruction, external compression (benign or malignant), or stricture. They provide support during healing following ureteral injury or new ureteral anastomosis.

Within the authors' institution, the two stents most commonly used are the Percuflex (Boston Scientific, Marlborough, MA, USA) and the Inlay (Bard Medical, Covington, GA, USA). According to the manufacturer websites, these stents both possesses several advantages: lubricious coating and tapered tips to allow for smooth placement, pusher and fluoroscopic markings to ensure accurate placement, stent material that softens at body temperature, and double pigtails to prevent migration. Different sizes are available with diameters ranging from 4.7 to 8 French (Inlay) and 4.8 to 8 French (Percuflex). In the authors' experience, a 6 French stent is used for benign pathology and a 7 French is used for malignant. Research has shown though that there is no statistically significant difference in ability to resist external compressive forces between the Percuflex 6 and 8 French stents [8]. Larger diameter stents, however, are less likely to accordion during placement due to increased rigidity; this can be helpful when the stent must bypass a tight obstruction. These double pigtail ureteric stents also have some other similarities including a short, clear plastic sheath that straightens the curl to allow easier loading of the stent over a wire. There is a nylon tether attached to the distal portion of the stent that is long enough to exit the urethra. This allows for the patient to remove the stent at home without the need for cystoscopy. At our institution it is common practice to remove the tether prior to placement to prevent inadvertent removal of the stent by the patient. There have been reports of patients removing the tether but not the stent, resulting in later encrustation and need for surgery [9]. Therefore, patients need to be educated on the appearance of both the stent and the attached tether if the patient is to remove the stent on their own.

10.4 Long-Term Use (Metal)

Polymer stents, when used for long-term stent placement, typically require exchange every 3-6 months due to encrustation. Metal ureteral stents, along with the potential for great resistance to collapse with extrinsic pressure, were developed with the goal of longer indwell time. Such a stent may be of particular benefit in patients with malignant obstruction who will often require ongoing stent changes during their therapy.

A metal stent that has been well studied is the Resonance metallic ureteral stent (Figure 10.1), which has a manufacturer recommended dwell time of 12 months. During the writing of this chapter, there was no safety or outcomes data available to support this dwell time in the human urinary tract. Several studies have shown this stent to be a safe and viable option for managing chronic ureteral obstruction [10–12]. Liatsikos reported a 100% patency rate in patients with malignant obstruction, but only 44% in patients with benign causes [12]. Kadlec *et al.* reported on a five-year experience including 47 patients. The failure rate of the metallic stent in this sample was 28% [11], which is relatively similar to the failure rate of polymer stents [13]. When the metallic stent failed, it was found to occur within the first few weeks [12] to months of placement [11].

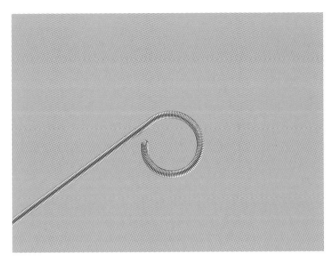

Figure 10.1 Resonance metallic ureteral stent. Reproduced with permission of Cook Medical Incorporated, Bloomington, Indiana.

In a single institution cost analysis, the Resonance stent was found to be more expensive to place initially relative to polymer stents, but when the more frequent changes of polymer stents required are factored in, the Resonance stent provides a potential annual cost savings of 47–74% [14]. The Resonance stent has been found to possess drawbacks though. It does not appear to be a viable option in children, as it was reported to fail sooner relative to adults [15]. Patients with a history of radiation therapy were found to have a lower ureteral patency rate relative to patients without a radiation history [10]. The metal stent is susceptible to encrustation as well, with 12 out of 54 stents showing signs of this as reported by Liatsikos *et al.* [12].

Modi *et al.* described several findings with their use of the Cook Resonance stent in a multi-center retrospective experience. When placed in patients who have failed plastic stents for management of ureteral obstruction, the Cook Resonance stent failed in 38% of patients at an average time of 2.2 months. This shows that early follow-up is vital instead of simply placing the metal stent and having the patent return in 12 months for exchange. The optimal follow-up timeline is not known, but the authors of this study recommended ultrasound or CT scan at 4 weeks post-placement to assess for presence of hydronephrosis. Furthermore, 41% of patients had their metal stent removed by 4.75 months due to stent symptoms, infection, obstruction, or migration. In these situations, KUB (Figure 10.2) was accurate in diagnosing stent migration but was unable to accurately diagnose stent encrustation as diagnosed in patients on cystoscopy following a negative KUB. This was believed to be due to the high radiopacity of the metal stent obscuring the encrustation [16].

As evidenced by the history of stents, design modifications typically arise out of a need, such as improvements related to anchoring, patient comfort, ease of passage, resistance to obstruction, and encrustation. Despite the ease of use and popularity of existing double-J ureteral stents, modifications continue to be developed within several different areas. There is a wealth of research that exists, reporting on modifications aimed at optimizing the ureteral stent. These typically fall within a set of subcategories including prevention of infection, patient comfort, improved drainage, and long-term use.

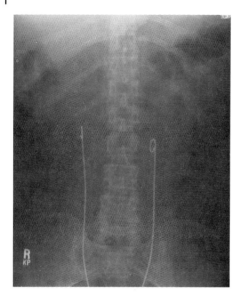

Figure 10.2 Abdominal x-ray of resonance metallic ureteral stent. Reproduced with permission of Bodo Knudsen, MD, Columbus, OH.

10.5 Comfort/Convenience

Double pigtail stents are known for causing bothersome symptoms. Joshi *et al.* carried out a study of 85 patients with indwelling ureteral stents and found that 80% experienced pain [17, 18]. Several factors have been found independently to have a negative impact on patient comfort: positive urine culture at time of stenting, proximal curl in a calyx instead of renal pelvis, distal curl crossing to the contralateral side of the bladder, and longer stenting duration [19].

Stent material has been targeted as a possible area of improving patient comfort. In a study comparing a firm stent (Percuflex, Boston Scientific) versus a soft stent (Contour, Boston Scientific) made by the same company with a similar stent design, there was no significant difference in patient comfort level [20].

It has been theorized that reducing the amount of total material present in the bladder may reduce bothersome symptoms. Loop stents were created to test this hypothesis, and these loop stents consist of a thin loop in place of the distal J-curl. Two loop stents with differing lengths were compared to standard ureteral stents, the Polaris™ and Percuflex Plus® stents [21]. Differences in subjective symptoms were measured via the Ureteric Stent Symptoms Questionnaire (USSQ), a validated questionnaire [17, 18]. This study was terminated early, however, as at the time of interim analysis no statistically significant difference was noted between the four stents. The authors did not discuss removal of the loop stents, but our own experience has been that the small diameter distal loops were more difficult to visualize at the time of cystoscopic removal.

The dual-durometer stent was designed to provide a softer distal end for increased comfort while keeping the firm proximal end for to maintain the stent in proper position. In a prospective, randomized study, patients received either the Bard Inlay ("standard") stent (Figure 10.3) or the Polaris (Boston Scientific, Marlborough, MA, USA) dual durometer stent (Figure 10.4). Patients then completed USSQ evaluations.

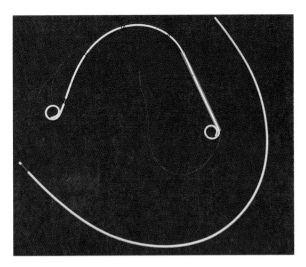

Figure 10.3 Bard inlay ureteral stent (green) and stent pusher (orange). Reproduced with permission of Chad Gridley, MD,Columbus, OH.

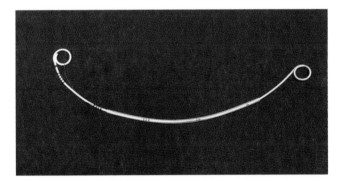

Figure 10.4 Boston Scientific dual durometer stent. Reproduced with permission of Chad Gridley, MD, Columbus, OH.

Following analysis of the data, no significant difference was found in terms of pain or urinary symptoms [22].

The Tail Stent (Boston Scientific, Marlborough, MA, USA) is constructed in a way that proximally the stent is identical to a standard 7 F pigtail stent but then tapers to a lumen-less 3 F distal point. This stent aims to reduce the irritative voiding symptoms through use of a softer distal segment. Dunn *et al.* completed a study of 60 patients comparing the tail stent to the Percuflex double pigtail stent. There was a noted statistically significant 20% reduction in overall irritative voiding symptoms, with most of the effect due to reduction in frequency and incontinence [23]. At present, this stent is not currently commercially.

There has also been research done to decrease the discomfort of stent retrieval. Taylor *et al.* reported on the use of magnets to assist with stent removal, eliminating the need for cystoscopy. Successful stent removal was completed in 29/30 patients but still required transurethral access [24], which is an aspect of the procedure that patients are often the most fearful of. The use of magnetic stents has not been widely adopted but they do remain commercially available.

10.6 Dissolvable Stent

There have been countless reports of patients who fail to follow up after stent placement. These stents can become forgotten and can encrust, often requiring a complex procedure for removal. Dissolvable stents is an area of research aimed at eliminating this complication. Lingeman *et al.* researched the TUDS (temporary ureteral drainage stent) manufactured by Boston Scientific [25, 26]. The Phase I trial showed that the stent was safe and provided 48 hours of drainage as intended [25]. Phase II testing showed a 78% effectiveness rate defined as providing drainage for 48 hours and maintaining good position. However, three patients retained stent fragments beyond 3 months requiring extracorporeal shockwave lithotripsy or ureteroscopy to remove the retained fragments [26]. The TUDS stent is currently not commercially available.

The Uriprene stent is another biodegradable stent that is being evaluated, and several studies have been done in an animal model [27–29]. Chew *et al.* showed that the Uriprene stent was biocompatible and caused less hydronephrosis compared to conventional polymer stents [28, 29]. The Phase I trial has recently been completed.

10.7 Drainage

The double-lumen stent was created to address stent failure in the setting of malignant external ureteral obstruction at times when two ureteral stents will be placed within a single ureter. In a comparison study, the dual-lumen stents studied provided superior drainage to single lumen stent [30]. Two separate single lumen stents placed together provided the greatest drainage.

In a head to head animal model trial, the standard 7Fr pigtail, the 14/7Fr endopyelotomy stent, and the 7/3Fr Tail stents had statistically similar flow rates [31]. All three provided superior ureteral drainage relative to a control. The Spirastent appeared to provide inferior drainage.

With regards to resisting external forces, metallic stents generally possess greater ability to resist tensile and compressive forces relative to plastic stents. Christman *et al.* showed that both the Resonance metallic stent (Cook Medical, Bloomington, IN, USA) and the coil-reinforced polymeric double-pigtail Silhouette stent (Applied Medical, Rancho Santa Margarita, CA, USA) possessed significantly greater ability to resist compressive forces compared to plastic stents [8]. The Resonance stent was shown to resist external compression of 31 pounds along the length of the ureter. The Silhouette stents varied among different diameters but were able to resist external compression of 10–17 pounds. In contrast, tradition common plastic stents were shown to collapse and compress with no more than 5 pounds of pressure [8].

10.8 Anti-Reflux

Ureteral stents cross the ureteral orifice, inhibiting the natural anti-refluxing mechanism of this anatomical structure. It has been hypothesized that this occurrence can increase the risk of irritative symptoms, renal injury, and urinary tract infection. Battaglia *et al.* looked at this effect on kidney transplant patients and randomized 44 patients to receive either a non-refluxing stent or a conventional stent [32]. No statistically significant difference was noted with regards to vesicoureteral reflux, urinary tract infection, or graft outcome.

Soria *et al.* studied the effectiveness of a self-retaining, anti-reflux stent that is placed in the ureter but does not cross the ureterovesical junction. A significant difference was found on ultrasound at 3 and 6 weeks while the stents were in place with there being more renal dilation in animals with the conventional stent. This difference resolved by the fifth month of follow-up after the stents had been removed [33]. Of note, the anti-refluxing stent requires intraureteral removal, making removal more complex than office cystoscopy.

10.9 Self-Expanding

The Wallstent (Boston Scientific, Marlborough, MA, USA) endoprosthesis is a cylindrical tube made of crossing filaments of superalloy wire with a tantalum core that expands once the outer sheath is removed [34]. Early on, this stent was noted to have difficulty with becoming obstructed due to tissue ingrowth [34]. This stent has been used in Europe in patients for several decades but has never achieved widespread use in North America. In a large study in the Netherlands, Campschroer *et al.* reported their experience with the Wallstent and showed a primary patency rate of 41% over an average of 37 months [35]. The Allium stent (Allium LTD, Caesarea, Israel) consists of a nickel-titanium self-expanding scaffold wrapped in a biocompatible polymer with an intravesical anchor. Moskovitz *et al.* have done the largest study investigating the use of this stent, and within their population of 49 ureter units in 40 patients, 98% of the units maintained initial lumen patency. At an average follow-up time of 21 months, only 1 occlusion occurred and this was at 11 months. Stent migration was noted in 7 patients and occlusion in 1, which necessitated removal. In 8 patients who had scheduled stent removal at a mean of 11 months, all continued to have patent ureters at follow-up that ranged from 6-45 months [36].

10.10 Thermo-Expanding

The Memokath 051 ureteral stent (PNN Medical, Denmark) is a thermo-expandable stent in the shape of a spiral and is constructed of nickel-titanium. The thermo-expandable component causes the stent to be flaccid at a cool temperature of 10 degrees Celsius and return to a preformed shape at a temperature closer to 50 degrees Celsius [37]. This allows for easy insertion. Additionally, the tight spiral is believed to decrease the amount of tissue ingrowth [37]. Klarskov *et al.* showed the stent to be safe option in patients with incurable ureteral obstruction [38]. Agrawal *et al.* described their 11-year follow-up and found the Memokath 051 to be a suitable option for long-term management of ureteral obstruction. Of patients with malignant obstruction, 89% maintained upper tract decompression at a mean of 16 months. They did note an 18% migration rate that required reinsertion at an average of 7 months [39].

10.11 Spiral Stent

Ureteral stents have been shown to undergo significant movement with changes in body position [40]. A spiral cut double-J stent (Percuflex Helical, Boston Scientific, Marlborough, MA, USA) was created to address the hypothesis that colic experienced with an indwelling ureteral stent is, at least in part, due to the stiffness of the stent and limited ability to conform to a patient's ureter. Mucksavage *et al.* carried out an animal study comparing this stent to a standard double-J stent, and found similar flow rates between the two stents [41]. Clinical trials are needed to assess affect on patient comfort. Currently this stent is not commercially available.

Along a similar vein, the addition of a spiral ridge has been studied as to its ability to improve drainage. Using a mechanical ureteric model, Stoller *et al.* showed that a spiral-ridged JJ stent (Spirastent, Urosurge, Coralville, IA, USA) provided superior flow relative to smooth-walled JJ stents [42]. This stent was also studied for the potential to increase stone clearance rates following ESWL. Gerber *et al.* compared a spiral double-J stent (SpiraStent, Urosurge, Coralville, IA, USA) to a standard double-J stent (Percuflex Plus, Boston Scientific, Marlborough, MA, USA). The rate of stone fragment passage following extracorporeal shockwave lithotripsy was compared and found to have no statistically significant difference [43]. The spiral stent was noted to be more difficult to insert and was more likely to become displaced.

10.12 Film-Anchoring Stent

The 3F Microstent (PercSys, Palo Alto, CA, USA) is a stent that works on the theory that occupying a smaller percentage of ureteral lumen will allow the best chance for a calculus to pass. The Microstent possesses a proprietary film anchoring system that is deployed proximal to an obstructing stone and a distal 3 French distal anchoring bladder curl. Lange *et al.* carried out a study in a simulated urinary model and in an ex vivo porcine urinary model, comparing the flow rates through an obstructed ureter using the 3F Microstent and a 4.7F Double-J stent [44]. Their results showed no significant difference in flow rate between the Microstent and the double-J stent human trials are needed to assess the tolerability of this novel stent.

10.12.1 Infection/Biofilm

Properties that decrease the occurrence of urinary tract infection and inhibit the formation of bacterial biofilms are mostly within the realm of bacterial coating, which is described in another chapter.

10.13 Future Directions

While it is difficult to predict the future, it is likely new technologic innovations will be leveraged to develop the next generation of ureteral stents. Tissue engineering may hold promise in this regard. Amiel *et al.* successfully created tissue engineered ureteral stents by seeding bovine chondrocytes onto polymer mesh cylinders [45]. Future work assessing the functional ability tissue engineered stents within the urinary tract will help determine if such technology holds promise.

Drug-eluting ureteral stents, utilizing technology developed for cardiac stents, is a new developing area of stent design. Krambeck *et al.* carried out a study evaluating the effectiveness of a ketorolac-loaded stent with measured endpoints of unscheduled physician contact, change in pain medication, early stent removal, and medication use [46]. There was no significant difference noted though between the ketorolac stent and the control. Perhaps future designs will produce a more comfortable stent.

As shown, existing ureteral stents, although well functioning and well tolerated, still have room for improvement. There have been many variations in stent design but no significant single design has proven to be more comfortable and efficacious to date. New technologies coupled with new stent design may hold the key to the future in terms of developing an "ideal" stent that is both effective at draining the collecting system but also minimizing patient discomfort.

References

[1] Bloom DA, *et al.* Stents and related terms: a brief history. Urology. 1999;54(4):767–771.

[2] Bitschay J, Brodny ML. A History of Urology in Egypt. New York: Riverside Press, 1956, 76.

[3] Herman JR. Urology: A View Through the Retrospectroscope. Hagerstown, Maryland, Harper & Row, 1973.

[4] Tulloch WS. Restoration of continuity of the ureter by means of polyethylene tubing. Br J Urol. 1952;24(1):42–45.

[5] Zimskind PD, Kelter TR, Wilkerson SL. Clinical use of long-term indwelling silicone rubber ureteral splints inserted cystoscopically. J Urol 1967;97(5):840–844.

[6] Gibbons RP, Mason JT, Correa RJ Jr. Experience with indwelling silicone rubber ureteral catheters. J Urol 1974;111(5):594–599.

[7] Finney RP. Experience with new double J ureteral catheter stent. J Urol 1978;120(6):678–681.

[8] Christman MS, L'esperance JO, Choe CH, Stroup SP, Auge BK. Analysis of ureteral stent compression force and its role in malignant obstruction. J Urol 2009;181:392–396.

[9] van Diepen S, Grantmyre J. Broken retrieval string leads to failed self-removal of a double-J ureteral stent. Can J Urol. 2004;11(1):2139–2140.

[10] Wang HJ, Lee TY, Luo HL, Chen CH, Shen YC, Chuang YC, *et al.* Application of resonance metallic stents for ureteral obstruction. BJU Int 2011;108:428–432.

[11] Kadlec AO, Ellimoottil CS, Greco KA. Five-year experience with metallic stents for chronic ureteral obstruction. J Urol 2013;190:937–941.

[12] Liatsikos E, Kallidonis P, Kyriazis I, Constantinidis C, Hendlin K, Stolzenburg JU, *et al.* Ureteral obstruction: Is the full metallic double-pigtail stent the way to go? Eur Urol 2010;57:480–486.

[13] Chung SY, Stein RJ, Landsittel D, Davies BJ, Cuellar DC, Hrebinko RL, *et al.* 15-year experience with the management of extrinsic ureteral obstruction with indwelling ureteral stents. J Urol 2004;172:592–595.

[14] Taylor ER, Benson AD, Schwartz BF. Cost analysis of metallic ureteral stents with 12 months of follow-up. J Endourol 2012;26:917–921.

[15] Gayed BA, Mally AD, Riley J, Ost MC. Resonance metallic stents do not effectively relieve extrinsic ureteral compression in pediatric patients. J Endourol 2013;27:154–157.

[16] Modi AP, Ritch CR, Arend D, *et al*. Multicenter experience with metallic ureteral stents for malignant and chronic benign ureteral obstruction. J Endourol 2010;24:1189–1193.

[17] Joshi HB, Newns N, Stainthorpe A, MacDonagh RP, Keeley FX, Jr, Timoney AG. Ureteral stent symptom questionnaire: development and validation of a multidimensional quality of life measure. J Urol 2003a;169:1060.

[18] Joshi HB, Stainthorpe A, MacDonagh RP, Keeley FX, Jr, Timoney AG, Barry MJ. Indwelling ureteral stents: evaluation of symptoms, quality of life and utility. J Urol 2003b;169:1065–1069.

[19] El-Nahas A, El-Assmy A, Shoma A, Eraky I, El-Kenawy M, El-Kappany H. Self-retaining ureteral stents: analysis of factors responsible for patients' discomfort. J Endourol 2006;20(1):33–37.

[20] Joshi HB, Chitale SV, Nagarajan M, *et al*. A prospective randomized single-blind comparison of ureteral stents composed of firm and soft polymer. J Urol 2005;174(6):2303–2306.

[21] Lingeman JE, Preminger GM, Goldfischer ER, *et al*. Assessing the Impact of Ureteral Stent Design on Patient Comfort. J Urol 2009;181(6):2581–2587.

[22] Davenport K, Kumar V, Collins J, Melotti R, Timoney AG, Keeley FX, Jr. New ureteral stent design does not improve patient quality of life: a randomized, controlled trial. J Urol 2011;185:175–178.

[23] Dunn MD, Portis AJ, Kahn SA, *et al*. Clinical effectiveness of new stent design: randomized single-blind comparison of tail and double-pigtail stents. J Endourol 2000;14:195.

[24] Taylor WN, McDougall IT. Minimally invasive ureteral stent retrieval. J Urol. 2002;168(5):2020–2023.

[25] Lingeman JE, Schulsinger DA, Kuo RL. Phase I trial of a temporary ureteral drainage stent. J Endourol 2003a;17(3):169–171.

[26] Lingeman JE, Preminger GM, Berger Y, Denstedt JD, Goldstone L, Segura JW, *et al*. Use of a temporary ureteral drainage stent after uncomplicated ureteroscopy: results from a phase II clinical trial. J Urol 2003b;169(5):1682–1688.

[27] Hadaschik BA, Paterson RF, Fazli L, Clinkscales KW, Shalaby SW, Chew BH. Investigation of a novel degradable ureteral stent in a porcine model. J Urol. 2008;180(3):1161–1166.

[28] Chew BH, Lange D, Paterson RF, *et al*. Next generation biodegradable ureteral stent in a Yucatan pig model. J Urol 2010;183(2):765–771.

[29] Chew BH, Paterson RF, Clinkscales KW, Levine BS, Shalaby SW, Lange D. In vivo evaluation of the third generation biodegradable stent: a novel approach to avoiding the forgotten stent syndrome. J Urol 2013;189(2):719–725.

[30] Hafron J, Ost MC, Tan BJ, Fogarty JD, Hoenig DM, Lee BR, *et al*. Novel dual-lumen ureteral stents provide better ureteral flow than single ureteral stent in ex vivo porcine kidney model of extrinsic ureteral obstruction. Urology 2006;68(4):911–915.

[31] Olweny EO, Portis AJ, Afane JS, *et al*. Flow characteristics of 3 unique ureteral stents: investigation of a Poiseuille flow pattern. Journal of Urology. 2000;164(6):2099–2103.

[32] Battaglia M, Ditonno P, Selvaggio O, Palazzo S, Bettocchi C, Peschechera R, *et al.* Double J stent with antireflux device in the prevention of short-term urological complications after cadaveric kidney transplantation: single-center prospective randomized study. Transplantation Proceedings 2005;37(6):2525–2526.

[33] Soria F, Morcillo E, Serrano A, *et al.* Preliminary Assessment of a New Antireflux Ureteral Stent Design in Swine Model. Urology 2015;86(2):417–422.

[34] Pollak JS, Rosenblatt MM, Egglin TK, Dickey KW, Glickman M. Treatment of ureteral obstruction with the Wallstent endoprosthesis: Preliminary results. J Vasc Interv Radiol 1995;6:417–425.

[35] Campschroer T, Lock MT, Lo RT, Bosch JL. The Wallstent: long-term follow-up of metal stent placement for the treatment of benign ureteroileal anastomotic strictures after Bricker urinary diversion. BJU Int. 2014;114(6):910–915.

[36] Moskovitz B, Halachmi S, Nativ O. A new self-expanding, large-caliber ureteral stent: results of a multicenter experience. J Endourol 2012;26(11):1523–1527.

[37] Staios D, Shergill I, Thwaini A, Junaid I, Buchholz NP. The Memokath stent. Expert Review of Medical Devices 2007;4(2):99–101.

[38] Klarskov P, Nordling J, Nielsen JB. Experience with Memokath 051 ureteral stent. Scandinavian Journal of Urology and Nephrology 2005;39(2):169–172.

[39] Agrawal S, Brown CT, Bellamy EA, Kulkarni R. The thermo-expandable metallic ureteric stent: an 11-year follow-up. BJU International 2009;103(3):372–376.

[40] Chew BH, Knudsen BE, Nott L, Pautler SE, Razvi H, Amann J, *et al.* Pilot Study of Ureteral Movement in Stented Patients: First Step in Understanding Dynamic Ureteral Anatomy to Improve Stent Discomfort. J Endourol 2007;21:1069–1075.

[41] Mucksavage P, Pick D, Haydel D, *et al.* An in vivo evaluation of a novel spiral cut flexible ureteral stent. Urology 2012;79:733–737.

[42] Stoller ML, Schwartz BF, Frigstad JR, Norris L, Park JB, *et al.* An in vitro assessment of the flow characteristics of spiral-ridged and smooth-walled JJ ureteric stents. BJU Int 2000;85(6):628–631.

[43] Gerber R, Nitz C, Studer UE, Danuser H. Spiral stent versus standard stent in patients with midsize renal stones treated with extracorporeal shock wave lithotripsy: which stent works better? A prospective randomized trial. J Urol 2004;172(3):965–966.

[44] Lange D, Hoag NA, Poh BK, *et al.* Drainage characteristics of the 3 F MicroStent using a novel film occlusion anchoring mechanism. J Endourol 2011;25:1051–1056.

[45] Amiel GE, Yoo JJ, Kim BS, Atala A. Tissue engineered stents created from chondrocytes. J Urol 2001;165:2091–2095.

[46] Krambeck AE, Walsh RS, Denstedt JD, Preminger GM, Li J, Evans JC, et al. A novel drug eluting ureteral stent: a prospective, randomized, multicenter clinical trial to evaluate the safety and effectiveness of a ketorolac loaded ureteral stent. J Urol 2010;183:1037–1042.

11

Coated and Drug-Eluting Stents

Thomas O. Tailly[1] and John D. Denstedt[2]

[1] Division of Urology, Department of Surgery, Ghent University Hospitals, Ghent, Belgium
[2] Professor of Urology Division of Urology, Department of Surgery, Schulich School of Medicine & Dentistry-Western University, London, Ontario, Canada

11.1 Introduction

The development of the double-J stent by Finney has initiated an immense expansion of the endourological surgical potential [1]. Like many other foreign bodies, due to lack of biocompatibility, indwelling double-J stents are fraught with complications such as pain, hematuria, encrustation, and urinary tract infections, having a tremendous impact on quality of life [2]. Encrustation is a very common problem with approximately 9–27% of stents demonstrating a degree of encrustation within 6 weeks of implantation and an increasing incidence with indwelling time (Figure 11.1) [3,4]. Despite antibiotic prophylaxis in children stented for 3 weeks following ureteral reimplantation, almost half of the stents appeared to be colonized at stent extraction [5]. Riedl *et al.* demonstrated that virtually all stents from chronically stented patients show bacterial colonization on the surface [6]. Although alpha-blockers can reduce stent-related symptoms, they are not able to completely eliminate stent associated symptoms [7].

Many research groups have put their efforts toward new stent designs, biomaterials, and coatings with the goal of increasing biocompatibility, thus reducing stent-related symptoms and complications [8]. This chapter provides an overview of the wide array of stent coatings, such as lubricating, antimicrobial, anti-fouling (preventing deposition of conditioning film constituents), or drug-eluting coatings that have been and are being studied to this purpose.

11.2 Stent Coatings

11.2.1 Hydrophilic Coatings

Hydrogel is composed of hydrophilic polymers that absorb water, thus increasing the elastic properties and reducing surface friction. This would theoretically render a hydrogel-coated stent easier to insert and more biocompatible. Despite this promising premise, in vitro tests have not been consistently in favor of hydrogel coatings. In comparison

Ureteric Stenting, First Edition. Edited by Ravi Kulkarni.

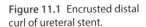

Figure 11.1 Encrusted distal curl of ureteral stent.

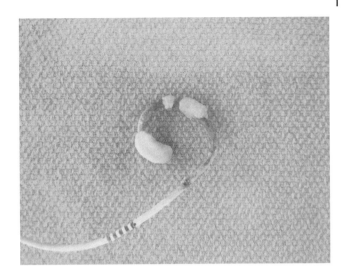

to uncoated stents, results have ranged from decreased to increased rates of biofilm formation and encrustation [9–11].

John *et al.* demonstrated the efficacy of hydrogel-coated antibacterial-impregnated stents in vitro [12]. When comparing the inhibitory capacity of hydrogel-coated and uncoated stents that were dipped in ciprofloxacin, gentamicin, or cefazolin, hydrogel-coated stents demonstrated a significantly longer antibacterial activity [12].

Polyvinyl pyrrolidone (PVP) coated stents are available as the Bard Inlay® stent. Tunney and Gorman demonstrated that this hydrophilic coating renders a stent more lubricious compared to uncoated polyurethane and silicone stents [13]. The PVP-coated stents additionally showed a decreased bacterial adherence of *E. coli* compared to silicone stents and of *E. faecalis* compared to polyurethane stents [13]. These promising results were corroborated by Khandwekar et al who surface engineered Tecoflex® stents to contain PVP-Iodine (PVP-I) [14]. The in vitro results of these PVP-I coated stents showed increased lubricity, reduced encrustation deposits and a decreased bacterial adherence with *P. aeruginosa* and *S. aureus* as compared to regular Tecoflex® stents [14].

11.2.2 Phosphorylcholine

As phosphorylcholine (PC) is naturally present on the outer membrane of erythrocytes [15], it is hypothesized that applying a PC-coating to a surface would increase biocompatibility. After testing PC-coated stents in 44 patients who were stented for 12 weeks, Stickler *et al.* demonstrated that the PC-coated stents had fewer encrustations and reduced biofilm and bacterial adherence when compared to 28 uncoated stents that were previously removed from the same patient cohort [16].

11.2.3 Diamond-Like Carbon

Another strategy to improve biocompatibility, that has previously been applied to vascular, orthopedic, and other implants, is an amorphous diamond-like carbon (DLC) coating [17]. Polyurethane surfaces coated with a DLC layer of 100–200 nm thickness have a dramatically decreased surface friction, resulting in significantly reduced stent encrustation and bacterial adherence [18]. Laube *et al.* implanted DLC-coated stents in 10 patients known to be very prone to stent encrustation and demonstrated significantly reduced encrustation and bio-film formation, compared to previously used stents in these patients [19]. The DLC-coated stents were significantly better tolerated than uncoated stents.

11.2.3.1 *Oxalobacter formigenes*–Derived Enzymes

The link between *Oxalobacter formigenes* and calcium oxalate stone formation has been well established, with a lack of *O. formigenes* colonization in the gut increasing the risk of calcium oxalate stone disease [20]. This observation had inspired Watterson *et al.* to coat stent surfaces with *O. formigenes*–derived oxalate degrading enzymes [21]. Although the coated silicone surfaces were less encrusted as compared to uncoated surfaces in an in vivo rabbit model, these findings were not statistically significant [21].

11.2.4 Glycosaminoglycans

Glycosaminoglycans (GAGs) are well-known inhibitors of calcium oxalate crystal growth, with heparin, although not naturally present in human urine, being the strongest inhibitor [22].

Whereas heparin-coated surfaces were demonstrated to resist encrustations, a decrease in bacterial adherence could not be identified in comparison to uncoated devices in an in vitro model [23,24].

Results from small in vivo human studies supported these findings, with heparin-coated stents demonstrating reduced encrustation in contrast to uncoated stents, even after up to 12 months indwelling time [25,26]. With this potential of longer indwelling times, necessitating fewer stent exchanges, Tenke and colleagues advocated that heparin coated stents, although more expensive than regular uncoated stents, can be cost-effective [27].

Pentosan polysulphate (PPS), a semi-synthetic GAG, has been shown to inhibit calcium oxalate crystallization in vitro and in vivo [28,29]. Evaluating PPS-coated and uncoated silicone disks that had remained in a rabbit bladder for 50 days, Zupkas *et al.* identified that the coated disks had significantly fewer encrustations than the uncoated disks [30].

11.2.5 Antibiotic Coatings

Until recently, antibiotic-impregnated stent coatings were still in a preliminary test phase. An Italian research group demonstrated that a combination of systemic antibiotics with antibiotic-coated stents is more effective in the prevention of biofilm formation than either alone [31,32]. Clarithromycin-coated stents prevent *P. aeruginosa* adherence more effectively in combination with systemic Amikacin, whereas the *E. faecalis* biofilm reducing abilities of Rifampin-coated stents were improved with the aid of systemically administered Tigecycline in a rat model [31,32]. The first in-human randomized study with antibiotic (silver sulfadiazine) coated stents has been registered with http://www.clinicaltrials.gov (NCT02266368) and is currently recruiting participants. Although commonly used in indwelling catheters, this is only the second report of a silver-based coating being applied on ureteral stents. The first report was by Multanen *et al.*, who demonstrated that a silver nitrate and ofloxacin coating decreased stent surface encrustation and accelerated stent degradation of a biodegradable poly-L-lactic acid stent [33].

11.2.6 MPEG-DOPA

Ko *et al.*, inspired by marine fauna, tested a novel copolymer mPEG-DOPA, that anchors the anti-fouling component polyethylene glycol to the stent surface with 3,4-dihydroxyphenylalanine, a mussel adhesive protein allowing the marine mussel to attach to any surface [34]. Building on the promising results of the in vitro work by Ko *et al.*, Pechey *et al.* demonstrated in an in vivo rabbit model that a cross-linked DOPA-anchored copolymer resisted adherence with *E. coli* and biofilm formation better than uncoated or unlinked mPEG-DOPA–coated stents [35]. Further investigations are ongoing.

11.3 Drug-Eluting Stents

11.3.1 Triclosan

Triclosan, often used in deodorants, soap, and many other consumer products, exhibits antibacterial and antifungal capacities. Triclosan-eluting stents (Triumph®) have demonstrated reduced surface attachment and growth inhibition of several uropathogens in vitro and in vivo in comparison to uncoated Percuflex® stents [36,37]. Further studies in human subjects showed reduced symptomatic urinary tract infections resulting in decreased antibiotics use in long-term stented patients [38]. The stents significantly reduced stent-related pain and urinary symptoms in short-term stented patients without, however, influencing biofilm formation, encrustation, or infection rate [39].

11.3.2 Ketorolac

A prospective double-blind randomized trial demonstrated that a *Ketorolac-eluting stent (Lexington®)* reduced the need for analgesia, an effect most apparent in men and patients younger than 45 years old [40]. However, the primary endpoint of intervention for pain was not significantly different for the Lexington stent versus the control stent, a Percuflex Plus® Double J stent [40].

11.3.3 Chlorhexidine

The most recent developments on stent coatings report the use of a sustained release varnish containing chlorhexidine (CHX-SVR). After promising in vitro results with stents coated with a 2% chlorhexidine concentration, CHX-SVR coated catheters have been studied in vivo in a dog model, confirming the inhibitory effects on bacterial growth and reduced biofilm formation [41,42]. Phuengkam *et al.* proposed a new approach to CHX coatings by using CHX-loaded nanosphere [43]. CHX-nanoparticle coated stents demonstrated a sustained release of CHX up to 15 days and significant antibacterial effect against common uropathogens in an in vitro environment [43].

11.3.4 Metal Drug-Eluting Stents

Due to the long indwelling time, metal mesh stents are commonly plagued by complications such as migration, encrustation, and tissue hyperplasia growing into the stent [44–46]. Drawing from endovascular stent experience, a paclitaxel-eluting metal mesh ureteral stent has been developed and compared in vivo in a porcine model to a bare metal stent (BMS), demonstrating reduced inflammation and surrounding tissue hyperplasia [47]. Similarly, a Zotarolimus-eluting stent showed a significantly reduced hyperplastic reaction; however, without influencing tissue inflammation when compared to a BMS in an animal model [48].

11.4 Conclusion

Current pharmacological treatments are unable to eliminate stent encrustation, device associated infection, and stent-related symptoms. A wide array of stent coatings have been reported with promising in vitro results. However, only few coatings were actually tested in animal models or human trials. Further research is warranted to pursue in vivo studies of already developed coatings and to continue the search for the ideal stent that is biocompatible, resists encrustation and infection, causes no stent-related symptoms, and is easy to insert.

References

[1] Finney RP. Experience with new double J ureteral catheter stent. J Urol 1978;120:678–81.

[2] Joshi HB, Stainthorpe A, MacDonagh RP, Keeley FX, Timoney AG, Barry MJ. Indwelling ureteral stents: evaluation of symptoms, quality of life and utility. J Urol 2003;169:1065–1069.

[3] el-Faqih SR, Shamsuddin AB, Chakrabarti A, Atassi R, Kardar AH, Osman MK, et al. Polyurethane internal ureteral stents in treatment of stone patients: morbidity related to indwelling times. J Urol 1991;146:1487–1491.

[4] Kawahara T, Ito H, Terao H, Yoshida M, Matsuzaki J. Ureteral stent encrustation, incrustation, and coloring: morbidity related to indwelling times. J Endourol 2012;26:178–182.

[5] Uvin P, Van Baelen A, Verhaegen J, Bogaert G. Ureteral stents do not cause bacterial infections in children after ureteral reimplantation. Urology 2011;78:154–158.

[6] Riedl CR, Plas E, Hübner WA, Zimmerl H, Ulrich W, Pflüger H. Bacterial colonization of ureteral stents. Eur Urol 1999;36:53–59.

[7] Lamb AD, Vowler SL, Johnston R, Dunn N, Wiseman OJ. Meta-analysis showing the beneficial effect of α-blockers on ureteric stent discomfort. BJU Int 2011;108:1894–1902.

[8] Lange D, Bidnur S, Hoag N, Chew BH. Ureteral stent-associated complications-where we are and where we are going. Nat Rev Urol 2015;12:17–25.

[9] Gorman SP, Tunney MM, Keane PF, Van Bladel K, Bley B. Characterization and assessment of a novel poly(ethylene oxide)/polyurethane composite hydrogel (Aquavene) as a ureteral stent biomaterial. J Biomed Mater Res 1998;39:642–649.

[10] Tunney MM, Keane PF, Jones DS, Gorman SP. Comparative assessment of ureteral stent biomaterial encrustation. Biomaterials 1996;17:1541–1546.

[11] Desgrandchamps F, Moulinier F, Daudon M, Teillac P, Le Duc A. An in vitro comparison of urease-induced encrustation of JJ stents in human urine. Br J Urol 1997;79:24–27.

[12] John T, Rajpurkar A, Smith G, Fairfax M, Triest J. Antibiotic pretreatment of hydrogel ureteral stent. J Endourol 2007;21:1211–1216.

[13] Tunney MM, Gorman SP. Evaluation of a poly(vinyl pyrollidone)-coated biomaterial for urological use. Biomaterials 2002;23:4601–4608.

[14] Khandwekar AP, Doble M. Physicochemical characterisation and biological evaluation of polyvinylpyrrolidone-iodine engineered polyurethane (Tecoflex(®)). J Mater Sci Mater Med 2011;22:1231–1246.

[15] Chen H, Yuan L, Song W, Wu Z, Li D. Biocompatible polymer materials: Role of protein–surface interactions. Prog Polym Sci 2008;33:1059–1087.

[16] Stickler DJ, Evans A, Morris N, Hughes G. Strategies for the control of catheter encrustation. Int J Antimicrob Agents 2002;19:499–506.

[17] Roy RK, Lee K-R. Biomedical applications of diamond-like carbon coatings: a review. J Biomed Mater Res B Appl Biomater 2007;83:72–84.

[18] Jones DS, Garvin CP, Dowling D, Donnelly K, Gorman SP. Examination of surface properties and in vitro biological performance of amorphous diamond-like carbon-coated polyurethane. J Biomed Mater Res B Appl Biomater 2006;78:230–236.

[19] Laube N, Kleinen L, Bradenahl J, Meissner A. Diamond-like carbon coatings on ureteral stents--a new strategy for decreasing the formation of crystalline bacterial biofilms? J Urol 2007;177:1923–1927.

[20] Knight J, Deora R, Assimos DG, Holmes RP. The genetic composition of Oxalobacter formigenes and its relationship to colonization and calcium oxalate stone disease. Urolithiasis 2013;41:187–196.

[21] Watterson JD, Cadieux PA, Beiko DT, Cook AJ, Burton JP, Harbottle RR, et al. Oxalate-degrading enzymes from Oxalobacter formigenes: a novel device coating to reduce urinary tract biomaterial-related encrustation. J Endourol 2003;17:269–274.

[22] Angell AH, Resnick MI. Surface interaction between glycosaminoglycans and calcium oxalate. J Urol 1989;141:1255–8.

[23] Lange D, Elwood CN, Choi K, Hendlin K, Monga M, Chew BH. Uropathogen interaction with the surface of urological stents using different surface properties. J Urol 2009;182:1194–1200.

[24] Hildebrandt P, Sayyad M, Rzany A, Schaldach M, Seiter H. Prevention of surface encrustation of urological implants by coating with inhibitors. Biomaterials 2001;22:503–507.

[25] Riedl CR, Witkowski M, Plas E, Pflueger H. Heparin coating reduces encrustation of ureteral stents: a preliminary report. Int J Antimicrob Agents 2002;19:507–510.

[26] Cauda F, Cauda V, Fiori C, Onida B, Garrone E. Heparin coating on ureteral Double J stents prevents encrustations: an in vivo case study. J Endourol 2008;22:465–472.

[27] Tenke P, Riedl CR, Jones GL, Williams GJ, Stickler D, Nagy E. Bacterial biofilm formation on urologic devices and heparin coating as preventive strategy. Int J Antimicrob Agents 2004;23 Suppl 1:S67–S74.

[28] Martin X, Werness PG, Bergert JH, Smith LH. Pentosan polysulfate as an inhibitor of calcium oxalate crystal growth. J Urol 1984;132:786–788.

[29] Norman RW, Scurr DS, Robertson WG, Peacock M. Inhibition of calcium oxalate crystallisation by pentosan polysulphate in control subjects and stone formers. Br J Urol 1984;56:594–598.

[30] Zupkas P, Parsons CL, Percival C, Monga M. Pentosanpolysulfate coating of silicone reduces encrustation. J Endourol 2000;14:483–488.

[31] Minardi D, Cirioni O, Ghiselli R, Silvestri C, Mocchegiani F, Gabrielli E, et al. Efficacy of tigecycline and rifampin alone and in combination against Enterococcus faecalis biofilm infection in a rat model of ureteral stent. J Surg Res 2012;176:1–6.

[32] Cirioni O, Ghiselli R, Silvestri C, Minardi D, Gabrielli E, Orlando F, et al. Effect of the combination of clarithromycin and amikacin on Pseudomonas aeruginosa biofilm in an animal model of ureteral stent infection. J Antimicrob Chemother 2011;66:1318–1323.

[33] Multanen M, Tammela TLJ, Laurila M, Seppälä J, Välimaa T, Törmälä P, et al. Biocompatibility, encrustation and biodegradation of ofloxacine and silver nitrate coated poly-L-lactic acid stents in rabbit urethra. Urol Res 2002;30:227–232.

[34] Ko R, Cadieux PA, Dalsin JL, Lee BP, Elwood CN, Razvi H. First prize: Novel uropathogen-resistant coatings inspired by marine mussels. J Endourol 2008;22:1153–1160.

[35] Pechey A, Elwood CN, Wignall GR, Dalsin JL, Lee BP, Vanjecek M, et al. Anti-adhesive coating and clearance of device associated uropathogenic Escherichia coli cystitis. J Urol 2009;182:1628–1636.

[36] Cadieux PA, Chew BH, Knudsen BE, DeJong K, Rowe E, Reid G, et al. Triclosan Loaded Ureteral Stents Decrease Proteus Mirabilis 296 Infection in a Rabbit Urinary Tract Infection Model. J Urol 2006;175:2331–2335.

[37] Chew BH, Cadieux PA, Reid G, Denstedt JD. In-vitro activity of triclosan-eluting ureteral stents against common bacterial uropathogens. J Endourol 2006;20:949–958.

[38] Cadieux P a, Chew BH, Nott L, Seney S, Elwood CN, Wignall GR, et al. Use of triclosan-eluting ureteral stents in patients with long-term stents. J Endourol 2009;23:1187–1194.

[39] Mendez-Probst CE, Goneau LW, MacDonald KW, Nott L, Seney S, Elwood CN, et al. The use of triclosan eluting stents effectively reduces ureteral stent symptoms: a prospective randomized trial. BJU Int 2012;110:749–754.

[40] Krambeck AE, Walsh RS, Denstedt JD, Preminger GM, Li J, Evans JC, et al. A novel drug eluting ureteral stent: a prospective, randomized, multicenter clinical trial to evaluate the safety and effectiveness of a ketorolac loaded ureteral stent. J Urol 2010;183:1037–1042.

[41] Zelichenko G, Steinberg D, Lorber G, Friedman M, Zaks B, Lavy E, et al. Prevention of initial biofilm formation on ureteral stents using a sustained releasing varnish containing chlorhexidine: in vitro study. J Endourol 2013;27:333–337.

[42] Segev G, Bankirer T, Steinberg D, Duvdevani M, Shapur NK, Friedman M, et al. Evaluation of urinary catheters coated with sustained-release varnish of chlorhexidine in mitigating biofilm formation on urinary catheters in dogs. J Vet Intern Med 2013;27:39–46.

[43] Phuengkham H, Nasongkla N. Development of antibacterial coating on silicone surface via chlorhexidine-loaded nanospheres. J Mater Sci Med 2015;26:5418.

[44] Chung KJ, Park BH, Park B, Lee JH, Kim WJ, Baek M, et al. Efficacy and safety of a novel, double-layered, coated, self-expandable metallic mesh stent (Uventa^{TM}) in malignant ureteral obstructions. J Endourol 2013;27:930–935.

[45] Liatsikos E, Kallidonis P, Kyriazis I, Constantinidis C, Hendlin K, Stolzenburg J-U, et al. Ureteral Obstruction: Is the Full Metallic Double-Pigtail Stent the Way to Go? Eur Urol 2010;57:480–487.

[46] Agrawal S, Brown CT, Bellamy EA, Kulkarni R. The thermo-expandable metallic ureteric stent: an 11-year follow-up. BJU Int 2009;103:372–376.

[47] Liatsikos EN, Karnabatidis D, Kagadis GC, Rokkas K, Constantinides C, Christeas N, et al. Application of paclitaxel-eluting metal mesh stents within the pig ureter: an experimental study. Eur Urol 2007;51:217–223.

[48] Kallidonis P, Kitrou P, Karnabatidis D, Kyriazis I, Kalogeropoulou C, Tsamandas A, et al. Evaluation of zotarolimus-eluting metal stent in animal ureters. J Endourol 2011;25:1661–1667.

12

Coated and Drug-Eluting Ureteric Stents

Panagiotis Kallidonis[1], Wissam Kamal[2], Vasilis Panagopoulos[2] and Evangelos Liatsikos[3]

[1] Urology Specialist, Department of Urology, University Hospital of Patras, Patras, Greece
[2] Department of Urology, University Hospital of Patras, Patras, Greece
[3] Professor of Urology, Department of Urology, University Hospital of Patras, Patras, Greece

12.1 Introduction

Conventional bare metal stents (MSs) have been established as an invaluable tool in interventional cardiology and radiology during the performance of Percutaneous Transluminal Angioplasty (PTA) [1, 2]. MSs are small, tubular, wire mesh devices, which are loaded in a collapsed form onto the catheter balloon. The system composed of the stent and catheter is inserted over a guidewire through a vascular lesion, the balloon is inflated to dilate the obstruction, and the stent is released on the vascular wall. After the stent is expanded, it acts as a mechanical scaffold, which prevents elastic recoil and maintains vessel luminal patency. The stent is eventually incorporated to the vascular wall after a period of epithelization [3]. The use of MSs has also been investigated in urological practice for the long-term catheterization of the ureter and urethra [4, 5].

Ureteral MSs were efficient in alleviating mainly malignant ureteral obstructions [6]. Nevertheless, a number of complications were noted including infection, restenosis due to the urothelial luminal hyperplasia, stent migration, encrustation, infection, and difficulties in stent removal [5, 7]. As a result, the long-term experience was related to controversial results regarding the ureteral patency [7, 8]. The most common cause of restenosis for ureteral MSs was the hyperplastic reaction that developed through the stent struts. The latter issue represented also a complication of MSs placed in the vascular system. In an attempt to overcome it, the drug eluting stents (DESs) were developed and introduced in the clinical practice of interventional radiology and cardiology [1, 6]. The concept of DES in urology is similar to that used in the vascular system. The DESs aim to eliminate the hyperplastic reaction of the MSs. Coated metallic stents (CMSs) were also proposed to the urological field as a solution to avoid the in-growth of hyperplastic tissue through the stent struts. The CMSs usually a have polytetrafluoroethylene (PTFE) cover, which does not allow the tissue in-growth into the stent and maintains the patency of the stent. Chung *et al.* compared MSs with PTFE-CMSs and noticed that there was tissue in-growth into the stent lumen causing almost complete occlusion in the group with the MSs. Moreover, there was not obstruction from tissue in-growth in a group of CMSs [9].

Ureteric Stenting, First Edition. Edited by Ravi Kulkarni.
© 2017 John Wiley & Sons Ltd. Published 2017 by John Wiley & Sons Ltd.

12.2   Drug-Eluting Metal Stents

12.2.1   The Concept of Drug-Eluting Stents

DESs minimize the neointemal hyperplasia and reduce the re-stenosis rates when used in the vessels [1]. They release anti-proliferative pharmacological substances in a controlled fashion in the vessel lumen. Specifically, the anti-proliferative drug is coated onto the stent surface and is slowly released. These substances reduce the hyperplastic reaction by inhibiting the smooth muscle cell (SMCs) cycle and their proliferation [10, 11]. The SMCs of the ureteral wall are associated with collagen production, which is directly correlated to the re-stenosis phenomenon after the placement of MSs. The DESs could result in reduction of the hyperplastic reaction of the ureteral wall and eventually could reduce the lumen restenosis rates [6, 12].

12.2.2   Design and Structure of Drug-Eluting Stents

DESs are consisted by three components: the stent platform, the coating, and the active pharmaceutical substance. As newer generations of DES are developed, significant evolution in stent structure, polymer coating, and pharmaceutical substances is noted along with a promising lower morbidity and longer lasting outcome [3].

The proper design of stent platform is of high importance as it ensures the optimal stent geometry, maximum radial strength with minimal shortening, and radial recoiling. Biologically inert materials such as stainless steel, nickel-titanium, and cobalt-chromium are usually used for the stent platforms.

The stent platform of the DESs is covered by a polymeric coating, which is responsible for the controlled release of the drug. The polymeric material is selected to induce minimal reaction of the surrounding tissue and should be non-thrombotic, non-inflammatory, non-toxic, and hemocompatible (when referring to vascular stents). These properties are important for the prevention of thromboembolic events and facilitate the epithelization process of the stent. There are several categories of stent polymeric coatings for DESs [1, 3].

12.3   Pharmaceutical Substances

The selection of the most appropriate substance for a DES is based on the purpose of the stent. The drugs used on DESs usually inhibit one or more biochemical pathways related to the hyperplastic reaction and platelet aggregation and eventually prevent intraluminal restenosis. Pharmaceutical substances for potential use in DESs include a variety of mechanisms of action with the main effect to be immunosuppressive (tacrolimus), anti-inflammatory (sirolimus, biolimus A9, dexamethasone), anti-proliferative (sirolimus, everolimus, tacrolimus, zotarolimus, pimercolimus, biolimus A9, paclitaxel, actinomycin D), antibacterial agents (triclosan), and anti-thrombogenic (antiplatelet GP IIb/IIa antiboby) [6].

12.4   Drug-Eluting Stents in Urology

In an attempt to confront the above-mentioned complications of MSs, DESs have been investigated in experimental studies. Liatsikos *et al.* used a commercially available paclitaxel-eluting stent (TAXUS, Boston Scientific, Natick, MA, USA) in porcine ureters [13].

A DES was inserted in the one ureter and a MS (R-Stent,Orbus Medical Technologies, Hoevelaken, Netherlands) in the other ureter of each animal. During the 21-day follow-up period, most of the MSs were occluded, whereas the remaining stents were stenosed by hyperplastic reaction. DESs were all patent during the above follow-up period. The authors concluded that DESs induced less inflammation and ureteral tissue hyperplasia (responsible for ureteral occlusion) in comparison to the conventional MSs. Similar results were also presented by Kallidonis *et al.* evaluating the effect of zotarolimus-eluting stents (Endeavor, Medtronics, USA) in porcine and rabbit ureters [14]. A MS (R-Stent, Orbus Medical Technologies, Hoevelaken, Netherlands) was placed in the one ureter (control) and a DES in the other ureter of the same animal. The follow-up period was 4 and 8 weeks for the pigs and rabbits, respectively. Hyperplasia was revealed by the CT or IVP in both MSs and DESs. Seven porcine ureters with MSs were completely occluded. Despite the hyperplasia of their lumen, DESs were never obstructed. Two rabbit ureters stented by MS were obstructed, whereas ureters stented by DES were never occluded. The evaluation of the renal function (MAG3 scintigraphy) showed that seven porcine renal units and the one rabbit unit with obstructed stented ureter were significantly compromised. Optical coherence tomography (Figure 12.1) and histology (Figure 12.2) revealed increased hyperplastic reaction in the ureters stented by MSs in comparison to DESs.

(a)   (b)

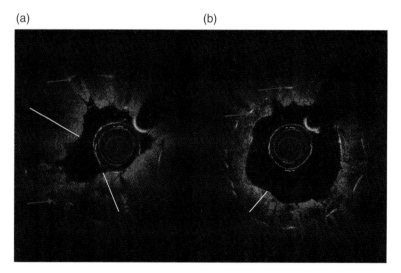

Figure 12.1 Optical coherence tomography (OCT) images from the stented ureters of the same pig. The OCT images were obtained after 4 weeks of follow-up. The struts of the stent are presented as illuminating sites with shadows behind them (red arrows). The struts mark the border between the urothelium and muscular layer of the ureter for either pigs or rabbits. a) A characteristic OCT presentation of a ureter with an implanted conventional MS. The tissue between a strut of the stent and the ureteral lumen can be observed and the extensive hyperplastic reaction of the urothelium extends inside the lumen of the ureter and compromises patency (white line). b) A respective image from a ureter stented with drug-eluting stent (DES). Notice the clearly less hyperplastic reaction in comparison to the conventional MS (white line).

(a)   (b)   (c)

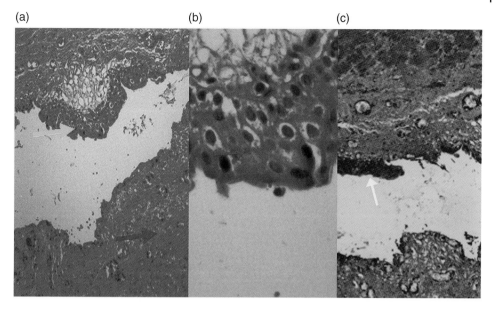

Figure 12.2 Ureter dilated by DEB and specimen removal after 24 h. a). The blue arrows show sites of reconstitution of the urothelial layer. The substantially less acute inflammation and granulation tissue formation are marked by the red arrows. H&E, 200x. b) Reconstitution of the urothelium and limited infammation (red arrow). H&E, 400x. c) Immunohistochemistry for paclitaxel and streptavidin-biotin peroxidase staining shows that paclitaxel is located in the superficial epithelial cells (yellow arrow) and in the muscularis propria (red arrow). The magnification used was 200x.

12.5   Coated Metallic Stents

12.5.1   The Concept of Coated Metal Stents

Another option for reducing the re-stenosis rates related to the hyperplastic reaction is the CMSs. The material covering the struts of the CMSs does not allow the protrusion of the hyperplastic reaction through the struts and consequently reduces the incidence of restenosis [15].

12.5.2   Coated Metal Stents in Urology

The use of vascular CMSs in the urinary tract showed unfavorable outcomes with high migration rates [7, 16, 17]. Recently, specially designed CMSs for the urinary tract have been introduced such as the Allium (Allium Medical Solutions Ltd, Caesarea, Israel) and the UVENTA (Taewoong Medical Co., Ltd, Gyeonggi-do, South Korea) [18, 19]. The above stents share a stent platform consisted of super-elastic nickel-titanium alloy (Nitinol), which is considered biocompatible, with high endurance to compression while remaining flexible. Moreover, a polytetrafluroethylene (PTFE) cover inhibits tissue in-growth into the stent lumen [20].

Table 12.1 Summary of the clinical experience with coated metallic stents.

Study	Stent	Number of Ureters	Etiology of obstructions	Stricture length	Follow Up Period	Patency Rate	Complications
Moskovitz et al. [18]	Allium	49	Malignant	Not reported	Mean 21 (1–63) months	98%	• Stent occlusion after one year (2%) • stent migration (14.2%)
Leonardo et al. [21]	Allium	12	Benign	Not reported	Median 10 months	100%	No Complications
Chung et al. [22]	UVENTA	71	Malignant	Mean 11.8 ± 6.4 cm	Median 308 (range 35–802) days	64% - primary 81.7% - overall	• Persistent Pain (15.5%) • LUTS (7%) • Acute Pyelonephritis (2.8%) • Stent Migration (2.8%) • Persistent hematuria (2.8%).
Kim et al. [19]	UVENTA	20	Malignant	Mean 10.6 (range 2–20) cm	Mean 7.3 (range 3–15) months	100%	• LUTS • abdominal pain • transient gross hematuria

The Allium comes in 10- and 12-cm lengths and two diameters of 24 F and 30 F. It is composed of Nitinol and covered with PTFE in order to avoid tissue in-growth inside its lumen and early encrustation. It has an intra-vesical anchor to prevent migration, which was an issue in the early experience with vascular CMSs [16, 17]. Moskovitz *et al.* inserted the Allium stent in 49 ureters in cases with history of malignant disease and no perioperative complications occurred. Over a mean follow up time of 21 (range 1–63) months, stent migration occurred in 14.2% and only one case of stent occlusion was observed [18]. Leonardo *et al.* treated 12 benign cases of ureteral obstruction with Allium and achieved patency in all cases during the follow-up period. The mean follow-up period was 10 months. No complications were encountered intra-operatively and during the follow-up period [21]. It should be noted that if a complication occurs during the follow-up of the patients, the Allium could be easily removed [18, 21].

The UVENTA stent has a PTFE membrane-covered metal mesh to avoid tissue in-growth and hence prevent obstruction. Moreover, the design of stent aims in preventing the migration of the stent [19]. Its length ranges between 6–12 cm with diameters of 7, 8, and 10 mm. Kim *et al.* used the UVENTA stent in 18 patients (20 ureters) with malignancy. During a mean follow-up of 7.3 (range 3–15) months, no obstruction of the stents occurred. In addition, hyperplastic reactions, migration or encrustation were not observed. Chung *et al.* published a series of 71 ureters managed by UVENTA for malignant obstruction. During a median follow-up of 308 (range 35–802) days, the overall success rate was 81.7%. The reasons of failure varied and included tumor progression beyond the stent segment, reactive hyperplasia, bladder invasion, and stent related pain [22]. A comparative study evaluated the efficacy of the UVENTA and the thermoexpandable metal alloy spiral stent (Memokath 051, PNN, Copenhagen, Denmark) and showed higher clinical success rate of UVENTA over the Memokath 051 in benign and malignant ureteral obstructions. The complication rates were similar for both stents [23]. A multicenter study compared the efficacy of UVENTA with double-J stent insertion for the management of 42 malignant ureteral obstructions. The study showed that the UVENTA was superior to the double-J stents in terms of technical success and patency [24]. A summary of the experience with CMSs is presented in Table 12.1.

12.6 Conclusions

The concept for the use of DES and CMSs in the urinary tract aimed in the reduction of luminal restenosis related to the tissue hyperplasia of the ureteral wall. Current experience with DES in the ureter is limited to experimental in vivo studies evaluating vascular DESs. Further investigations are deemed necessary in order to draw safe conclusions regarding their efficacy, safety and potential clinical use. The initial clinical experience of vascular CMSs in the urinary tract was unfavorable and the recently introduced specially designed for the urinary tract CMSs showed promising results. Large prospective trials with long follow-up periods are deemed necessary for the establishment of CMSs in the urological practice.

References

[1] Kukreja N, Onuma Y, Daemen J, Serruys PW. The future of drug-eluting stents. Pharmacological research: the official journal of the Italian Pharmacological Society 2008;57(3):171–180.

[2] Macdonald S. Carotid artery stenting trials: conduct, results, critique, and current recommendations. Cardiovascular and Interventional Radiology 2012;35(1):15–29.

[3] Khan W, Farah S, Domb AJ. Drug eluting stents: developments and current status. Journal of controlled release: official journal of the Controlled Release Society 2012;161(2):703–712.

[4] Liatsikos E, Kallidonis P, Stolzenburg J-U, Karnabatidis D. Ureteral stents: past, present and future. Expert review of medical devices 2009;6(3):313–324.

[5] Oosterlinck W. Treatment of bulbar urethral strictures a review, with personal critical remarks. The Scientific World Journal 2003;3:443–454.

[6] Kallidonis PS, Georgiopoulos IS, Kyriazis ID, Al-Aown AM, Liatsikos EN. Drug-eluting metallic stents in urology. Indian journal of urology: IJU: journal of the Urological Society of India 2014;30(1):8–12.

[7] Liatsikos EN, Karnabatidis D, Katsanos K, Kallidonis P, Katsakiori P, Kagadis GC, et al. Ureteral metal stents: 10-year experience with malignant ureteral obstruction treatment. The Journal of Urology 2009;182(6):2613–2617.

[8] Agrawal S, Brown CT, Bellamy EA, Kulkarni R. The thermo-expandable metallic ureteric stent: an 11-year follow-up. BJU International 2009;103(3):372–376.

[9] Chung HH, Lee SH, Cho SB, Park HS, Kim YS, Kang BC, et al. Comparison of a new polytetrafluoroethylene-covered metallic stent to a noncovered stent in canine ureters. Cardiovascular and Interventional Radiology 2008;31(3):619–628. PubMed PMID: 18214599. Epub 2008/01/25. eng.

[10] Alahmar AE, Grayson AD, Andron M, Egred M, Roberts ED, Patel B, et al. Reduction in mortality and target-lesion revascularisation at 2 years: a comparison between drug-eluting stents and conventional bare-metal stents in the "real world". International journal of cardiology 2009;132(3):398–404.

[11] McGinty S, McKee S, Wadsworth RM, McCormick C. Modelling drug-eluting stents. Mathematical medicine and biology: a journal of the IMA 2011;28(1):1–29.

[12] Liourdi D, Kallidonis P, Kyriazis I, Tsamandas A, Karnabatidis D, Kitrou P, et al. Evaluation of the distribution of Paclitaxel by immunohistochemistry and nuclear magnetic resonance spectroscopy after the application of a drug-eluting balloon in the porcine ureter. J Endourol 2015;29(5):580–589. PubMed PMID: 25441059. Epub 2014/12/03. eng.

[13] Liatsikos EN, Karnabatidis D, Kagadis GC, Rokkas K, Constantinides C, Christeas N, et al. Application of paclitaxel-eluting metal mesh stents within the pig ureter: an experimental study. Eur Urol 2007;51(1):217–223. PubMed PMID: 16814926. Epub 2006/07/04. eng.

[14] Kallidonis P, Kitrou P, Karnabatidis D, Kyriazis I, Kalogeropoulou C, Tsamandas A, et al. Evaluation of zotarolimus-eluting metal stent in animal ureters. Journal of endourology/Endourological Society 2011;25(10):1661–1667.

[15] Liatsikos EN, Siablis D, Kalogeropoulou C, Karnabatidis D, Triado[poulos A, Varaki L, et al. Coated v noncoated ureteral metal stents: an experimental model. J Endourol. 2001;15(7):747–751. PubMed PMID: 11697409. Epub 2001/11/08. eng.

[16] Barbalias GA, Liatsikos EN, Kalogeropoulou C, Karnabatidis D, Zabakis P, Athanasopoulos A, *et al*. Externally coated ureteral metallic stents: an unfavorable clinical experience. Eur Urol 2002;42(3):276–280. PubMed PMID: 12234513. Epub 2002/09/18. eng.

[17] Liatsikos EN, Kagadis GC, Barbalias GA, Siablis D. Ureteral metal stents: a tale or a tool? J Endourol 2005;19(8):934–939. PubMed PMID: 16253054. Epub 2005/10/29. eng.

[18] Moskovitz B, Halachmi S, Nativ O. A new self-expanding, large-caliber ureteral stent: results of a multicenter experience. J Endourol 2012;26(11):1523–1527. PubMed PMID: 22697886. Epub 2012/06/16. eng.

[19] Kim JH, Song K, Jo MK, Park JW. Palliative care of malignant ureteral obstruction with polytetrafluoroethylene membrane-covered self-expandable metallic stents: initial experience. Korean journal of urology 2012;53(9):625–631. PubMed PMID: 23061000. Pubmed Central PMCID: PMC3460005. Epub 2012/10/13. eng.

[20] Kulkarni R. Metallic stents in the management of ureteric strictures. Indian J Urol 2014;30(1):65–72. PubMed PMID: 24497686. Pubmed Central PMCID: PMC3897057. Epub 2014/02/06. eng.

[21] Leonardo C, Salvitti M, Franco G, De Nunzio C, Tuderti G, Misuraca L, *et al*. Allium stent for treatment of ureteral stenosis. Minerva urologica e nefrologica = The Italian journal of urology and nephrology. 2013;65(4):277–283. PubMed PMID: 24091480. Epub 2013/10/05. eng.

[22] Chung KJ, Park BH, Park B, Lee JH, Kim WJ, Baek M, *et al*. Efficacy and safety of a novel, double-layered, coated, self-expandable metallic mesh stent (Uventa) in malignant ureteral obstructions. J Endourol 2013;27(7):930–935. PubMed PMID: 23590584. Epub 2013/04/18. eng.

[23] Kim KS, Choi S, Choi YS, Bae WJ, Hong SH, Lee JY, *et al*. Comparison of efficacy and safety between a segmental thermo-expandable metal alloy spiral stent (Memokath 051) and a self-expandable covered metallic stent (UVENTA) in the management of ureteral obstructions. Journal of laparoendoscopic & advanced surgical techniques Part A 2014;24(8):550–555. PubMed PMID: 24918272. Epub 2014/06/12. eng.

[24] Chung HH, Kim MD, Won JY, Won JH, Cho SB, Seo TS, *et al*. Multicenter experience of the newly designed covered metallic ureteral stent for malignant ureteral occlusion: comparison with double J stent insertion. Cardiovasc Intervent Radiol 2014;37(2):463–470. PubMed PMID: 23925919. Epub 2013/08/09. eng.

13

Ureteric Stents: A Perspective from the Developing World

Ravindra Sabnis

Professor of Urology, Department of Urology, Muljibhai Patel Urological Hospital, Nadiad, Gujarat, India

13.1 Introduction

Ureteric stents were developed in late 1960s [1] but routine use of these devices by medical professionals began a few decades later. JJ stents became available in India by the mid-1980s and were adopted by all urologists during the mid-1990s. Five Indian companies manufacture JJ stents at present and about 20 distributors make these available in all parts of the country.

JJ stents have become an integral part of an urologist's armamentarium and are indispensible, although they come at a price of morbidity and other related complications.

The patterns of use of JJ stents in India are distinct and are a little different from the Western world. There is a great variability in the healthcare provisions in different parts of India and other developing countries. Some regions offer only the very basic facilities. Therefore, the indications for the use of JJ stents, patient follow-up, compliance, and complications differ.

This chapter outlines the indications, technicalities, problems, and complications that are unique to India.

13.2 Pattern of JJ Stent Usage in India

13.2.1 Common Indication of Usage

Percutaneous nephrolithotomy, uretroscopy, and retrograde intra-renal surgery are widely practiced all over India. Placement of a JJ stent after these procedures is the main indication.

Obstructive uropathy due to impacted calculi is a common presentation. A solitary kidney or bilateral ureteric stones often complicate it. JJ stent insertion to relieve obstruction is common method to de-obstruct the system.

Many ureters need to be dilated before an ureteroscopy or retrograde intra-renal surgery. The placement of a JJ stent is necessary after these procedures. The stents are usually left in for a few weeks.

Failure of dilatation of ureter is not uncommon. A JJ stent is often left in to allow passive dilatation before a definitive procedure. Open surgery for stones is still practiced in some areas where endo-urological facilities are not available. JJ stent insertion is a common practice after an open pyelo or uretero-lithotomy.

Ureteric injuries are not uncommon during open urological, gynecological, and laparoscopic surgery undertaken for other reasons. The use of JJ stents during the repair of such injuries is commonplace. Uretero-vaginal fistulae are primarily treated conservatively by JJ stent insertion.

Many centers have a protocol of JJ stent insertion after transplant surgery; however, some centers do not advocate its routine use.

Reconstructive laparoscopic and robotic reconstructive surgery is on a rise in India. Following reconstructive procedures, such as ureteric re-implantation, pyeloplasty, and uretero-ureterostomy, the placement of a JJ stent is routine.

The availability of small diameter stents in India has led to a rise in their use in pediatric urological surgery.

The use of JJ stents in less well-defined indications such as stone related pyo-nephrosis is higher in India. Insertion of a JJ stent is considered an "easy" option compared to the use of a nephrostomy, due to a lack of expertise and facilities.

13.2.2   Stent Placement

Several methods of placement of JJ stent are practiced. The most standard method is under fluoroscopy and endoscopy control. However, ureteroscopy is performed without fluoroscopy control in many centers. The insertion of JJ stent is also undertaken without a radiological control. The outcomes of such procedure are un-predictable. Inadvertent creation of a false passage and subsequent placement of a JJ stent outside the ureter or the pelvi-calyceal system has been reported [2, 3]. This complication is clearly preventable. A similar problem can occur during open procedures when ureteric injury necessitates the placement of a JJ stent. A lack of imaging facility may lead to incorrect placement of the JJ stent at either end.

The non-availability of the correct length or diameter stent can also lead to inadequate drainage and subsequent migration. It is not uncommon in India where general surgeons and gynecologists undertake this procedure when ureteric trauma is suspected. The lack of urological training leads to stent-related complications [4].

The stents are placed in retrograde as well as an antegrade manner when retrograde placement is not possible. In a series of 30 patients with secondary malignant involvement of ureter only 50% of the ureters could be stented by a retrograde route [5].

There is a great variation in the type of anesthesia for ureteric stenting. The procedure may be performed in local anesthesia with or without sedation, regional, or general anesthesia [3, 5].

13.3   Stent Types and Economics

Globalization and opening of economic boundaries has led to the availability of all varieties of stents in India. However, stents manufactured by multi-nationals, for example, Cook, Boston Scientific, and Bard are expensive compared to those made in India. Five indigenous companies manufacture stents locally. Typically, 90–95% stents used in

India are locally produced. This practice is driven by the difference in the cost: $2 to $8 for an indigenous as compared to $18 to $25 for the imported version. Commonly available stents in India are made from polyurethane as they are cheap and suitable for short-term use [4].

In the vast majority of patients, ureteric stents are left in situ for a short duration (6 weeks) [4]. Recurrent benign strictures and malignant ureteric obstruction require long-term stenting. The use of metallic or segmental stents is rare in the Indian sub-continent due to the prohibitive cost of such devices. Encrustation of stents is a common problem in India due to the lithogenic urine and a high incidence of concomitant uro-lithiasis [4].

Locally manufactured stents vary in size from 3FG to 8FG in diameter and lengths vary from 8 cm to 32 cm.

13.4 Stent Tracking and Removal

Most urologists instruct patients on discharge with a date for stent removal and expect them to turn up on that day. In most centers, stents are removed under local anesthesia, using rigid cystoscopes in both sexes. This is due to sparse availability of flexible cystoscopes. Use of stent with threads and patients removing stent themselves is rarely practiced in India.

13.5 Stent Register

A formal stent register to enable patient tracking is infrequent. A designated person gives a reminder to the patient, around their due date of JJ stent removal. Lack of communication is a major difficulty in contacting patients. Although many patients do understand that they have a JJ stent in situ, but a significant proportion fail to show up [6]. With increasing availability of mobile phones, this problem is reduced to a great extent. Many centers have policy of not charging patients for stent removal, as poor compliance is often cost related.

Indigenously developed computer-based stent register has been developed by the Christian Medical College hospital, Vellore, in Southern India. This program is connected to the hospital medical information system and reminds both, the urologist as well as the patients of the impending stent removal or change [7].

13.6 Forgotten JJ Stents (Figures 13.1–13.3)

A "forgotten" JJ stent is still major problem in India. This is due to the lack of stent tracking systems, lower literacy levels and improper communication on the part of treating clinician [6]. In a resent series from India of 33 patients with retained JJ stents, less than 50% were aware that they had a stent in situ [6]. Around 50% of the patients were not counseled about the stent and 30% had not attended high school [6]. The mean age of presentation in a series was 25 ± 1.06 years and majority of patients presented with UTI, pain, and hematuria [6].

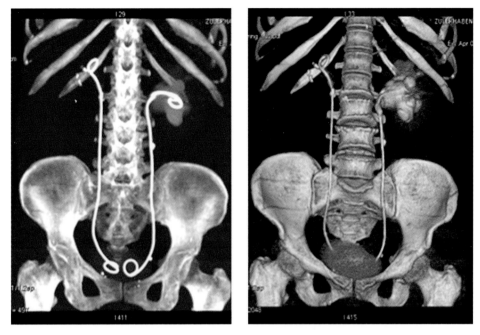

Figure 13.1 Fifty-three-year-old gentlemen admitted with retained stent inserted for obstructive uropathy three years ago.

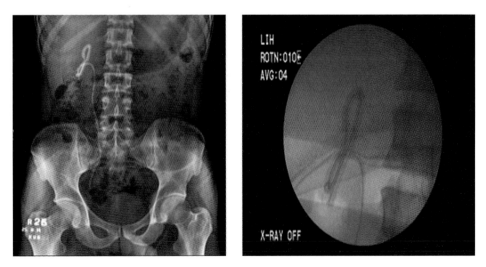

Figure 13.2 Retained stent for 10 years post open surgery for stone disease.

In a case series presented by Murthy *et al.* out of the 14 patients with retained stents, 7 patients had undergone open surgery, and 6 had a pyelolithotomy [8]. All the stents had been placed at different centers. This study suggests that a large number of stents are inserted by non-urologists, often after open surgical procedures and are forgotten due to the lack of knowledge on the part of the surgeon and the complications caused by retained stents [8].

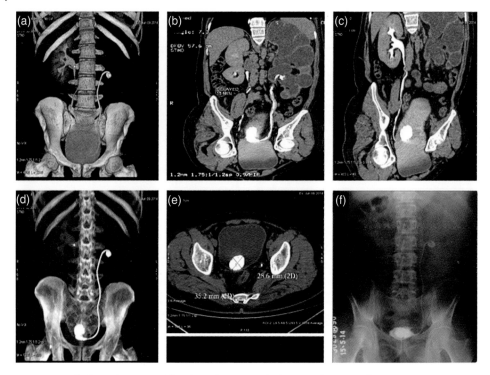

Figure 13.3a-f Thirty-four-year-old male with no comorbidities underwent left PCNL with DJ stenting 14 years ago, but DJ stent was not removed. SPCL with left PCN followed by laparoscopic left simple nephrectomy.

13.7 Why the Forgotten Stent is a Major Problem in India?

Uro-lithiasis is endemic in many parts of India [9]. A large number of endourological procedures, and therefore, JJ stent insertions are performed for stone-related problems. The risk of encrustation is high in patients with a history of uro-lithiasis [10]. Such patients are three times more likely to develop encrustation [10].

The combination of lithogenic urine, the delay in stent removal due to economical reasons in patients who have polyurethane stents, which have a higher propensity for encrustation makes this issue unique in India.

13.8 Trends in Management of Forgotten Stent

There is a significant variation in the trends of management across the country. Singh *et al.* proposed a sandwich therapy, which includes extracorporeal shockwave therapy with cystoscopy-guided traction, followed by endourological management [11]. The same group described an encrustation burden >400 mm^2 as significant and requiring intervention [11].

The use of endourological methods for the removal of encrusted stents is rising in India. Ureteroscopy was necessary in patients in 9 out of 14 in a series published [8]. Ureteroscopy was used in 45% patients in a series of retained stents [3]. Six out of fourteen patients required cystolithotripsy in a study [8]. Five out of 14 patients required PCNL in the same series. In general, about 30% patients with retained stent required a PCNL [6].

The use of extracorporeal lithotripsy in the management of encrusted stents has been low in India [6, 8]. The lack of availability has been the prime reason. However, the use of this modality is declining even in the centers, which have a lithotripter. Fifty-seven and a half percent of patients were offered lithotripsy in management of retained stents at centers with availability of SWL facility, whereas open surgery is used in 5–7% cases [6, 8, 11].

A forgotten stent can lead to complications, which in some instances may be life threatening. Severe urosepsis and renal failure or loss of the renal unit has been reported (Figures 13.4–13.8). In a study published from India 2 out of the 14 patients

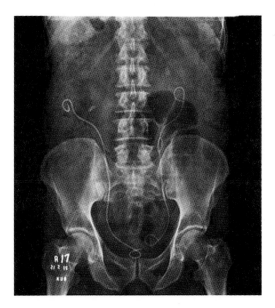

Figure 13.4 Extra anatomic placement of JJ stent.

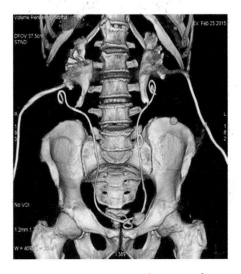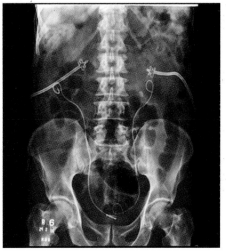

Figure 13.5 Extra anatomic placement of JJ stent with bilateral nephrostomy.

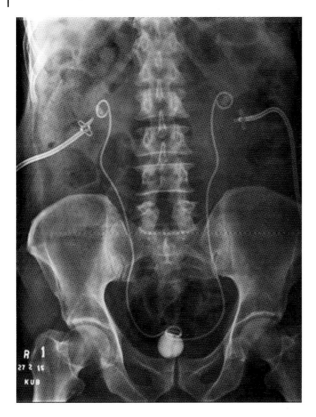

Figure 13.6 Repositioned stents after stone removal.

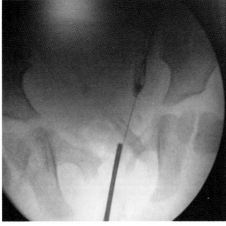
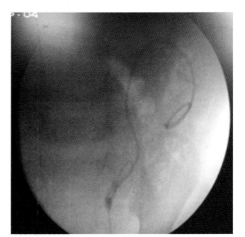

Figure 13.7 Migrated stent with entangled wire.

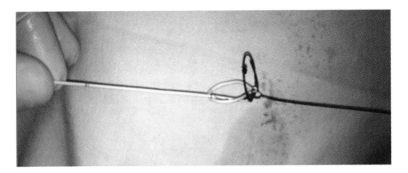

Figure 13.8 Stent knotted with wire.

developed severe complications. One patient with solitary functioning kidney developed renal failure and the second developed pyonephrosis and died due to sepsis [12].

13.9 JJ Stents Outside the Ureter and Pelvicalyceal System

Due to the non-availability of fluoroscopy, "blind" stent insertions are performed in many institutions. This often leads to misplaced stents, which may lie outside the ureter or the pelvi-calyceal system [13].

A case of an incorrect placement of a stent inserted accidentally in the common iliac vein, inferior vena cava, and finally into the right atrium has been reported. The stent was removed by an open surgical approach [2]. A 43-year-old female presented with acute recurrent colic due to lower ureteric stone. She was taken up for stone removal. Procedure was done without fluoroscopy. Guidewire went in with difficulty. Ureter could not be dilated, and hence, ureteroscopy was abandoned and only JJ stenting was done. In spite of stenting, she had persistent colic. When further evaluated, it was found that the stent had perforated the ureter and gone into the iliac vein. The upper end was lying in the atrium and the lower end in the exterior iliac vein. She was referred to our center for further management. Ureterorenoscopy with stone removal was done and JJ stent was placed. A stent in vascular system was removed by open surgery by opening the external iliac vein [2].

The above case report highlights the importance of using fluoroscopy with cystoscopy for JJ stent placement.

Extra anatomical placement of a JJ stent is relatively rare, but can have serious complications such as urosepsis and obstructive uropathy. This may lead to the development of a retroperitoneal urinoma or an abscess [7]. Patients with extrinsic compression caused by pelvic malignancies, radiation or retroperitoneal fibrosis are more prone to extra anatomic stent migration [12]. A large case series with 165 antegrade stenting patients reported anatomic stent migration in 5 patients (3%). The patients in this series presented with delayed complication such as urinoma, retroperitoneal abscess, ureterorectal fistula and ureterovaginal fistula [13].

13.10 Tips and Tricks for the Management of Migrated and Misplaced Stents

The lack of fluoroscopy control during stent insertion is the leading cause of mal-positioning or migration of ureteric stents (Figure 13.9). The risk factors associated with extra-anatomic misplacement of a JJ stent are pelvic malignancy, previous ureteric surgery, pelvic radiotherapy, or major pelvic surgery [9].

The use of a semi-rigid or flexible ureteroscope is the most effective method of retrival or re-positioning of such misplaced stents. Antegrade removal may be necessary if the ureteroscope fails to reach the lower end of the stent.

13.11 Recommended Protocol for the Repositioning of Incorrectly Placed Stents

Imaging and initial drainage: A CT scan is the preferred method of imaging to get the most accurate information (Figure 13.9). Insertion of a percutaneous nephrostomy is advantageous, especially if the system is dilated (Figure 13.10).

A hydrophilic guide wire is inserted in the ureter. This is likely to succeed as the misplaced stent will block the ureteric perforation.

Removal of the stent followed by a retrograde study is recommended if the above procedure fails. The contract should be injected nearer the expected site of perforation of the ureter. A duel-lumen ureteric catheter is very useful as one channel can be used for contrast while the other can accommodate a suitable guide wire.

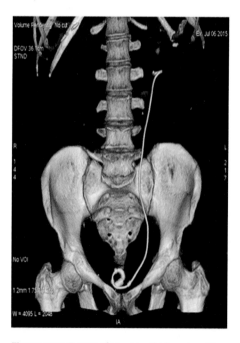

Figure 13.9 Twenty-five-year-old female with retained stent.

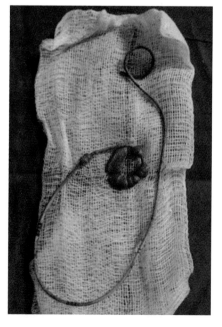

Figure 13.10 Retained encrusted stent in a 25-year-old female.

The use of a semi-rigid ureteroscope is often useful to help negotiate a guidewire past the traumatized segment of the ureter.

The use of the nephrostomy tube for the placement of a guidewire from above may prove useful if retrograde manipulations fail. The combination of retro and antegrade access and judicious use of methylene blue may help to locate ureteric lumen and a guide wire can then be passed. Once patient is stabilized, a procedure for stone extraction can be done in an antegrade or retrograde manner as per the merit of the case (Figure 13.11).

In the event of failure of all the above maneuvers, an open corrective procedure may be necessary (Figures 13.12 and 13.13).

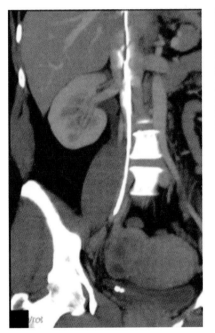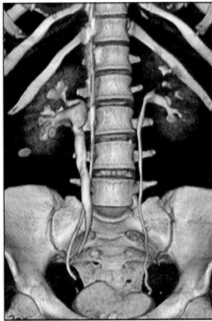

Figure 13.11 Stent placed into external iliac vein, IVC and right atrium.

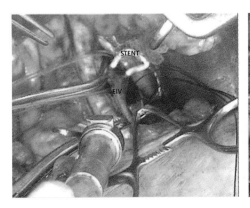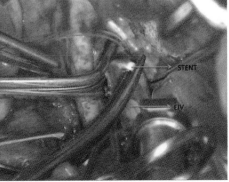

Figure 13.12 Stent placed into external iliac vein, IVC and right atrium, intraoperative picture.

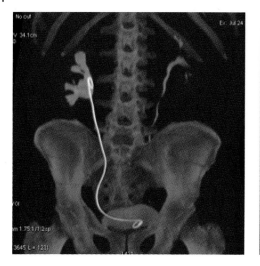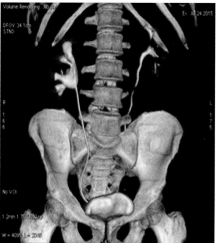

Figure 13.13 Heavy encrustation on a forgotten stent.

References

[1] Zimskind PD, Fetter TR, Wilkerson JL. Clinical use of long-term indwelling silicone rubber ureteral splints inserted cystoscopically. J Urol. 1967;97(5):840–844.

[2] Sabnis RB, Ganpule AP, Ganpule SA. Migration of double J stent into the inferior vena cava and the right atrium. Indian Journal of Urology: IJU: Journal of the Urological Society of India. 2013;29(4):353–354.

[3] Adamo R, Saad W, Brown D. Management of Nephrostomy Drains and Ureteral Stents. Tech Vasc Interv Radiol. 2009;12:193–204.

[4] Singh I. Indwelling JJ ureteral stents-A current perspective and review of literature. Indian J Surg 2003;65:405–412.

[5] Uthappa MC, Cowan NC. Retrograde or antegrade double-pigtail stent placement for malignant ureteric obstruction? Clin Radiol 2005;60:608–612.

[6] Patil SM, Magdum PV, Shete JS, Nerli RB, Hiremath MB. Forgotten dj stent—a source of morbidity: is stent registry a need of the hour? International Journal of Recent Scientific Research 2015;6(2):2674–2676.

[7] Sabharwal S, Macaden AR, Abrol N, Mukha RP, Kekre NS. A novel computer based stent registry to prevent retained stents: Will patient directed automated short message service and letter generator help? Indian J Urol. 2014;30(2):150–152.

[8] Kusuma M, Reddy VR, Jayaram S, Prasad DV. Endourological Management of Forgotten Encrusted Ureteral Stents. Int. braz j urol. [Internet]. 2010 [cited 2015 July 26];36(4):420–429.

[9] Singh PP, Barjatiya MK, Dhing S, Bhatnagar R, Kothari S, Dhar V. Evidence suggesting that high intake of fluoride provokes nephrolithiasis in tribal populations. Urological Research 2001;29(4):238–244.

[10] Vanderbrink BA, Rastinehad AR, Ost MC, Smith AD. Encrusted urinary stents: evaluation and endourologic management. J Endourol 2008;22(5):905–912.

[11] Singh I, Gupta NP, Hemal AK, Aron M, Seth A, Dogra PN. Severely encrusted polyurethane ureteral stents: management and analysis of potential risk factors. Urology 2001;58(4):526–531.

[12] Singh I. Indwelling JJ ureteral stents: A current perspective and review of literature. Indian J Surg 2003;65:405–412.

[13] Rao AR, Alleemudder A, Mukerji G, Mishra V, Motiwala H, Charig M, Karim OM. Extra-anatomical complications of antegrade double-J insertion. Indian J Urol. 2011;27(1):19–24.

14

Ethical Issues in Ureteric Stenting

Ravi Kulkarni

Consultant Urological Surgeon, Ashford and St Peter's Hospitals NHS Foundation Trust, Chertsey, Surrey, UK

Inserting a stent in the ureter is a common procedure performed frequently by urologists all over the world. Relieving upper tract obstruction with an uncomplicated device with anticipated improvement in symptoms and renal function is an appealing concept.

A JJ stent is inserted in the ureter for a variety of reasons. This has been addressed in another section of this book. Benign conditions causing ureteric obstruction, such as edema, after instrumentation, require short-term stenting. Recurrent benign strictures require corrective surgery to resolve the underlying pathology for a satisfactory long-term outcome. However, this may not be feasible in a cohort of patients due to severe comorbidity, anatomical difficulties, recurrence after such procedures, or patient choice. These patients are rendered stent dependent if definitive corrective surgery is not feasible. Morbidity of stenting in this group of patients can be significant and the impact on the quality of their life cannot be under-estimated.

Upper tract obstruction caused by a malignant process leading to renal impairment is a frequent event especially in pelvic malignancies of gynecological, colorecal or urological primaries. It can be caused by the compression of the ureter by the primary tumor or lymph nodal metastases. A direct invasion of the ureteric orifices will also lead to obstruction in malignancies of the prostate, bladder, cervix, or rectum.

Left untreated, this will invariably result in patient's demise due to progressive renal failure. Apart from the life-prolonging benefits of JJ stent insertion, it may open the door for possible adjuvant treatments for the underlying primary malignancy after the renal function improves.

However, the decision to relieve malignant ureteric obstruction is seldom easy. This chapter addresses some of the ethical dilemmas faced by the team that gets involved in the care of patients with malignant ureteric obstruction. The circumstances are not dissimilar in some patients with recurrent benign obstruction, especially if they have significant comorbidity.

14.1   Clinical Presentation

Hospitalization due to renal failure caused by malignancy often occurs into a medical facility nearer to the patient's home. This may not necessarily be the main site of patient's oncological care [1]. The medical (or surgical) team involved in the emergency care of the patient may not have access to the full details of the underlying condition or the treatment nor its success or failure. There often is a lack of information about the definitive long-term plans already in place in the management of such patients.

This invariably leads to an emergency decompression of the obstructed renal unit (often bilateral) in the form of nephrostomy tube insertion or JJ stenting.

The benefits from such intervention need careful consideration as the desire to prolong life as well as the perception of an improvement in the quality of life varies from patient to patient. The purported improvement may not necessarily materialize [2] and can lead to disappointment. For instance, a failure of ureteric stents to decompress upper tracts is not uncommon [9]. This may lead to the insertion of nephrostomy tubes. The patient may find the morbidity associated with JJ stents or the nephrostomy tube unacceptable.

The ethics behind the decision to decompress the obstructed upper urinary tract needs to be questioned and debated. Prolongation of life may not be the patient's desired option. The patient may not be able to communicate his or her desire due to the drowsiness caused by uremia. Failed oncological treatments might have led to a decision of "not to treat" with further intervention. This information is often not available to the team managing the emergency situation [1] and may lead to an unwelcome prolongation of the agony of the patient as well as the family.

End-of-life care for advanced malignant disease has been debated for decades. Consideration needs to be given to several factors before embarking on ureteric stenting.

14.2   Salvage Therapy Options

Recurrent malignant tumours that have become refractory to treatment, often present with ureteric obstruction. This could be the terminal event in this group of patients. A frank discussion with the patient and the family is essential before relief of obstruction is considered. This is pertinent in the cohort of patients in whom no further salvage therapeutic options are envisaged.

However, in a sizable proportion of patients, ureteric obstruction may be the first presenting feature of an underlying malignancy. The improvement in renal function and optimising the associated complications can open the door for adjuvant therapies and improve survival [3]. The severity of renal failure may disguise the reversibility and a nihilistic pathway may be adopted in error.

Morbidity associated with the conventional options such as JJ stenting or nephrostomy tube insertion may put the patient off and refusal may result in patient demise. However, segmental stents have significant advantages over both these traditional methods of ureteric decompression and should be offered to the patient if palliation and limited prolongation of life is a considered appropriate.

14.3   Patient Desire

Patient's own desire can vary from "stopping any further intervention" to try "everything that is possible." The expression of this desire may not be evident to the treating medical team and can result in an inappropriate pathway undertaken due to sheer ignorance. The patient's and the family's perceptions change. The original decision might be reversed due to changes in family circumstances. The lack of involvement of the primary care team with is conversant with the patient and family circumstances can result in uncomfortable end points.

14.4   Patient Status, Family and Social Issues

Drowsy or semi-conscious patients cannot be relied upon to express their desire or give full details of their underlying pathology. Careful consideration should be given to the wishes of the patient prior to their deterioration. Legal aspects and family issues also need attention to avoid inappropriate action or inaction.

The patient and the family may express a desire to extend the life in extenuating circumstances. This should be respected. A nephrostomy tube or insertion of a JJ stent will prolong life, albeit for a limited period. However, the morbidity associated with either of these options can be considerable. Both, the patient and the family must be fully aware of these before embarking on intervention [4].

As an opposite point of view, demanding withholding all treatment also needs to be evaluated and respected. Complex family dynamics, inter-personal relationships, and pecuniary interests of the parties concerned need to be taken into account [5].

Any decision taken should be documented and if necessary, witnessed to avoid future legal implications.

14.5   Ethical Issues in Benign Ureteric Obstruction

Patients with severe comorbidity, extremes of age, and other intractable untreatable conditions may present with recurrent benign ureteric obstruction. Once again, renal failure can be a presenting feature in this complex group of patients.

Aggressive intervention is often initiated by the emergency team, as benign etiology is perceived as treatable. Quality of life at the time of presentation, anticipated improvement before and after intervention, patient's own desire, comorbidity, and the feasibility of corrective surgery should be assessed before a decision to intervene is taken.

14.6   Role of Palliative Care Teams

The vast majority of patients who present in the above clinical scenarios have a long history. They are managed by multiple teams, which often include palliative care physicians and nurses. The input of these teams is vital in the decision-making process. They often know the patient and the family background better than most emergency care teams.

14.7 A Multidisciplinary Approach

The decision to undertake any form of intervention in the form of stenting or nephrostomy prior to stenting should be taken by a multi-disciplinary team [6]. Senior members of each team must be involved to ensure a sensible and appropriate path is chosen. Not infrequently, these patients are admitted under a non-surgical speciality under emergency circumstances. A senior urologist must be the member of the multidisciplinary team, as the urology team will undertake the subsequent management. A full review of prognostic factors should be undertaken in the light of the clinical features, underlying pathology and patient circumstances to ensure selection of an appropriate pathway [7].

14.8 Other Considerations

Insertion of a JJ stent does not necessarily result in adequate decompression of upper tract obstruction. Such inadequate drainage may necessitate further interventions [8, 9].

Stent-related morbidity adds to the distress caused by the underlying pathology [10]. It is therefore important to offer adequate information and counsel the patient before embarking on intervention.

A nephrostomy tube insertion is more effective in relieving ureteric obstruction than a JJ stent. However, the morbidity related to a nephrostomy is significantly higher than that of a JJ stent. Pain, infections, accidental dislodgement resulting in loss of access, difficulties in re-insertion, and the sheer practical inconvenience of having a tube sticking out of one's loin (in many patients, both sides), can be unacceptable to many patients. However, once inserted, the patient may end up living with such tubes for the rest of their life.

A frank discussion with the patient and the family is essential before nephrostomy insertion is considered [11–14].

14.9 Summary

The decision to undertake upper urinary tract decompression with a JJ stent or a nephrostomy in patients with malignant ureteric obstruction and complex benign strictures needs careful consideration. Such intervention may be appropriate in the vast majority of patients and will lead to an improvement of the patient [15]. However, the same decision may turn out to be undesirable in a cohort of patients and may lead to prolongation of life without an improvement in the quality. Therefore, all decisions need to be carefully evaluated. An open and frank discussion with the patient and close family members is essential and management plans should be tailor-made [16–18]. There is a perception that palliative care, especially nearer the end of life, is becoming more aggressive [19]. Therefore, it is more imperative that all aspects of the patient care are fully evaluated before intervention is undertaken [20]. Patient's own involvement cannot be overstressed [21]. Those involved in the care of such patients are equally important [22].

Ureteric stents have made invaluable contribution to the management of ureteric obstruction regardless of the etiology. This knowledge should be combined with the wisdom of when and when not to use them.

References

[1] Gill TM, Gahbauer EA, Han L, Allore HG. The role of intervening hospital admissions on trajectories of disability in the last year of life: prospective cohort study of older people. BMJ 2015;350:h2361.

[2] Woodhouse CR. Supra-vesical urinary diversion and ureteric re-implantation for malignant disease. Clin Oncol (R Coll Radiol) 2010;22(9):727–732.

[3] Jones OM, John SK, Lawrance RJ, Fozard JB. Long-term survival is possible after stenting for malignant ureteric obstruction in colorectal cancer. Ann R Coll Surg Engl 2007;89(4):414–417.

[4] Lapitan MC, Buckley BS. Impact of palliative urinary diversion by percutaneous nephrostomy drainage and ureteral stenting among patients with advanced cervical cancer and obstructive uropathy: a prospective cohort. J Obstet Gynaecol Res 2011;37(8):1061–1070.

[5] Clint Parker J, Goldberg DS. A Legal and Ethical Analysis of the Effects of Triggering Conditions on Surrogate Decision-Making in End-of-Life Care in the US. HEC Forum 2015 Jun 18. [Epub ahead of print]

[6] Liberman D, McCormack M. Renal and urologic problems: management of ureteric obstruction. Curr Opin Support Palliat Care 2012;6(3):316–321.

[7] Cordeiro MD, Coelho RF, Chade DC, Pessoa RR, Chaib MS, Colombo-Júnior JR, Pontes-Júnior J, Guglielmetti GB, Srougi M. A prognostic model for survival after palliative urinary diversion for malignant ureteric obstruction: a prospective study of 208 patients. BJU Int 2014 Oct 18. doi: 10.1111/bju.12963. [Epub ahead of print]

[8] Allen DJ, Longhorn SE, Philp T, Smith RD, Choong S. Percutaneous urinary drainage and ureteric stenting in malignant disease. Clin Oncol (R Coll Radiol) 2010;22(9):733–739.

[9] Docimo SG, Dewolf WC. High failure rate of indwelling ureteral stents in patients with extrinsic obstruction: experience at 2 institutions. J Urol 1989; 142(2 Pt 1):277–279.

[10] Monsky WL, Molloy C, Jin B, Nolan T, Fernando D, Loh S, Li CS. Quality-of-life assessment after palliative interventions to manage malignant ureteral obstruction. Cardiovasc Intervent Radiol 2013;36(5):1355–1363.

[11] Muruganandham K, Kapoor R. Malignant ureteral obstruction: Whether decompression really improves patient outcomes and quality of life? Indian J Urol 2008;24(1):127–128.

[12] Wilson JR, Urwin GH, Stower MJ. The role of percutaneous nephrostomy in malignant ureteric obstruction. Ann R Coll Surg Engl. 2005;87(1):21–24.

[13] Friedlander JI, Duty BD, Okeke Z, Smith AD. Reviews in Endourology: Obstructive Uropathy from Locally Advanced and Metastatic Prostate Cancer: An Old Problem with New Therapies. J Endourol 2012;26(2):102–109.

[14] Kouba E, Wallen EM, Pruthi RS. Management of Ureteral Obstruction Due to Advanced Malignancy: Optimizing Therapeutic and Palliative Outcomes. The Journal of Urology, Volume 2008;180(2):444–450.

[15] Wu JN, Meyers FJ, Evans CP. Palliative care in urology. Surg Clin North Am 2011;91(2):429–444.

[16] Lee OT, Wu JN, Meyers FJ, Evans CP. Genito-urinary Aspects of Palliative Care. In: Oxford Textbook of Palliative Medicine, 5th Edition, pp 443–446, 2015.

[17] Chung SY, Stein RJ, Landsittel D, Davies BJ, Cuellar DC, Hrebinko RL, Tarin T, Averch TD. 15-year experience with the management of extrinsic ureteral obstruction with indwelling ureteral stents. J Urol 2004;172(2):592–595.

[18] Gasparini M, Carroll P, Stoller M. Palliative percutaneous and endoscopic urinary diversion for malignant ureteral obstruction. Urology. 1991;38(5):408–412.

[19] Earle CC, Neville BA, Landrum MB, Ayanian JZ, Block SD, Weeks JC. Trends in the aggressiveness of cancer care near the end of life. J Clin Oncol. 2004;22(2):315–321.

[20] Singer PA, Martin DK, Kelner M. Quality end-of-life care: patients' perspectives. JAMA. 1999;281(2):163–168.

[21] Wright AA, Mack JW, Kritek PA, Balboni TA, Massaro AF, Matulonis UA, Block SD, Prigerson HG. Influence of patients' preferences and treatment site on cancer patients' end-of-life care. Cancer. 2010;116(19):4656–4663.

[22] Steinhauser KE, Christakis NA, Clipp EC, McNeilly M, McIntyre L, Tulsky JA. Factors considered important at the end of life by patients, family, physicians, and other care providers. JAMA. 2000;284(19):2476–2482.

15

Equipment and Technical Considerations During Ureteric Stenting

Jonathan Cloutier[1] and Olivier Traxer[2]

[1] Consultant Urologist, Department of Urology, University Hospital Center of Quebec City, Saint-François d'Assise Hospital, Quebec City, Canada
[2] Professor of Urology, Department of Urology, Tenon University Hospital, Pierre & Marie Curie University, Paris, France

15.1 Introduction

A safe ureteral access is mandatory before an endourological procedure. This chapter gives an overview of the accessories that can be used and are helpful during a routine or more complicated ureteral stenting. Specific technical tips will be suggested in the chapter according to certain situations that could be encountered during vesico-ureteral manipulations.

15.2 Equipment

15.2.1 Cystoscope

Cystoscopy is the first step before gaining a ureteral access. A complete inspection of the bladder is mandatory to avoid missing a bladder tumor, bladder stone, or a complete ureteral duplication not diagnosed with the preoperative imaging.

Taking a look to the ureteral orifice could give information regarding the possibility of encountering difficulties during the insertion of the instruments or accessories into the ureter (Figure 15.1).

The guidewire placement can be done with a rigid or a flexible cystoscope. In a prospective randomized trial, Tepeler *et al.* have evaluated the feasibility of placing a ureteral catheter before percutaneous nephrolithotomy. They found that a flexible cystoscope shortens the preparation period and minimizes the discomfort of the operational staffs associated with the patient positioning and transfer [1].

However, if a flexible cystoscope is used for the placement of the guidewire in the treatment of a ureteral pathology, a decrease of straightening can be felt secondary to the flexibility of the scope compared to a rigid cystoscope. In this situation, it is advisable to leave in place the guidewire just below the point of ureteral resistance and deploy a ureteral or a dual-lumen catheter to assist the passage of the guidewire or for injecting contrast for a better evaluation of the ureteral anatomy. A more slippery guidewire could also be used to pass the obstruction. One advantage of the rigid cystoscope is to give

Ureteric Stenting, First Edition. Edited by Ravi Kulkarni.
© 2017 John Wiley & Sons Ltd. Published 2017 by John Wiley & Sons Ltd.

Figure 15.1 Ureteral orifice, which has a "tent," is more compliant.

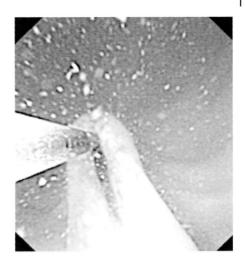

strength when a double-J ureteral stent has to go through an impacted stone or a stricture, which offer resistance to the passage of the stent. The rigid cystoscope will prevent the chance of forming an unwanted loop into the bladder or a loss of force in the urethra.

15.2.2 Fluoroscopy Guidance

As stated in the guidelines, fluoroscopy should be used during all endourological procedures. However, some groups have demonstrated the feasibility and safety without fluoroscopy or with its minimal use [2–4].

To further reduce radiation exposure with fluoroscopy during ureteral stenting and ureteroscopy, the concept of as-low-as-reasonably achievable (ALARA) should be kept in mind. However, this principle should not compromise the surgeon's need to use fluoroscopy while gaining ureteral access in complex situations. "Manipulation feeling" is an important aspect to endourology, and fluoroscopy time will decline with the increase of surgical expertise [5].

15.2.3 Guidewires

Guidewires are essential for ureteral access and stenting. Their use is helpful for placing a ureteral catheter, ureteral access sheath, or ureteroscope in a tortuous ureter. They are a vital tool during an endoscopic ureteral or renal surgery. The insertion of a double-J ureteral stent can be rapidly achieved if a working (safety) wire is in place during an unexpected event.

There are many types of guidewires. Most wires are 150 cm long and have a 0.035" or 0.038" (=1 mm) diameter. The optimal guidewire should have enough shaft rigidity ("stiff type") to allow the advancement of instruments, require minimal force to flex the tip in response to an obstruction or resistance along the ureter, and need a large force before causing tissue perforation – a feature that enhances safety. Currently, there are a variety of guidewires with a different combination of these features. The variations are 3 to 5 cm floppy tip, straight or curved tip, PTFE or hydrophilic-coated, hybrid, and stiff shaft.

Many investigators have evaluated these guidewires to determine the force required to perforate the ureter, the tip bending force, the amount of friction, and the force needed to achieve shaft deformation [6–9]. In most cases, the conclusions remain almost the same: each guidewire may have its usefulness depending on the situation. The ideal guidewire still does not exist, and no specific guidewire can be recommended. It is advisable to maintain a variety of guidewires in the armamentarium of the urologist. Consequently, expensive combination guidewires are not recommended when a simple, inexpensive PTFE-coated guidewire will suffice.

It should be borne in mind that the size of the guidewire is a useful tool to estimate the size of stone fragments. This helps to decide if they should be actively removed or if they are suitable for free passage and, therefore, can be left in place. The authors recommend using stiff hydrophilic wires, whose first 3 to 5 cm are completely floppy and less traumatic and the shaft is stiff (Figure 15.2). Standard floppy tip polytetrafluoroethylene (PTFE) can also be used, but the hydrophilic wire has shown its superiority over the standard PTFE in gaining access to renal cavities by passing ureteral stones [6,9]. However, the hydrophilic wire must be kept moist before its use and before the passage of accessories over it. The tip of guidewires can be straight, angled or "J" tip, and the surgeon has to use his experience to decide when to use an angled rather than a straight tip wire (Figure 15.3).

When two wires are used, and the flexible ureteroscope is placed over the working wire, it is recommended to use a hydrophilic wire or a two floppy tip wires to protect the working channel of the scope. Going up into the ureter directly over the wire facilitates

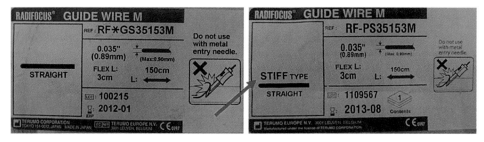

Figure 15.2 Hydrophilic straight soft and stiff guidewires.

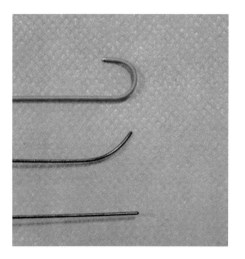

Figure 15.3 Different tips of guidewires.

the scope placement into pelvis and the calyces. The authors strongly recommend the use of a safety wire even though the literature suggests the feasibility of flexible ureteroscopy without a safety wire [10–13].

The safety wire could be a standard PTFE type, which is less expensive. However, with this guidewire, a polyurethane double-J ureteral stent needs to be placed. If the urologist chooses to insert a silicone JJ stent at the end of the procedure, a hydrophilic guidewire is needed as the friction with the PTFE wire is excessive and stent placement will prove difficult.

In the presence of severe uretero-hydronephrosis, the dilated ureter may develop a complete 360-degree loop. It is often difficult to realign the ureter with a standard guidewire despite the placement of a ureter catheter. To avoid the risk of perforation, we recommend the use of a complete hydrophilic guidewire with a "soft" shaft. It is often less traumatic and once in the renal pelvis, advancement of a ureteral catheter and changing of the guidewire to a stiffer variety is easier (Figure 15.4).

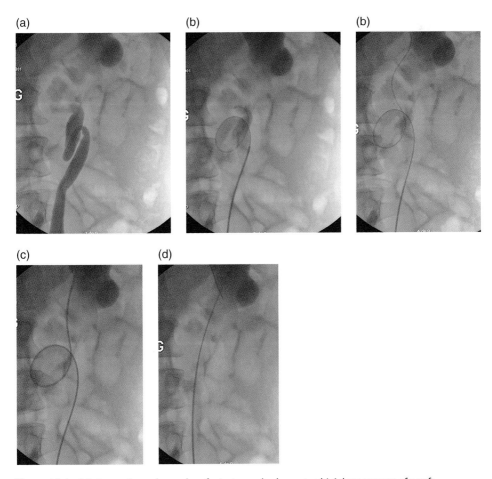

Figure 15.4 a) Retrograde pyelography of a tortuous hydroureter. b) Advancement of a soft hydrophilic guidewire toward the ureteral loop and up to the renal pelvis. c) Advancement of the ureteral catheter into the renal pelvis. d) Changing the soft guidewire for a stiffer one will facilitate the realignment of the tortuous ureter.

15.2.4 Ureteral Catheters

There are different types and sizes of ureteral catheters (Figure 15.5). If difficulties are encountered while placing the guidewire with the cystoscope, a 5 to 7 F open-end ureteral catheter can facilitate the insertion of a guidewire into the ureter. This catheter is made of polyurethane. Its usage is not obligatory, but it helps to perform a retrograde pyelogram to define the ureteral anatomy. Also, a selective urinary sample for cytology or culture can be obtained.

The deployment of a ureteral catheter is also useful if a soft hydrophilic guidewire is used to pass an impacted stone. At this point, the ureteral catheter (5 F) can be advanced proximal to the stone. This will allow the collection of a urine sample for culture in an obstructed kidney and to place a stiffer wire. The latter will facilitate the placement of a ureteral stent if necessary in patients with an impacted stone.

A ureteral catheter should also be employed when a false passage has been encountered during the ureteral orifice cannulation. In this situation, a whistle-tip ureteral catheter with an angled-tip guidewire can help to find the way into the distal ureter (Figure 15.6). With a false passage on the right ureter, the correct way into the lumen will be found by orienting the open end and the angle-tip guidewire at 11 o'clock at the ureteral orifice. On the left side, it should be orientated at 2 o'clock.

15.2.5 Coaxial Dilators

The 8/10 FG coaxial dilators allow a progressive dilation of the ureteral orifice with the 8 F stylet that is placed over a guidewire and followed by the 10 F sheath (Figure 15.7). Next, the 8 F stylet is removed, and placement of a second guidewire could be performed (Figure 15.8). However, this catheter does not allow injection of contrast with a guidewire in situ if an adapter is not used.

One of the advantages of this catheter is the 10 F sheath that can be placed up to the distal ureteral and facilitate the placement of a double-J ureteral stent by aligning the

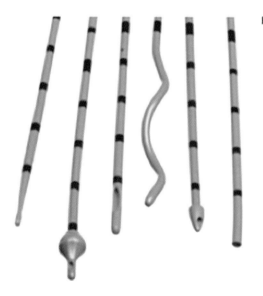

Figure 15.5 Different tips of ureteral catheter.

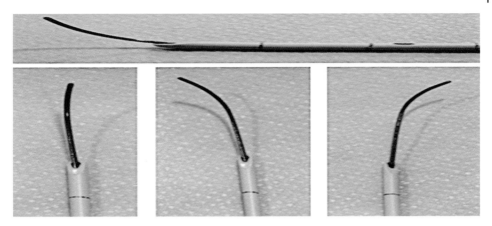

Figure 15.6 Advantage of using a whistle tip ureteral catheter with a curve tip guidewire, particularly to facilitate ureteral cannulation even with a distal ureter hooked.

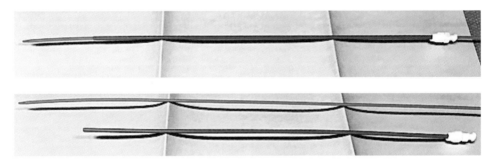

Figure 15.7 8/10 coaxial dilators.

(a)   (b)

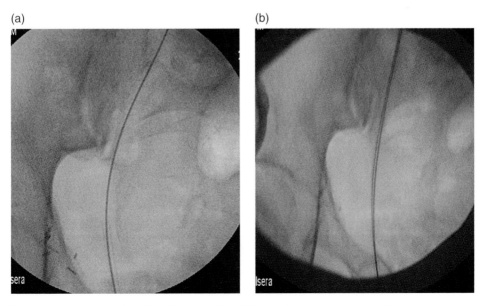

Figure 15.8 a) Low opacity of the distal tip of the 10 F stylet into the distal ureter. b) Placement of a second guidewire into the 10F stylet.

urethra up to the distal ureter. It avoids kinking into the urethra or bladder when resistance is encountered during the stent placement. When the double J is in place, the 10 F sheath is partially removed into the urethra while maintaining the pusher of the double J in the right position. When the 10 F sheath is in the urethra, the guidewire can be removed to confirm the appropriate position of the double J into the bladder.

15.2.6 Dual-Lumen Catheter

A dual-lumen catheter is not used during all surgical procedures, but it can be very useful to place a second guidewire, or while contrast injection is needed. The main advantage is to keep the safety guidewire in situ (Figure 15.9). With its progressive a-traumatic 6 F distal tip up to 10 F maximal proximal diameter, it can also dilate the ureter slightly, and make the access to the upper tract with the flexible ureteroscope easier. Guidewires of 0.038" diameter can be passed into each lumen of this catheter. The dual-lumen catheter is placed over a guidewire under fluoroscopic guidance.

The new ureteral access sheath by Rocamed has a variation with its two lumens that are accessible from the end of the ureteral access sheath. If the surgeon prefers to use a ureteral access sheath for specific cases, this sheath will avoid using a dual-lumen catheter if felt necessary (Figure 15.10).

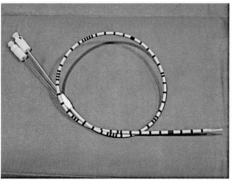 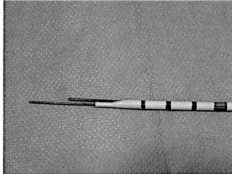

Figure 15.9 Dual-lumen catheter.

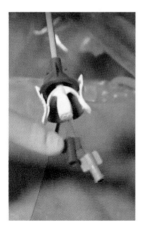 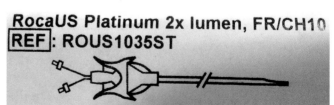

Figure 15.10 Rocamed ureteral access sheath with two distal lumens usable.

15.2.7 Contrast

Contrast is often needed when a difficult ureteral access is encountered. One will never regret the use contrast to define better the ureteral anatomy, tortuosity, perforation and intrarenal anatomy. If ureteroscopy is being performed for a suspected upper tract urothelial carcinoma, it is mandatory to collect urine sample for cytology before contrast is injected.

15.2.8 High-Pressure Catheters and Balloon Dilators

In the presence of a tight ureteral stricture, that prevents access to the upper urinary tract (even after an initial double-JJ stent placement for 5–7 days), a retrograde balloon ureteral dilation can be deployed (Figure 15.11) [14]. It should be inserted over the working guidewire and then inflated under fluoroscopic control up to 12–18 atmospheric pressure until reaching an adequate ureteral dilation to relieve stricture and to facilitate the placement of larger instruments. Balloon catheters of various length (4–10 cm) and inflated diameter (4–10 mm) are commercially available. Although these devices almost always allows getting access to the renal cavities, the possibility of a long-term success can vary according to the length and the nature of the strictures. For instances, ischemic stenosis is a poor prognostic factor for durable success [15]. However, we strongly recommend against the practice of primary dilatation the ureteral strictures. We suggest that a JJ stent should be placed as an initial step and to return one or two weeks later for a definitive ureteroscopy. An unexplained stenosis should always be subjected to a biopsy to rule out urothelial carcinoma.

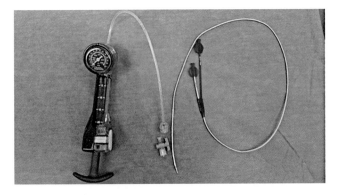

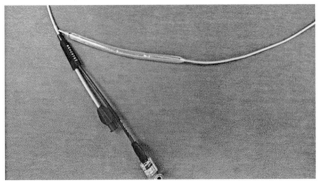

Figure 15.11 Ureteral balloon dilator.

15.2.9 "Hockey Stick" KMP or Imager II Catheters

The KMP catheter or Imager II is most of the time use during a percutaneous nephro-lithotomy to facilitate an antegrade placement of the guidewire into the ureter. However, a longer catheter (up to 100 cm) is also available for retrograde access. It can be useful particularly when a partial ureteral duplication is present, and difficulties are encountered to cannulate one of the ureters. This catheter allows performing retrograde pyelography to define the ureteral anatomy and can be followed by the placement of a guidewire into the correct ureter. It could admit placement of a stent, a dual-lumen catheter or to advance a flexible ureteroscope over the wire (Figure 15.12).

15.2.10 Ureteral Stent

The ureteral catheter or double-J stent (of different size, shape, and materials) may be placed at the end of the endoscopic procedure to guarantee the drainage of renal cavities and avoid post-operative complications. It is especially advisable after a long procedure, in the presence of residual fragments or ureteral lesion, and when a ureteral access sheath has been used for a prolonged period of time [16]. The conventional JJ stent is an autostatic catheter with a pig tail shaped curls present at both ends which hold the tube in place and prevent migration (Figure 15.13).

The authors recommend the removal of the JJ stent within 8–10 days, as prolonged placement of a JJ stent will hamper the passage of fragments. The use of stents on a string, to be removed by the patient at home has been recommended. Data suggest that there are no adverse events. It also reduces the need of consultation to the emergency room related to the stent [17–20].

In patients who have undergone an uncomplicated ureteroscopy with no residual fragments, stenting should be avoided as it is found to be associated with higher postoperative morbidity [21–23]. Routine stenting is not recommended before ureteroscopy, although it may facilitate ureteroscopic management of stones and improve the stone-free rate [24].

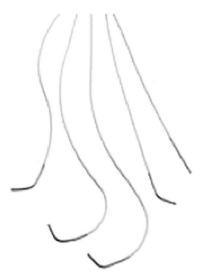

Figure 15.12 Different tips of KMP catheters. It could be helpful to place a guidewire into a ureter of a partial ureteral duplication or a transureteroureterostomy.

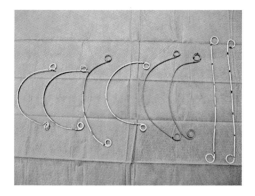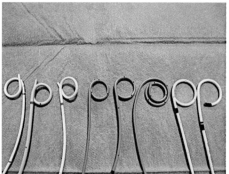

Figure 15.13 Different types of ureteral stents.

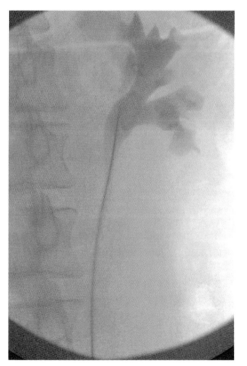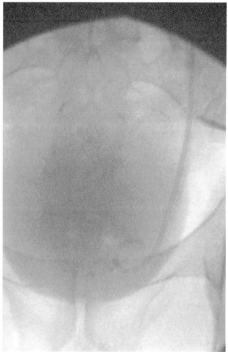

Figure 15.14 Ideal placement of a JJ ureteral stent. Proximal loop into the pelvis and distal loop not longer than the midline of the coccyx.

However, an initial double-J stent placement can be performed to obtain a progressive dilation of a naive ureter when the insertion of the ureteroscope is difficult, despite the uses of a narrow access sheath or a small flexible ureteroscope. For this purpose, stenting for a period of five days is adequate. A second attempt of ureteroscopy results in a high rate of success.

Some authors recommend the optimal position of the JJ stent into the renal pelvis and bladder to avoid morbidity related to the stent. Placing the proximal loop into the renal pelvis, and the distal loop not longer than the sacrum could decrease the urinary symptoms related to the stent (Figure 15.14) [25]. However, controversies remain [26].

One other questions related to the stent is the material used. Currently, most stents are made of polyurethane that is easily inserted over a PTFE guide-wire. However, as presented at the WCE in 2015, there is evidence to suggest that a silicone JJ stent could reduce stent-related symptoms [27]. One of the disadvantages of silicone stent is the friction when they are inserted over a PTFE guidewire. It is, however, very easy and safe to insert over a stiff hydrophilic guidewire. The questions of a higher stent cost should also be considered as in a vast majority of the patients, a double-J stent has a short indwelling time.

15.3 Tips and Tricks

When resistance is encountered during JJ placement, some tricks can facilitate its insertion.

1) The guidewire is held straight by the assistant.
2) Use the 8/10 F coaxial dilators. The 10 F will align the urethra with the distal ureter, and it will avoid any loss of strength into the urethra.
3) Insertion of the JJ stent with direct endoscopic vision into a rigid cystoscope. This tip will assure to have as much strength as you need directing into the ureter.
4) If the insertion is still not feasible, combined the above tricks with a smaller diameter JJ stent.
5) If stenting is still unsuccessful, leave the guidewire with the proximal tip into the renal cavities, re-attempt stenting after 24 or 48 hours later. It will create a passive dilation that would be enough to place the stent.

15.4 Conclusion

A large variety of ancillary equipment and accessories are available in the field of endourology. However, an adequate knowledge of all this equipment is essential to achieve success the ureteral access even in special situations as a partial ureteral duplication or a severe tortuous ureter. The urologist should always continue to keep be familiar with the new devices as well as the tip and tricks of different endourologist for specific situations.

References

[1] Tepeler A, Silay MS, Akman T, *et al.* Comparison of flexible and rigid cystoscopy-assisted ureteral catheter insertion before percutaneous nephrolithotomy: a prospective randomized trial. J Endourol 2013; 27(6):722–726.
[2] Türk C, Knoll T, Petrik A, *et al.* Guidelines on Urolithiasis 2015. Available at: Uroweb. org [accessed July 1, 2016].
[3] Hsi R, Harper J. Fluoroless ureteroscopy: Zero-dose fluoroscopy during ureteroscopic treatment of urinary-tract calculi. J Endourol 2013; 27(4):432–437.
[4] Deters L, Dagrosa L, Herrick B, *et al.* Ultrasound guided ureteroscopy for the definitive management of ureteral stones: A randomized controlled trial. J Urol 2014; 192(6);1710–1713.

[5] Sfoungaristos S, Lorber A, Gofrit ON, *et al*. Surgical experience gained during an endourology fellowship program may affect fluoroscopy time during ureterorenoscopy. Urolithiasis. 2015; 43(4):369–374.

[6] Clayman M, Uribe C, Eichel L, *et al*. Comparison of guide wires in urology. Which, when and why? J Urol 2004; 171:2146–2150.

[7] Sarkissian C, Korman E, Hendlin K, Monga M. Systematic evaluation of hybrid guidewires: shaft stiffness, lubricity, and tip configuration. Urology 2012; 79:513–517.

[8] Torricelli F, De S, Sarkissian Carl, Monga M. Hydrophilic guidewires: evaluation and comparison of their properties and safety. Urology 2013; 82:1882–1886.

[9] Liguori G, Antoniolli F, Trombetta C, *et al*. Comparative experimental evaluation of guidewire use in urology. Urology 2008; 72:286–290.

[10] Rizkala ER, Monga M. Controversies in ureteroscopy: Wire, basket, and sheath. Indian J Urol 2013; 29(3):244–248.

[11] Patel SR, McLaren ID, Nakada SY. The ureteroscope as a safety wire for ureteronephroscopy. J Endourol 2012; 26(4):351–354.

[12] Dickstein RJ, Kreshover JE, Babayan RK, Wang DS. Is safety wire necessary during routine flexible ureteroscopy? J Endourol 2010; 24(10):1589–1592.

[13] Ulvik O, Wentzel-Larsen T, Ulvik NM. A safety guidewire influences the pushing and pulling forces needed to move the ureteroscope in the ureter: a clinical randomized, crossover study. J Endourol 2013; 27(7):850–855.

[14] Holden T, Pedro RN, Hendlin K, *et al*. Evidence-based instrumentation for flexible ureteroscopy: A review. J Endourol 2008; 22:1423–1426.

[15] Schöndorf D, Meierhans-Ruf S, Kiss B, *et al*. Ureteroileal strictures after urinary diversion with an ileal segment-is there a place for endourological treatment at all? J Urol. 2013;190(2):585–590. doi: 10.1016/j.juro.2013.02.039. [Epub 2013 Feb]

[16] Rapoport D, Perks AE, Teichman JM. Ureteral access sheath use and stenting in ureteroscopy: effect on unplanned emergency room visits and cost. J Endourol 2007; 21(9):993–997.

[17] Kim DJ, Son JH, Jang SH, *et al*. Rethinking of ureteral stent removal using an extraction string: what patient feel and what is patients' preference? A randomized controlled study. BMC Urol 2015; 15(1):121.

[18] Barnes KT, Bing MT, Tracy CR. Do ureteric stent extraction strings affect stent-related quality of life or complications after ureteroscopy for urolithiasis: a prospective randomized control trial. BJU Int. 2014; 113(4):605–609.

[19] Bockhotl NA, Wild TT, Gupta A, Tracy CR. Ureteric stent placement with extraction string: no strings attached? BJU Int. 2012; 110:E1069–E1073.

[20] Loh-Doyle JC, Low RK, Monga M, Nguyen MM. Patient experiences and preferences with ureteral stent removal. J Endourol 2015; 29(1):35–40.

[21] Song T, Liao B, Zheng S, Wei Q. Meta-analysis of postoperatively stenting or not in patients underwent ureteroscopic lithotripsy. Urol Res. 2012 Feb; 40(1):67–77.

[22] Haleblian G, Kijvikai K, de la Rosette J, Preminger G. Ureteral stenting and urinary stone management: a systematic review. J Urol. 2008 Feb; 179(2):424–30.

[23] Nabi G, Cook J, N'Dow J, *et al*. Outcomes of stenting after uncomplicated ureteroscopy: systematic review and meta-analysis. BMJ. 2007; 334(7593):572.

[24] Rubenstein RA, Zhao LC, Loeb S, *et al*. Prestenting improves ureteroscopic stone-free rates. J Endourol 2007; 21(11):1277–1280.

[25] Lee SJ, Yoo C, Oh CY, *et al.* Stent position is more important than a-blockers or anticholinergics for stent-related lower urinary tract symptoms after ureteroscopic ureterolithotomy: a prospective randomized study. Korean J Urol 2010; 51(9):636–641.

[26] Abt D, Mordasini L, Warzinek E, *et al.* Is intravesical stent position a predictor of associated morbidity? Korean J Urol 2015; 56(5):370–378.

[27] Traxer O. Effects of silicone hydrocoated double loop ureteral stent on symptoms and quality of life in patients undergoing F-URS for kidney stone: a comparative randomized multicentre clinical study. WCE ePoster Library. Oct 4, 2015. Available at: http://wce.multilearning.com/wce/2015/eposters/112720/olivier.traxer.effects.of. silicone.hydrocoated.double.loop.ureteral.stent.on.html?f=p6m2e874o11128 [accessed July 1, 2016].

16

Extra-Anatomic Stent Urinary Bypass

Stuart Nigel Lloyd

Consultant Urological Surgeon, Hinchingbrooke Park, Huntingdon, UK

16.1   Introduction

This chapter describes the use of a method of bypassing ureteric obstruction or injury by a subcutaneous route using a specifically designed stent. This can be a temporary or permanent solution for patients with a nephrostomy.

Living life with one or two nephrostomy tube drains is something that none of us would wish for, but they are usually placed when no alternative option is available. Nephrostomy tubes are plagued by problems such as blockage, displacement, infection, the need for frequent attention to dressings, bags, and the need for regular replacement (Figure 16.1). For most patients, extra-anatomic stent drainage is an alternative (Figure 16.2a, b). Conversion of a nephrostomy to a subcutaneous urinary stent using the native bladder as the reservoir is a quick and simple procedure. The technique was first proposed by Ahmadzadeh in 1991 for malignant obstruction [1]. This technique was later popularised by Mr. Peter Paterson (urologist) and Dr. Patrick Forrester (radiologist) at Glasgow Royal Infirmary [2]. Since then, the author has performed over 300 such procedures for a variety of indications, providing the national referral centre for such cases [3, 4]. The technique has been modified and the applications extended to benign and malignant diseases for both short- and long-term use. This procedure dramatically enhances the quality of life rather than cures the condition. In cases of urinary fistula it has been used to enable the fistula to dry up and buy time for the patient to be better prepared for reconstructive surgery. A shorter, similar 8FG Flexima 24 cm Boston Scientific stent was used to bypass an ischemic stricture where ureteric re-implantation was not possible post renal transplant [5].

This technique is a procedure that in most situations the only alternative is long-term nephrostomy drainage. This stent is suitable for the majority of my cases despite some deficiencies with stent design. The fixed length and the tapered tip that reduces the internal diameter of the lumen are limitations. The long length in some means excess coil within the bladder and the tapered tip needs excising before delivery. There are no plans to modify the Paterson-Forrester stent. Initially, the stent was manufactured by Boston and subsequently by Cook initially in a kit. After a temporary withdrawal of production of the product, it is now produced on its own.

Ureteric Stenting, First Edition. Edited by Ravi Kulkarni.
© 2017 John Wiley & Sons Ltd. Published 2017 by John Wiley & Sons Ltd.

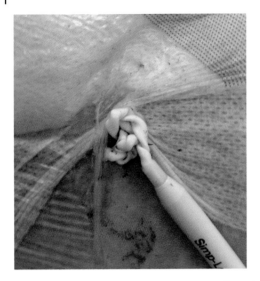

Figure 16.1 Complications of nephrostomy tubes – kinking.

(a)   (b)

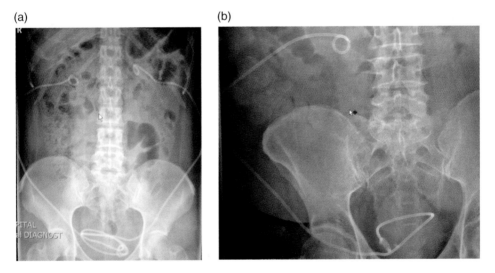

Figure 16.2 a) Bilateral subcutaneous extra-anatomic stent b) Unilateral subcutaneous stent.

16.2 Indications

The indications for this type of stent are best considered as temporary or permanent. This procedure does not preclude subsequent reconstruction and it can be used pending more definitive repair or treatment. The scale of surgery is minor and can be considered in almost any type of ureteric obstruction. The majority of patients have a permanent nephrostomy due to malignant obstruction. Most patients either have had a conventional JJ ureteric stent that repeatedly blocks or it may be that a stent could not be passed across the obstruction. Ureteric obstruction can be due to direct tumor invasion or extrinsic compression. Pelvic malignancies such as gynecological, large-bowel or prostate but also metastatic diseases such as breast cancer are usual causes. Benign conditions such as post-irradiation stricture or ureteric trauma secondary to vascular or bowel surgery are also suitable indications.

16.3   Contraindications

The only requirement is that the bladder functions sufficiently that the patient maintains continence and that there is no local tumor invasion directly into the bladder. Thus a bladder fistula, intravesical tumor and poorly compliant bladder are all contraindications. However, if the patient has an indwelling catheter along with nephrostomy drainage the diversion could still be considered.

The technique of insertion and change of the Paterson-Forrester stent will be described including details of the additional instruments and consumables needed to carry out the procedure. The potential complications and issues and the techniques of managing these will be discussed.

16.4   The Paterson Forrester Stent

This is an 8.5FG 65 cm stent produced by Cook (Figure 16.3). What makes it unusual is that it is longer than a conventional stent and only has a few side hole at the coils of the pig tail, thus there are no side holes throughout the length of the stent. There is a lumen, a flat end, and a tapered end to the stent. One significant flaw in the design is the tapered end, which was designed to aid placement but it actually results in premature blockage due to the impact of reducing the functional lumen. After placement of the tapered end into the bladder, the tip is extracted per urethra and the distal 2 mm of the tapered tip is excised to enhance the functional lumen. Another issue is the small diameter of the

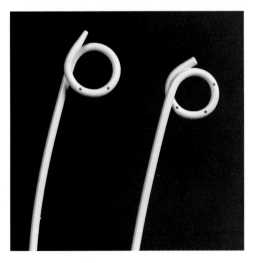

Figure 16.3 Pigtail of the Paterson-Forrester subcutaneous stent.

stent, which reduces its functional longevity. The stent is made from polyurethane and has a promoted life of 3 months although with consent from the patient, the stent can be left in place for 12 months or longer, thus reducing the need for change and hospitalization. In cases of terminal illness, the stent can be left in place without a plan for change unless occlusion occurs.

The stent sits in the subcutaneous layer of the abdomen between the kidney and the bladder. Within a few weeks, a fibrous sheath forms around the stent like a new ureter making subsequent change easy. Urine only drains though the stent lumen of and not along the outside as seen in conventionally sited ureteric stents. The stent is retained in the renal pelvis by the pigtail coil. The stent only comes in one length and thus any excess length of stent sits in the bladder with surprisingly few symptoms. The excess length does aid the process of stent change.

16.5   Stent Placement

The position of the nephrostomy tube is not critical but a lower or mid-calyceal transparenchymal puncture is preferred with a more anteriorly or laterally placed puncture if possible to make positioning on the operating table easier and also to reduce the likelihood of kinking or compression. Placement as a primary procedure by placing the proximal coil into the kidney through an 11 FG peel-away sheath (Cook), but it is easier and safer to have a preliminary nephrostomy tube in place for a week before placement to reduce the risk of loosing control of the puncture track.

Urine cultures should be sterile and the procedure covered with appropriate prophylactic antibiotics covering gram-negative organisms (i.e., Gentamicin 2–4 mg/Kg). The procedure is normally under general anesthesia, but it can be performed under local anesthesia with to without sedation or regional anesthesia, or depending on the fitness and preference of the patient and anesthetist. The ipsilateral side of the nephrostomy tube needs to be elevated on sandbags or bags of fluid (usually two x 3 liters bags of fluid, one under the shoulder the other under the pelvis. The legs are best supported in a Lloyd-Davies cystoscopy position and iodine skin preparation is used (Figure 16.4). Separate side and top drapes are used. If the procedure is a bilateral insertion then

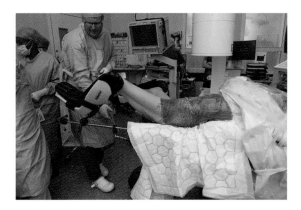

Figure 16.4 Semi-lateral positioning of the patient with two 3-liter bags of saline to elevate the ipsilateral side and a Lloyd-Davis cystoscopy position.

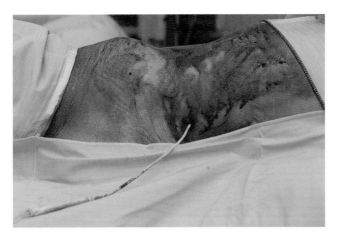

Figure 16.5 Iodine skin and nephrostomy tube preparation plus draping.

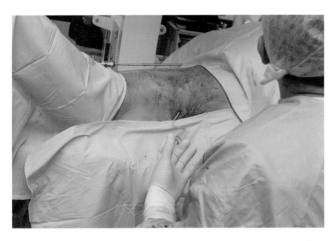

Figure 16.6 The operator sits and injects neat contrast (Urografin 150) to outline the collecting system.

two separate drapes are required but if the procedure is a bilateral exchange this can be performed in a supine position with a single draping.

The operator stands on the side of the nephrostomy with the x-ray C arm opposite and the monitor to the foot end of the table and the endoscopy monitor near the head end of the operating table (Figure 16.5).

16.6   Top End Aspect of Stent Insertion Procedure (Kidney Aspect)

After contrast is injected into the system a floppy tip, stiff core guidewire is passed into he collecting system and the nephrostomy removed over the wire (Figure 16.6). It is important to excise an ellipse of skin at the nephrostomy exit site to allow the subcutaneous track to be created under the skin edges (Figure 16.7). A minor open surgical tray is needed for this part of the procedure and a separate trolley (Figure 16.8).

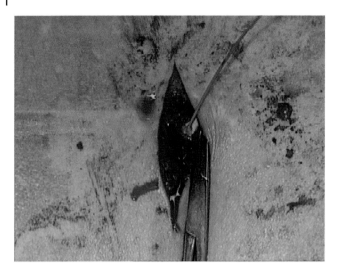

Figure 16.7 A sensor wire is placed through the nephrostomy tube and a skin ellipse cut to excised the skin puncture site of the nephrostomy site. The skin edges are also undermined.

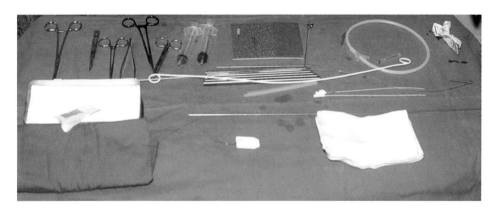

Figure 16.8 A minor open surgical tray is used to prepare for the skin excision and tunneling procedure.

It is best to make a 2-cm incision. X-ray screening is needed to check the position of the renal end of the PF stent and subsequently to check that the stent is not kinked in placement along the subcutaneous tunnel. The non-tapered end of the stent is advanced into the collecting system and positioned into the renal pelvis.

16.7   Tunneling Procedure

The metal Alken percutaneous puncture dilators are ideal for the procedure – size numbers 1, 2, and 4. If you miss out number 3, it is possible to pull the central core either way after number 4 is placed (Figure 16.9). The stent in the subcutaneous layers using the dilators in a series of small (12 cm) jumps avoiding acute angles. The route of

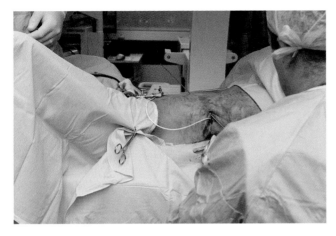

Figure 16.9 A series of subcutaneous jumps are made to tunnel the stent using the Alken dilators.

the stent is dependant upon scars, stomas, skin quality, fat folds and bony prominences. The tunneling stops supra-pubically just lateral to the midline above the pubic bone. It is best to infiltrate local anesthesia to the proposed puncture sites before the stent is placed in case of stent puncture.

16.8 Lower Aspect of Stent Insertion Procedure (Bladder Puncture)

An assistant distends the bladder while looking at the bladder vault with the cystoscope rotated using a 30- or 70-degree lens. Alternatively, a flexible cystoscope can be used. Bladder puncture is performed with a percutaneous puncture needle (Cook or Boston) size 16 gauge and then the wire is passed into the bladder followed by an 11FG short peel-away sheath and remove the wire (Figure 16.10). It is important to cystoscopically monitor the placement of the needle, the wire, the peel-away sheath and then the stent. In patients with abdominal scars, the addition of ultrasound scanning and open placement will reduce but not eliminate hollow viscous damage. Alternatively, an open cut-down method may be used. Prior to bladder stent placement it is important to cut off the distal tapered tip of the stent to functionally widen the stent lumen. The excess stent is coiled in the bladder and the peel-away sheath removed. The skin incisions with 4/0 Vicryl Rapide No. 9971 (Ethicon) and cyanoacrylate skin adhesive rather than dressings to all wounds (Figure 16.11). It is best to leave a 12 FG Foley two-way catheter for a few hours to ensure that there is no significant hematuria and to check that the stent or stents are draining well. The patient is typically treated as a day case or short stay setting.

16.9 The Technique of Stent Changes

The stent needs changing when it blocks, or ideally, before this happens. The stent can remain patent for varying times in different or the same patient. Surprisingly, calcification rarely occurs despite the length of stent in the bladder, but biofilm formation can

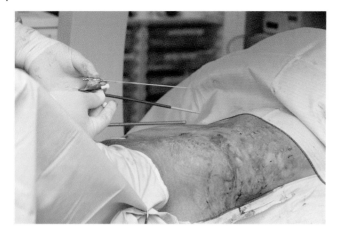

Figure 16.10 The bladder puncture procedure includes a nephrostomy type needle (16 Gauge) and a short size 11 FG peel-away sheath.

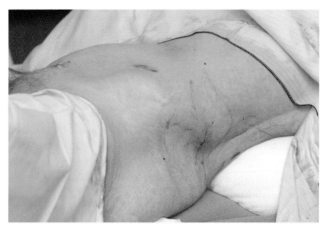

Figure 16.11 Skin closure with inverting 4/0 Vicryl Rapide sutures (9971) and cyanoacrylate glue as a sealant and dressing.

result in stent occlusion. It is best to perform the first change at 6 months and make a valued judgment as to the timing of subsequent changes, ideally at 12 months.

The change is much more simple than insertion. The patient can be positioned in the supine position and this can be done under local or general anesthesia as no tunneling is needed. With the help of x-ray control, a suitable position for incision is identified over the midpoint of the stent usually in the iliac fossa. This position allows easy access and control to exchange the upper part over a wire. Changing the stent entirely cystoscopically has been possible on occasion, but the risk is loss on control of the proximal coil. Thus there is more control through an open incision and cystoscopic control to aid placement of the distal loop.

A 2-cm incision is needed so it is possible to insert a finger to palpate the stent. A right-angle clip is passed under the stent and sheath and the shaft of the clip is used to secure the stent. After a careful longitudinal incision through the fibrous sheath, the

(a)   (b)

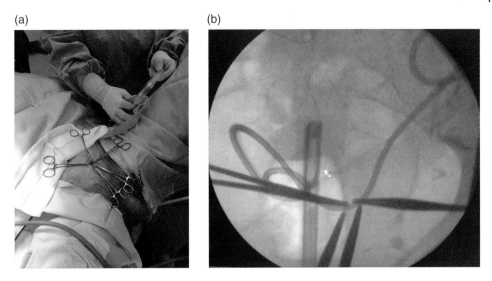

Figure 16.12 a) Secure the subcutaneous stent with mosquito clips to open the fibrous track. In this case an extra-anatomic stent in a transplant is being replaced b) X-ray screening is used to control the stent.

stent is secured and divided. The distal end is clamped with a mosquito clip and while the proximal end of the stent is changed first (Figures 16.12a, b). Contrast is injected through the stent to outline the system and then a stiff core wire is passed up the proximal end of the stent into the collecting system, the old stent removed over the wire, and the new stent replaced and positioned in the renal pelvis. The lower end of the stent is retrieved through the urethra while controlling the cut end at the incision point. A stiff core wire is the passed through the lower end and the distal end of the old stent can be retrieved either through the skin incision or the urethra.

The distal end of the new stent is then passed over wire through the fibrous sheath and into the bladder. It is best to pass the stent down the urethra and control the loop of stent in the incision. The stent can then be pushed back along the wire into the bladder after pulling the wire nearly fully out. The stent can also be pushed back with a clip in women or cystoscopy biopsy forceps in men.

The position of the stent is checked with x-ray screening and the wound closed with absorbable sutures and glue or a dressing. There is no need for a catheter with changes. The alternative method of placing the lower end of the stent is as a new stent with a repeat tunneling procedure.

16.10 Complications and How to Deal With Them

16.10.1 Early Issues

Misplacement of stent and kinking can occur (Figure 16.13). In very thin patients and where multiple scars are present and small bladder capacity. It is possible to cause bowel injury if the bladder puncture is more lateral and in patients with previous abdominal

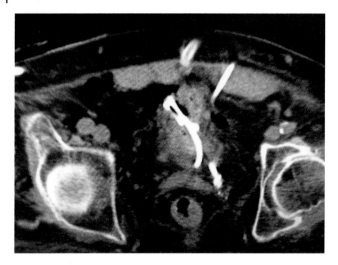

Figure 16.13 Misplaced stent – on CT scanning the coil of left extra-anatomic stent can be seen behind the bladder. This required repositioning under cystoscopic and radiological control.

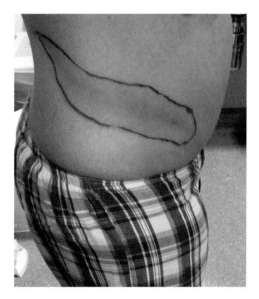

Figure 16.14 Early complications can include superficial cellulitis along the track. Treatment with IV antibiotics can resolve this in a freshly placed stent.

surgery. If concern is present postoperatively, a CT scan is the key to assess injury and plan management. Cellulitis can occur along the line of the stent, which can be resolved with IV antibiotics (Figure 16.14).

16.10.2 Late Issues

16.10.2.1 Stent Obstruction

This will happen if the stent is left in too long before replacement. Warning signs may be redness along the subcutaneous track of the stent and erosion (Figure 16.15).

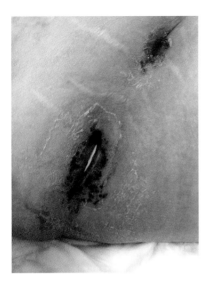

Figure 16.15 Skin erosion due to infection along the track occurs in patients when the stent is blocked or needs changing.

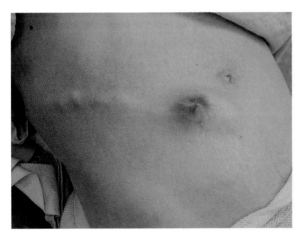

Figure 16.16 Cancer cells can seed along the subcutaneous track if the lower of the stent passes through pelvic cancer and thus active bladder involvement is contraindication for this technique.

An alternative may include placement of a nephrostomy and cystoscopic removal of the stent or exteriorization of the stent by incision over the stent above the infection or at the site of infection and then withdrawal of lower end of the stent into the incision. The lower part of the stent may be placed into a stoma bag or it may be feasible to change the upper part of the stent over a guidewire and either leaving the lower end draining into a bag or rerouting the lower end away from the site of infection.

In cases of advanced pelvic malignancy, there has been a case where tumor seeded along the track (Figure 16.16).

16.11   Future Developments

There are a few modifications, which would improve the functionality of the stent and improve its take-up. There should be a larger range of sizes potentially a 14-18FG. This may prolong the duration between changes. The Detour stent offers a long-term option but this is not without risk of complications and the method of insertion is a more complex and major surgical procedure.

References

[1] Ahmadzadeh M. Clinical experience with subcutaneous urinary diversion: new approach using a double pigtail stent. Br J Urol 1991; 67:596–599.

[2] Lingam K, Paterson PJ, Lingam MK, Buckley JF Forrester A. Subcutaneous urinary diversion: an alternative to percutaneous nephrostomy. J Urol 1994; 152:70–72.

[3] Minhas S, Irving HC, Lloyd SN, Eardley I, Browning AJ, Joyce AD. Extra- anatomic stents in ureteric obstruction: experience and complications. BJU Int 1999; 84:762–764.

[4] Lloyd SN, Kimuli M, Sciberras J. Extra-anatomic urinary drainage for urinary obstruction. In: Monica G, (ed), Chronic Kidney Disease. Available at: http://www.intechopen.com/redirector/articles/extra-anatomic-urinary-drainage-for-urinary-obstruction [accessed July 1, 2016].

[5] Tahir W, Hakeem, A, White A, Irving HC, Lloyd SN, Ahmad, N. Extra-anatomic stent (EAS) as a salvage procedure for transplant ureteric stricture. Am J Transplantation 2014; 14(8):1927–1930.

17

Detour Extra-Anatomical Ureteric Stent

Graham Watson

Consultant Urologist and Chairman, Medi Tech Trust, BMI The Esperance Hospital, Eastbourne, UK

17.1   Introduction

An extra-anatomic stent is a tunnel-like device, which extends further than a standard nephrostomy (Figure 17.1).

In 1991, Ahmadzadeh [1] described the use of a stent, which ran from the kidney to the bladder via a tunnel in the subcutaneous fat. It was basically an extra long JJ stent of 11FG diameter, which was inserted as a nephrostomy, tunneled in the subcutaneous tissues, and then inserted via a suprapubic puncture into the bladder. The stents had side holes in the standard manner but were long enough for this greater distance around the body. He used this device on eight patients and found that the hydronephrosis improved in seven (Figures 17.2–17.7). These stents were changed on a tri-monthly basis.

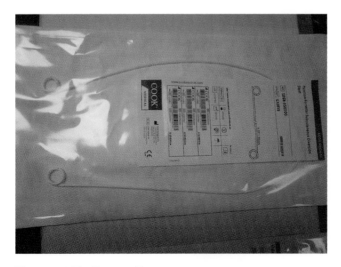

Figure 17.1 The Paterson-Forrester stent.

Ureteric Stenting, First Edition. Edited by Ravi Kulkarni.
© 2017 John Wiley & Sons Ltd. Published 2017 by John Wiley & Sons Ltd.

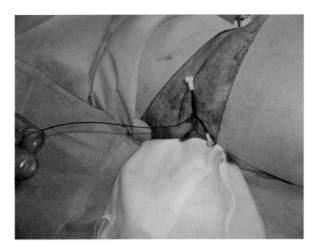

Figure 17.2 A peel-away sheath into the pelvicalyceal system is used to insert the proximal coil of the Paterson-Forrester stent.

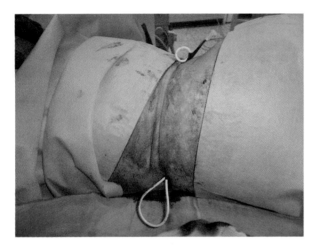

Figure 17.3 A peel-away sheath is then used to tunnel the Paterson-Forrester stent to the iliac fossa and the distal coil will then be inserted into the bladder.

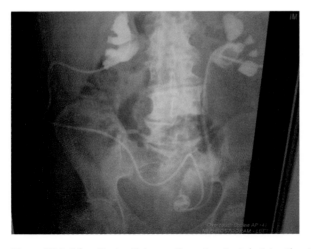

Figure 17.4 A functioning Paterson-Forrester stent draining the right kidney to the bladder. The patient has a left ureteric JJ stent and left Foley catheter nephrostomy in place. Both kidneys drained via the left nephrostomy.

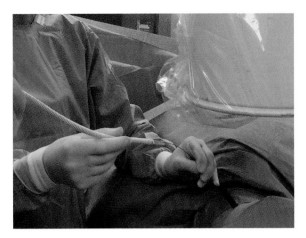

Figure 17.5 The detour stent being passed over a guidewire into the pelvicalyceal system via 32 F Amplatz sheath. Note the section lying in the renal pelvis is 20 F soft silicone, there is then a yellow teflon section, which anchors to the renal cortex. A PTFE 28 F section protects the extra anatomic section of the stent.

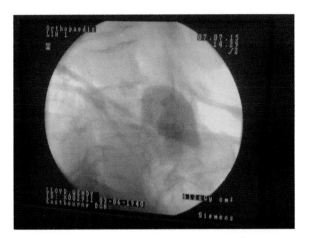

Figure 17.6 The detour stent has been inserted through the Amplatz sheath into the renal pelvis but the Teflon-coated section corresponding to the metallic ring needs withdrawing 2 cm to lie within the renal cortex. This is best accomplished by reinserting the Amplatz sheath over the tube rather than pulling on the Detour stent.

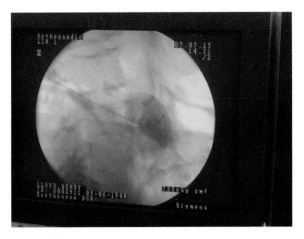

Figure 17.7 After passing an Amplatz sheath over the Detour stent and withdrawing the stent 2 cm the teflon ring is lying closer to the renal cortex. One further correction was made to get the positioning optimized.

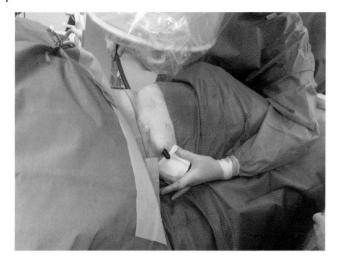

Figure 17.8 A hollow plastic dilator with a removal nose cone is used to make a subcutaneous tunnel.

A further development made by Desgrandschamps and coworkers [2] was the development of a larger caliber dual-lumen tube with a silicone core of 20Ch and an external PTFE portion giving an outer diameter of around 28FG. This device is marketed as the Detour stent (Coloplast Ltd). It is inserted in the renal pelvis via a 32FG Amplatz sheath and requires an open procedure to anastomose the PTFE outer sheath to the outer wall of the bladder leaving a length of silicone to lie within the bladder lumen. The Detour stent does not need routine changing (Figure 17.8).

17.2 The Need for an Extra-Anatomic Drainage

The reason that the extra-anatomic stent initiative was so important was that patients with an external nephrostomy or worse with bilateral nephrostomies have a limited lifestyle revolving around urine leakage, restricted movement, and unpredictable and frequent admissions for nephrostomy replacement. It is not only indicated for those patients where an indwelling JJ stent cannot be passed but also for those cases where the JJ stent can be passed but fails to resolve the obstruction. This is much more common an event than might be supposed. Ramsay *et al.* (1985) and Payne and Ramsay (1988) have shown that JJ stents in the normal pig ureter cause a degree of obstruction, which is more severe in the acute stage and is largely prevented by draining the bladder [3,4]. A number of studies have shown that even when correctly placed a JJ stent may not relieve obstruction. Hubner *et al.* (1992) studied 20 patients with JJ stents and nephrostomy tubes [5]. In 17 of these patients, flow only occurred at a mean renal pelvic pressure of 19.9 cm of water. In three of the patients there was no flow even at much higher pressures. We know from studies on the chronically obstructed kidney that the intra-pelvic pressures generated may be much lower than in health (Figures 17.9 and 17.10). So, even these relatively mild obstructions become functionally important (Vaughan *et al.*, 1970) [6]. Docimo and Dewolf (1989) looked at the functioning of polyurethane and silicone JJ stents and subdivided the patients into intrinsic and extrinsic obstruction. Intrinsic obstruction (principally

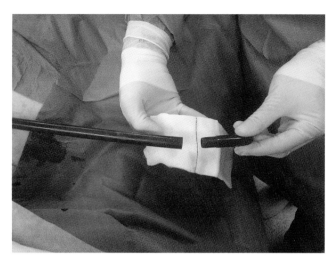

Figure 17.9 After passing the track dilator subcutaneously the nose cone is removed and the Detour stent passed through the hollow tube.

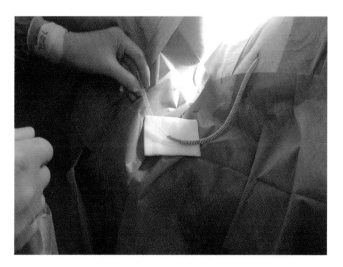

Figure 17.10 The Detour stent has been passed through the tunneler. Methylene blue plus contrast injected back through the Detour stent is used to check free communication with the pelvicalyceal system.

secondary to stones) drained well in 100% of cases [7]. In extrinsic compression the stent failed to resolve the obstruction in 20 out of 46 patients. Chung *et al.* (2004) studied patients on long-term stent management; there were 101 patients with 138 stents of which 58 (42%) failed to resolve the obstruction [8]. Predictors of stent failure were malignancy (where only 56% were successful compared to 91% in benign disease) and renal impairment. This data argues for early review of all patients having JJ stent insertion with at least a follow-up ultrasound and check of renal function at 6 weeks post-insertion. If the hydronephrosis has not improved then in many patients, a renography and possibly a change of drainage strategy is indicated (Figure 17.11).

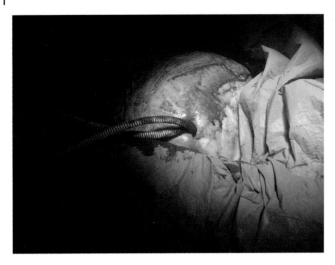

Figure 17.11 Both Detour stents have now been brought out to the anterior abdominal wall at the site for siting the drainage bag.

17.3 Prerequisites for Extra-Anatomic Stenting

The extra-anatomic JJ stent can only be used where there is a functioning bladder but the Detour stent has been tried in cases where there is no bladder. Although this use lies outside of the product license for the device, it will be discussed in this chapter with the understanding that for some patients a careful discussion about the pros and cons is warranted (Figure 17.12).

17.4 Experience with the Extra-Anatomic JJ Stent

Following on from the experience of Ahmadzadeh with an 11FG JJ stent, Minhas *et al.* reported on their experience from Leeds, UK, using a 50 cm 8FG double-pigtail stent [9]. The tunneling was accomplished using a triple incision technique, one for a nephrostomy puncture, one for a suprapubic puncture, and one midway for easier tunneling through the subcutaneous fat. These stents were replaced every six months by cutting down onto the subcutaneous tunnel under local anesthesia and passing guidewires through the lumen and then inserting a new stent. Minhas reported on 13 patients: 3 had infection leading to erosion through the skin and they were converted back to nephrostomy drainage; in the remaining patients the stents tided them through till death which in 2 patients was after more than 12 months (Figures 17.13–17.16).

The latest commercial device is the Paterson-Forrester stent, which is 8FG silicon tubing of approximately 50-cm length (Cook, Ireland Ltd). It can even be inserted under local anesthesia. A peel-away sheath is used for nephrostomy, tunneling, and suprapubic insertion. A minimum of two small incisions is required. By the time the stent is due for change at 6 months, an established track has formed around the stent and this allows change of the stent over guidewires after cutting down onto the track under local anesthesia. Problems occur with changing if the stent becomes encrusted

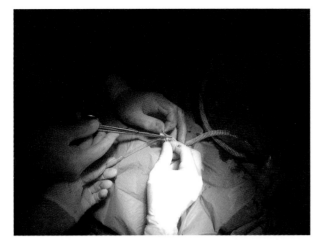

Figure 17.12 The PTFE coating around the inner silicone tubing is carefully cut back to 2 cm deep to the skin making sure that the silicone tube is not inadvertently punctured.

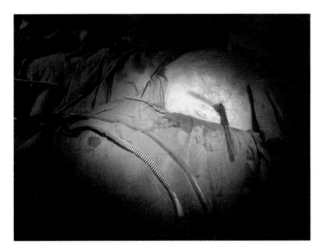

Figure 17.13 The silicone tubes have now been exposed and shortened.

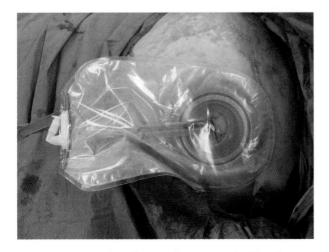

Figure 17.14 The tubing has now been covered with an ileostomy bag.

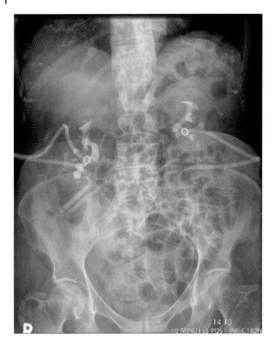

Figure 17.15 An IVU 10 minutes post injection showing unobstructed pelvicalyceal systems draining into a bag in the right iliac fossa via bilateral extra anatomic Detour stents.

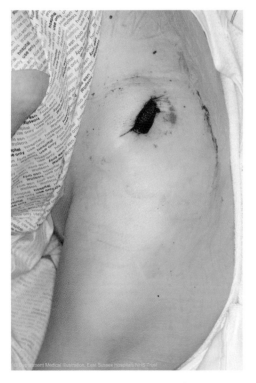

Figure 17.16 This patient had bilateral Detour stents inserted 6 months previously and now has eroded the detour stent through the skin at the site of the nephrostomy puncture.

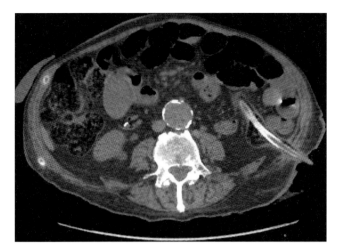

Figure 17.17 A CT scan on the same patient showing that the initial puncture had passed through the descending colon. Amazingly, the Detour stent had functioned without any problem for 6 months.

so that one cannot introduce a guidewire through its lumen and any calcification on the stent can damage the delicate track that has formed around it. Encrustation may lead to earlier stent change, which compounds the problem. Compared to a Detour stent, the Paterson-Forrester stent is cheaper and easier to insert but has the disadvantage of being more likely to fail due to obstruction or failure to exchange. One should think about this device over a Detour stent in patients with a very short life expectancy and where general anesthesia is contraindicated (Figure 17.17).

17.5   Experience With the Detour Stent

The first report of a clinical series with the Detour stent came from the Desgrandschamps' group [10] as early as 1995. In this report the authors described a series of 13 patients having 19 stents, which were described as pyelo-vesical but in addition there were 8 patients with 13 stents, which were brought out to skin where the tube or tubes drained into an ileostomy bag. The authors noted one patient in whom they failed to site the stent because the system was not dilated sufficiently. The mean follow-up of the group was 7.2 months and all the stented ureters were un-dilated. The same group published an abstract in 2001 by which time their numbers had only increased to 27 patients having a total of 35 stents. The authors reported that 19% were difficult to place. The stents had a mean follow-up of 6.3 months in the patients who had died of their underlying disease. The surviving patients had a mean follow-up of 47 months with the longest survivor having a stent working well at 84 months. Approximately 8.5% developed parietal complications, such as infection or erosion with leakage of urine, which is 2 patients. One stent had been removed because of erosion and two converted to a standard nephrostomy because of urine leakage. One might presume that this pioneering group had had some problems, assuming that they were reporting on their total experience each time, because the number of patients had only increased from 21 to 27 in 6 years. However, their results suggested that the concept and the device were both very encouraging. Apart from a recent publication from my unit there are only two other centers, which have published results. Jurczok *et al.* [11] reported on 10 patients with a nephro-vesical Detour stent and 8 patients with a nephro-cutaneous stent. The mean follow-up of the patients was 13.1 months by which time there were two patients developed complications. One stent became encrusted and a second became infected. Both occurred in the nephro-cutaneous group and both were removed with a return to a standard nephrostomy. Lloyd *et al.* (2007) from Leeds, UK, reported on an experience with 9 stents in 8 patients [12]. Interestingly, three had been converted from Paterson-Forrester stents because of problems with drainage. All the stents were pyelo-vesical and all were draining adequately with a mean follow-up of 17 months.

17.6   Personal Experience with Detour Stent

The series published by the author includes two cases of Paterson-Forrester stents, both of which failed within 6 months and were converted to Detour stents. The Detour stent experience from the author's unit consists of 35 patients with a total of 57 stents. The indications for surgery were bladder cancer in 19, prostate cancer in 4, retroperitoneal fibrosis in 1, bowel cancer obstructing the ureters in 3, advanced gynecological malignancy in 3, and 1 for benign stricture of the ureter. Seven patients with 8 stents had stenting to the ileal conduit. All of these patients have survived to the present. All of the stents have had to be removed after a mean of 20.5 months. The cause for removal was infection and erosion of the infected stent through the skin wall. All were converted back to nephrostomy tubes. Even though the Detour stents survived a useful length of time, we have abandoned this route and now prefer to implant the distal end of the Detour to skin even if a conduit exists. Only 9 patients had bladders suitable for receiving a Detour stent and we have sited a total of 13 stents in this group. In 1 patient in this group, the stent was encrusted and interestingly it proved possible to pass a flexible ureteroscope up the stent and the calcification was cleared using a holmium laser. One patient with two stents suffered from fistulation at the suprapubic incision and these were exteriorized. Seven of these patients have died of their malignant disease with their stents functioning satisfactorily. The mean survival in this group is 13.3 months. The largest group has been diverted to skin in the author's series. This group consists of 19 patients receiving a total of 36 stents. Four patients have had their stents removed because of erosion through the skin secondary to infection. Thirteen of the patients have died of their malignancy leaving 6 patients still alive. The longest surviving stent has been in place for 32 months. All of the patients were delighted with the improvement in their quality of life compared to life with a nephrostomy. While the Detour stent was in place all the patients had a collapsed pelvicalyceal system. Only one patient developed an obstruction and this was the patient who encrusted his stent and in whom it proved possible to dis-obstruct the stent using a flexible ureteroscope and holmium laser. In those cases, where there was advanced pelvic malignancy with only partial ureteric obstruction there was still some drainage of urine via the bladder and so insertion of the stent for diversion of urine is only partially successful.

In one patient who had had nephrostomy tubes prior to diversion stenting, the patient had fecal drainage from the site of his nephrostomy puncture but this only became apparent 6 months after the stent insertion. The patient was terminal from his malignant disease and the fistulation was not thought to have contributed to his poor clinical state. We had dilated the existing nephrostomy track having no idea that it had presumably been inserted through the colon before draining the kidney. Based on this event, there should be a low threshold for making a new puncture into the collecting system if the nephrostomy has been sited relatively anteriorly, even if there has been no obvious visceral damage.

17.7   The Technique

As with any percutaneous procedure, it is advisable to start the procedure if possible by inserting ureteric catheters and a urethral catheter. This can be done on the trolley before placing the patient on the operating table or it can be performed in a standard lithotomy position. In those patients where a ureteric catheter cannot be passed, a puncture to the collecting system will need to be performed under ultrasonic guidance. One can perform the procedure using a standard prone position but since the majority of procedures involve bilateral stenting, the author prefers a supine procedure with sandbags under the hip and scapula in order to access the kidney.

This position is preferred for the insertion of a Paterson-Forrester or the Detour stent. With the Detour stent, however, there is no possibility of performing the procedure under local anesthesia. Start by dilating a track into the collecting system through an incision of about 5 cm in the loin. The track is dilated to take a 32FG Amplatz sheath, which comes with the Detour stent set. Position the detour stent in the pelvicalyceal system and run in a mixture of methylene blue and contrast to check positioning. Contrast will run back through the Amplatz sheath but one can get enough opacification of the collecting system to position the metallic ring at the proximal portion of the stent at the level of the renal cortex. Now, withdraw the Amplatz sheath making sure that the position of the metallic ring does not alter. The metallic ring corresponds to a short section of Teflon, which adheres to the renal cortex and makes it hold fast. If you want to make an adjustment to the position of the stent then pass the Amplatz back over the detour stent; do not just pull on the stent or it becomes misshapen.

The creation of the subcutaneous tunnel again will often require dividing the track into two and aiming for some halfway point before bringing the stent out at the suprapubic incision. The tunneling is achieved using a plastic tube with a removable cap. The stent can then be passed through the tube and the tube withdrawn. Again take care that the detour stent does not make too severe an angulation so that it does not kink. At the suprapubic incision make an incision long enough so that the bladder can be accessed for an open insertion. Cut the detour stent so that it will lie without tension in the bladder and cut back the outer PTFE coat exposing 6 cm or so of silicone tubing. The bladder is filled using saline via a urethral catheter and the bare silicone tubing is inserted into the bladder and the PTFE coat is sewn to the serial layer of the bladder. If two detour stents are being placed then leave this part of the procedure to the end and place both stents into the bladder through separate small stab incisions. Leave the catheter for 48 hours so that there is enough time for the insertion sites to be leak-proof.

17.8   Alternative Techniques

In cases of pelvic malignancy it may not be prudent to insert the detour stent into the bladder and in some cases the bladder will have already been removed. In these cases there is an option of performing a pyelo-cutaneous detour stent. One simply chooses a site at which to have the stent exit on the anterior abdominal wall and bring both tubes (if performing a bilateral procedure) out at that point. It is important to have the PTFE outer coating cut back several centimeters deep to the skin level because the silicone tubing resists bacterial colonization, whereas infection of the PTFE coating will eventually result in the stent eroding through the skin. Take great care when cutting through the outer PTFE that the inner silicone tube is not damaged because leakage of urine can make management of the stent ileostomy very difficult due to urine leakage. Pyelo-cutaneous stents are more likely to become infected than pyelo-vesical stents but they still represent a significant advantage over life with a nephrostomy. It is vital, however, that there is full discussion with the patient beforehand and that the patient realizes that the device is being used outside its product license and that the stent may need adjustment in the future.

17.9   Complications

17.9.1   Infection

Infection of a stent is usually obvious. There is breakdown of the skin over the stent and the PTFE coating is exposed. It may be possible to expose the detour stent higher up in its course and place an ileostomy bag over the stent there (having cut back the PTFE so that only silicone tubing emerges beyond the skin). In one case, we have shortened the stent all the way back to the loin incision. The stent was still firmly anchored at the kidney and it has continued working as a nephrostomy. Infection makes removal of the stent extremely easy but uninfected portions of the stent remain anchored. Even anchored sections of the stent can be removed with more forceful traction.

17.9.2   Recurrent Obstruction

This too can become a real issue and will require a full evaluation and perhaps revision of the stent.

17.9.3   An Algorithm

There are a number of options when dealing with chronic obstruction of the upper urinary tract. These are long-term JJ stents, metallic stents, long-term Cope loop nephrostomies, Foley catheter nephrostomies, full reconstructive surgery, stented end ureterostomies, Paterson-Forrester extra anatomic stents and Detour stents (Tregunna and Watson, 2012) [13]. In a patient with a 5-year life expectancy or more then reconstruction should be considered as the ideal option. For the large number of patients with a limited prognosis or where reconstruction is considered too major an undertaking, then it is reasonable to work through the possible options. For many patients a JJ stent changed once or twice a year is acceptable and preserves the renal function. Too often, however, we do not consider other options and fail to pick up on a loss of renal function until it is too late. Ideally, any patient with an internal stent should be reviewed at 4 to 6 weeks post insertion along with an ultrasound of the kidneys and a measure of the renal function. This will reveal that the stent has failed to resolve the obstruction only when the renal dysfunction is irreversible. Extra-anatomic stents should be considered when ureteric stents fail or where the symptoms from the stent fail to resolve after a month. In the author's series, all Paterson-Forrester stents had to be converted to Detour stents and so the latter is used preferentially. Detour stents, however, do require a dilated percutaneous system in order to make a 32FG track into the renal pelvis. In those cases where this cannot be achieved then stented end ureterostomies should be considered.

17.9.4 Summary

The failure of rate of standard JJ stents in extrinsic compression (principally by malignancy) has been shown to be in the region of 40% This is often detected late this as there is an assumption that a stent is draining when it has been placed correctly. By the time the obstruction is detected, sufficient time has passed that one can assume that the stent had become blocked and the first action is to replace the stent. Therefore, patients should be reviewed at 4 to 6 weeks after stent placement to check on renal function and pelvicalyceal dilatation. In any case of obstruction of the upper tracts a decision must be made about whether to perform a complex reconstruction or to stent. Where there is a functioning bladder then ureteric stents and extra anatomic stents should be considered only for those patients in whom reconstruction is high-risk or the prognosis less than 5 years. In these cases, extra-anatomic stents should be considered early because they have an excellent success rate and are tolerated well by the patients (Table 17.1). Paterson Forrester stents have not proved as durable as Detour stents. Where there is no functioning bladder pyelo-cutaneous stenting using Detour stents do give a temporary solution and often this will be sufficient given the poor prognosis of the patient population we are treating. The pyelo-cutaneous option is not included in the product license of the stent and this must be disclosed to the patient in the preoperative discussions.

Table 17.1 The results of the Detour stent group showing the outcomes of the stents according to whether draining to bladder, skin or conduit. The results refer to the number of patients rather than the number of stents.

	total (patients)	Patient alive with intact stents	duration (months)	Patients died with intact stent	duration (months)	Stents removed	duration (months)
Detour stents to bladder	9	1	36	8	13.3	0	–
Detour stents to skin	19	6	17.5	9	4.5	4	11.5
Detour stents to conduit	7	0	–	0	–	7	20.5

References

[1] Ahmadzadeh M. Clinical experience with subcutaneous urinary diversion: New approach using a double pigtail Stent. Br J Urol 1991; 67:596–599.

[2] Desgrandschamps F, Cussenot O, Meria P, *et al.* Subcutaneous urinary diversions for palliativetreatment of pelvic malignancies. J Urol 1995; 154(2 Pt 1):367–370.

[3] Ramsay JW, Payne SR, Gosling PT, Whitfield HN, Wickham JE, Levison DA. The effects of double J stunting on unobstructed ureters. An experimental and clinical study. Br J Urol 1985;57(6):630–634.

[4] Payne SR, Ramsay JW, The effects of double J stents on renal pelvic dynamics in the pig. J Urol 1988;140(3):637–641.

[5] Hubner WA, Plas EG, Stoller ML. The double-J ureteral stent: in vivo and in vitro flow studies. J Urol 1992; 148(2 Pt 1):278–280.

[6] Vaughan ED Jr, Sorensen EJ, Gillenwater JY. The renal hemodynamic response to chronic unilateral complete ureteral occlusion. Invest Urol 1970;8(1):78–90.

[7] Docimo SG, Dewolf WC. high failure rate of indwelling ureteral stents in patients with extrinsic obstruction: experience at 2 institutions. J Urol 1989;142(2 Pt 1): 277–279.

[8] Chung SY, Stein RJ, Landsittel D, Davies BJ, Cuellar DC, Hrebinko RL *et al.* 15 year experience with the management of extrinsic ureteral obstruction with indwelling ureteral stents. J Urol 2004;172(2):592–595.

[9] Minhas S, Irving HC, Lloyd SN, Eardley I, Browning AJ, Joyce AD. Extra-anatomic stents in ureteric obstruction: experience and complications. BJU Int 1999;84(7):762–764.

[10] Jabbour ME, Desgrandschamps F, Angelescu E, Teillac P, Le Duc A. Percutaneous implantation of subcutaneous prosthetic ureters: long-term outcome. J Endourol 2001; 15(6):611–614.

[11] Jurczok A, Loertzer H, Wagner S, Fornara. Subcutaneous nephrovesical and nephrocutaneous bypass. Gynae Obstet Invest 2005;59(3):144–148.

[12] Lloyd SN, Tirukonda P, Biyani CS, Wah TM, Irving HC. The detour stent - a permanent solution for benign and malignant ureteric obstruction? Eur Urol 2007; 52(1):193–198.

[13] Tregunna R, Watson G. Algorithm of management for upper ureteric obstruction. British Journal of Medical and Surgical Urology 2012; 5S:S18–S23.

18

Tandem Ureteral Stents

David A. Leavitt[1], Piruz Motamedinia[2], Philip T. Zhao[2], Zeph Okeke[2] and Arthur D. Smith[3]

[1] The Smith Institute for Urology, Hofstra-North Shore-LIJ Health System, New Hyde Park, NY, USA
[2] The Smith Institute for Urology, Hofstra-North Shore-LIJ School of Medicine, New Hyde Park, NY, USA
[3] Professor of Urology, The Smith Institute for Urology, Hofstra North Shore-LIJ School of Medicine, New Hyde Park, NY, USA

18.1 Introduction

Ureteral stents are ubiquitous in urology and are most frequently placed to relieve upper urinary tract obstruction or to splint a newly created ureteral anastomosis. Unfortunately, single ureteral stents can become blocked or fail for various reasons. This is especially true in cases of malignant ureteral obstruction where single stents will eventually fail 20-60% of the time [1, 2]. In the past, these patients were left with the options of either percutaneous nephrostomy drainage or more invasive open urinary diversion procedures. Over the last few decades, alternatives have surfaced in the form of metallic stents and tandem, or ipsilateral, double ureteral stenting.

The aim of this chapter is to describe some of the limitations of single polymeric and metallic ureteral stents and to describe the rationale for tandem ureteral stents. An evaluation of the available literature on tandem ureteral stents is presented, including potential benefits, limitations, outcomes, and complications. Tandem ureteral stent usage is addressed in both malignant and benign etiologies of ureteral obstruction. The technique of tandem ureteral stent placement is also briefly described. Finally, the chapter will discuss cost considerations with tandem ureteral stents compared to metallic stents.

18.2 Mechanism of Ureteral Stent Failure and Corrective Measures

Single ureteral stents fail when urine flow both through and around the outside of the stent becomes completely obstructed. In the unstented, unobstructed state, urine travels down the ureter in discrete boluses. Introduction of an in-dwelling ureteral stent disrupts the normal coordinated peristaltic activity of the ureter and increases urothelial mucus production and cell sloughing [3]. This debris can temporarily or permanently obstruct the flow of urine through the stent and is thought to potentiate intraluminal ureteral stent encrustation. Thus, urine flow is preferentially directed around the ureteral stent.

Ureteric Stenting, First Edition. Edited by Ravi Kulkarni.

This becomes problematic in the setting of ureteral compression, either intrinsic or extrinsic, where the space between the inner ureteral wall and outside of the ureteral stent becomes compromised, and in some instances, completely obliterated. It is this combination of obstructed intra- and extra-luminal urine flow that results in ureteral stent failure and can manifest clinically as flank pain, hydronephrosis, and renal functional deterioration [4, 5].

Once a single ureteral stent has failed, options to rectify the situation include single ureteral stent exchange with the same stent material and dimensions, single ureteral stent exchange with different stent material and/or dimensions (e.g., larger bore stent, metallic stent), percutaneous nephrostomy drainage, more invasive urinary diversion operations, subcutaneous ureterovesical shunting, and tandem ureteral stenting.

None of these options is without its drawbacks. The considerable morbidity associated with invasive urinary diversions and subcutaneous ureterovesical shunting limits its widespread use in the current age of endourology, especially in patients with malignant ureteral obstruction in whom limited life expectancy is the norm. Indeed, expected 1-year survival for patients developing MUO is approximately 50% or less with median survival frequently reported at between 6 and 8 months [1, 6].

The trouble with single ureteral stents in MUO is that placement is unsuccessful in 10-30% of reported series and even when placed successfully, nearly half the time they are destined to fail [2]. Moreover, simple single ureteral stent exchange rarely provides any durable benefit as the newly placed single ureteral stent usually fails more rapidly than the originally placed one [7].

Metallic stents are designed to resist external compression better than polymeric stents, and this has been repeatedly shown on the bench top. However, in clinical practice, metallic ureteral stents also frequently succumb to ureteral stenosis, both from malignant and benign etiologies. Metallic stent failure rates in small, retrospective studies over the last decade have ranged from 20 to 100% [8–10]. In addition, metallic ureteral stents often require specialty ordering and are significantly more expensive than polymeric ureteral stents. Lastly, though touted to require stent exchanges only annually, many of these metallic stents require exchange before one year for a variety of reasons.

18.3 Tandem Ureteral Stents

Tandem ureteral stents were first described by Liu *et al.* almost 20 years ago to relieve persistent malignant ureteral obstruction despite prior single ureteral stent placement [11]. Tandem ureteral stents refers to the placement of two parallel, ipsilateral, double pigtail ureteral stents in-dwelling within the same ureter. These have been occasionally referred to as parallel or double ureteral stents, as well.

Conceptually, tandem ureteral stents are superior to single ureteral stents on two levels. First, the parallel stents have a higher tensile strength than a single stent and thus resist compression better. Second, and novel to tandem ureteral stents, is the fact that placing parallel stents within the same ureter provides an additional route for urinary drainage through the space created between the two stents (Figure 18.1). Though not fully known, it is hypothesized that this inter-stent space is more resistant to compression and may contribute to continued renal decompression even in the setting of completely occluded stents and tight external ureteral compression. Lending some credence to this hypothesis is at least one study showing tandem ureteral stents

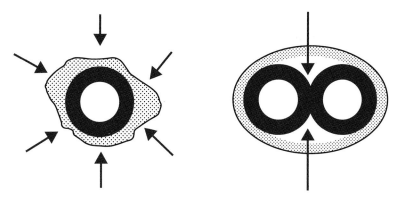

Figure 18.1 Pathway between tandem ureteral stents for extraluminal urine flow, even in the presence of extrinsic compression. *Source*: Fromer *et al.* [14] Reproduced with permission from Elsevier.

placed into pig ureters maintain improved flow characteristics (up to five times greater) in the setting of partial occlusion compared to partially occluded single plastic ureteral stents [12].

18.4 Technique

The technique for tandem ureteral stent placement follows readily from many of the maneuvers used during insertion of a single ureteral stent, making this technique easily adopted by those unfamiliar with the procedure. First described by Liu and Hrebinko in 1998, others have recapitulated the procedure since then, albeit with slight nuances [11, 13–15].

To place tandem ureteral stents, cystoscopy and retrograde pyelography is executed to delineate the ureteral stricture position and length, degree of hydronephrosis, and ureteral and pelvocalyceal anatomy. Subsequently, the ureteral orifice of the obstructed side is cannulated with a guidewire. Our institutional preference is to use the Sensor guidewire (Boston Scientific, Natick, MA, USA) as it has a floppy tip reducing potential injury to the ureteral wall, whereas the hydrophilic tip improves the likelihood of surpassing narrow or tortuous ureteral segments.

Once the initial wire is situated beyond the strictured area and seen to curl in the renal pelvis, a tapered 6 F/10 F dual lumen catheter is advanced over the guidewire. If need be, further retrograde pyelograms can be done through the second lumen. In addition, as it has a soft and tapered tip, the dual lumen catheter can be used to gently dilate areas of ureteral stenosis. An additional wire, often a super-stiff wife, is the passed up the open channel of the dual lumen catheter such that the tips of both wires are curled in the pelvocalyceal system.

The dual lumen catheter is then removed, leaving only the two wires within the ureter and renal pelvis. The final step is advancement of the two well-lubricated double pigtail ureteral stents. It is critical to advance the two stents simultaneously. If the stents are placed one after the other, advancement of the second stent may cause proximal migration of the initially inserted stent.

If ureteral stenosis precludes simultaneous placement of the ureteral stents, which can be estimated via the ease with which the dual-lumen catheter passes, then a few maneuvers may be entertained. Exchanging all wires out for super-stiff wires can improve successful stent placement by minimizing wire buckling during stent insertion. If stent insertion remains difficult, then ureteral dilation (e.g., radial balloon dilators) of the stenotic ureteral segment should be considered. Dilation pressures up to 20 atmospheres can be reached with some balloons, and this frequently will open the strictured area sufficiently to allow for subsequent insertion of tandem ureteral stents.

We prefer to place parallel 6 F or 7 F ureteral stents, however various size combinations have been described ranging from parallel 4.7 F stents to parallel 8 F stents [11, 14, 15]. Despite these measures, if parallel ureteral stent placement remains unsuccessful then a single ureteral stent should be inserted and an additional attempt at parallel stent placement can be attempted at the time of the next ureteral stent exchange.

18.5   Limited Evidence

Despite the seminal reports on tandem ureteral stents surfacing almost 20 years ago, there have been only limited small cases series and retrospective reports since. Nonetheless, when analyzing the data collectively, some common themes emerge. It appears tandem ureteral stent placement is safe, effective and a straightforward technique to perform even by those with limited prior experience with the technique. Tandem ureteral stents have proven effective for both malignant and benign ureteral obstruction, and in both men and women. They offer an excellent alternative to patients with terminal malignancy hoping to avoid percutaneous drainage bags or large urinary-diverting operations who have failed single in-dwelling ureteral stents. Furthermore, they also appear to be a good potential alternative when other single polymeric or metallic stents have failed. Though sparse, the evidence suggests lower urinary tract symptoms with tandem ureteral stents are no different than with single ureteral stents.

In their original report from 1998, Liu and Hrebinko describe the use of tandem 4.7 F double pigtail ureteral stents in four patients with non-urinary tract malignant ureteral obstruction [11]. All patients had failed prior single 6 F double pigtail ureteral stenting. All procedures were done under local and intravenous sedation. No intraoperative complications occurred and all stents were successfully changed at three months arbitrarily. Lower urinary tract symptoms were no worse than those caused by the solitary ureteral stent. All patients were considered clinical successes as evidenced by improved hydronephrosis, decreased serum creatinine and/or improved flank pain. Mean follow-up for this study was 5.8 months.

Shortly thereafter, Rotariu *et al.* [13] and Fromer *et al.* [14] described their experience with tandem ureteral stents for malignant ureteral compression in seven and five patients, respectively. In both studies, all patients had failed prior single ureteral stenting. Either tandem 8 F (Fromer), tandem 7 F (Rotariu) or a combination of an 8 F and a 6 F (Rotariu) double pigtail ureteral stents were used. Both of these studies highlighted the importance, and safety, of balloon dilating the ureter to facilitate placement of the larger caliber ureteral stents. Tandem ureteral stent insertion was successful in each patient. Stents were changed either every 2–3 months (Fromer) or every 4-6 months (Rotariu), and these time points were chosen arbitrarily rather than because of stent malfunction. Mean follow-up was between 12 and 16 months, and all patients tolerated tandem ureteral stents well with no noticeable increase in stent symptoms compared to single ureteral stents. Clinical improvement was appreciated in all patients as seen by diminished hydronephrosis, improved flank pain and, in the Rotariu study, a decline in mean serum creatinine from 3.2 mg/dL to 1.5 mg/dL.

More recently, Elsmara *et al.* have described their initial and updated experience with tandem ureteral stents for both benign (32 patients, 36 renal units) and malignant (40 patients, 49 renal units) ureteral obstruction [9, 15]. Mean follow-up was 25 months. Stent exchanges occurred at a mean of 4.8 months for benign ureteral obstruction patients and a mean of 4.3 months for malignant ureteral obstruction patients. Tandem ureteral stents failed (worsening hydronephrosis and flank pain or worsening renal function) in 6 renal units (12.2%) of those with malignant ureteral obstruction and none of those with benign obstruction. Four of the six failures were managed with simple tandem ureteral stent exchange. Balloon dilation was necessary in 36% of benign obstruction cases and 59% of malignant obstruction cases. When required, balloon dilation was usually only necessary during initial placement of the tandem ureteral stents, with subsequent exchanges rarely requiring additional balloon dilation.

18.6   Cost Considerations

Unlike metallic ureteral stents, for which many cost analyses have been done, none exist for tandem ureteral stents [16–20]. Most of these studies suggest metallic ureteral stents are anywhere from 10 to 20 times more expensive than polymeric ureteral stents, but because stent exchanges are less frequent, metallic stents potentially become cost-effect after approximately one to two years. The central theme to all these studies, and similarly the common flaw to them all, is the assumption that polymeric ureteral stents require stent exchanges every 3 months and metallic stents routinely last much longer and require stent exchanges only every 12 months. The truth of the matter is that most metallic ureteral stents require exchange prior to 12 months. Interestingly, in at least one report, tandem ureteral stents were used to successfully decompress a ureter with a failed metallic ureteral stent [9, 19].

Another problem with the existing cost studies is the joint analysis of both malignant and benign ureteral obstruction patients when reporting the results. This likely confounds the true success rates and time to stent exchange necessary in each of these very different patient populations. As has been suggested by Nagele *et al.* and Taylor *et al.*, in patients with long life expectancies, such as those with benign ureteral obstruction, metallic stents may become cost-effective over a longer period of time [16, 20]. However, in this scenario one often also considers an attempt at definitive stricture repair, thus obviating the need for ureteral stents altogether. Conversely, when looking at those with malignant ureteral obstruction, where average life expectancy is limited, the number of potential stent exchanges is few and the considerably more expensive cost of the metallic stents can rarely be "made up."

The frequency with which tandem ureteral stents require exchange is not known, but the scant available evidence shows changes every 4-5 months are very well tolerated with minimal problems. Furthermore, in at least one report, tandem ureteral stents remained in-dwelling for more than one year prior to successful exchange in two renal units, and more than 200 days in 14 renal units [9]. And, as operative duration, anesthetic requirement and recovery room duration and requirements are essentially no different for single and tandem ureteral stent placement, the main cost difference per given procedure boils down to the cost of the additional ureteral stent and wire, or approximately $100-$200 U.S. dollars at many centers. Therefore, tandem ureteral stents may actually be the most cost effective measure for long-term ureteral decompression.

18.7 Conclusion

The concept and use of tandem ureteral stents date back almost two decades. The technique of tandem ureteral stent insertion is easily adopted from that of single stent insertion and provides another means to preserve internal urinary drainage. Despite this, the evidence base surrounding tandem ureteral stents remains small and retrospective. Nonetheless, the collective experience with tandem ureteral stents appears favorable with very high, durable success rates, essentially no increase in urinary tract symptoms compared to single ureteral stents, and the potential for safe indwell durations of many months. Prospective, better-designed studies are necessary to address the many unanswered questions and help determine in which clinical settings and in which patients tandem ureteral stents benefit the most.

References

[1] Wong LM, Cleeve LK, Milner AD, Pitman AG. Malignant ureteral obstruction: outcomes after intervention. Have things changed? J Urol 2007;178:178–183.

[2] Docimo SG, Dewolf WC. High failure rate of indwelling ureteral stents in patients with extrinsic obstruction: experience at 2 institutions. J Urol 1989;142:277–279.

[3] Cormio L, Talja M, Koivusalo A, Mäkisalo H, Wolff H, Ruutu M. Biocompatibility of various indwelling double-J stents. J Urol 1995;153:494–496.

[4] Hübner WA, Plas EG, Stoller ML. The double-J ureteral stent: in vivo and in vitro flow studies. J Urol 1992;148:278–280.

[5] Ramsay JW, Payne SR, Gosling PT, Whitfield HN, Wickham JE, Levison DA. The effects of double J stenting on unobstructed ureters. An experimental and clinical study. Br J Urol 1985;57:630–634.

[6] Izumi K, Mizokami A, Maeda Y, Koh E, Namiki M. Current outcome of patients with ureteral stents for the management of malignant ureteral obstruction. J Urol 2011;185:556–561.

[7] Rosenberg BH, Bianco FJ, Wood DP, Triest JA. Stent-change therapy in advanced malignancies with ureteral obstruction. J Endourol 2005;19:63–67.

[8] Liatsikos E, Kallidonis P, Kyriazis I, *et al*. Ureteral obstruction: is the full metallic double-pigtail stent the way to go? Eur Urol 2010;57:480–486.

[9] Elsamra SE, Leavitt DA, Motato HA, Friedlander JI, Siev M, Keheila M, Hoenig DM, Smith AD, Okeke Z. Stenting for malignant ureteral obstruction: Tandem, metal or metal-mesh stents. Int J Urol 2015;22(7):629–636.

[10] Goldsmith ZG, Wang AJ, Banez LL, Lipkin ME, Ferrandino MN, Preminger GM, Inman BA. Outcomes of metallic stents for malignant ureteral obstruction. J Urol 2012;188:851–855.

[11] Liu JS, Hrebinko RL. The use of 2 ipsilateral stents for relief of ureteral obstruction from extrinsic compression. J Urol 1998;159:179–181.

[12] Hafron J, Ost MC, Tan BJ, *et al.* Novel dual-lumen ureteral stents provide better ureteral flow than single ureteral stent in ex-vivo porcine kidney model of extrinsic ureteral obstruction. Urology 2006;68:911–915.

[13] Rotariu P, Yohannes P, Alexianu M, *et al.* Management of malignant extrinsic compression of the ureter by simultaneous placement of two ipsilateral ureteral stents. J Endourol 2001;15:979–983.

[14] Fromer DL, Shabsigh A, Benson MC, Gupta M. Simultaneous multiple double pigtail stents for malignant ureteral obstruction. Urology 2002;59:594–596.

[15] Elsamra SE, Motato H, Moreria D, *et al.* Tandem ureteral stents for the decompression of malignant and benign obstructive uropathy. J Endourol 2013;27:1297–1302.

[16] Nagele U, Kuczyk MA, Horstmann M, *et al.* Initial clinical experience with full-length metal ureteral stents for obstructive ureteral stenosis. World J Urol 2008;26:257–262.

[17] Agrawal S, Brown CT, Bellamy EA, Kulkarni R. The thermo-expandable metallic ureteric stent: an 11-year follow-up. BJU Int 2008;103:372–376.

[18] Papatsoris AG, Buchholz N. A novel thermo-expandable ureteral metal stent for the minimally invasive management of ureteral strictures. J Endourol 2010;24:487–491.

[19] Lopez-Huertas H, Polcari AJ, Acosta-Miranda A, Turk T. Metallic ureteral stents: a cost-effective method of managing benign ureteral obstruction. J Endourol 2010;24:483–485.

[20] Taylor ER, Benson AD, Schwartz BF. Cost analysis of metallic ureteral stents with 12 months of follow-Up. J Endourol 2012;26:917–921.

19

Biodegradable Ureteric Stents

David I. Harriman[1] and Ben H. Chew[2,3]

[1] Department of Urologic Sciences, University of British Columbia, Vancouver, BC, Canada
[2] Assistant Professor of Urology, University of British Columbia, Vancouver, BC, Canada
[3] Director of Clinical Research, The Stone Centre at Vancouver General Hospital, Vancouver, Canada

19.1   Introduction

Ureteral stenting is one of the most common procedures performed by urologists. Despite their usefulness and necessity, ureteral stents are fraught with numerous complications and drawbacks including patient discomfort, hematuria, infection, vesicoureteral reflux (VUR), stent encrustation, stent migration, and the need for a repeat procedure for removal should the retention suture not be left externalized [1]. Recognizing these potential harms, biomedical companies and clinical researchers have attempted to develop a stent that overcomes these issues through advancements in stent design, composition and coating.

No stent or material has proven superior at eliminating complications to date. Ideally, a ureteric stent would be composed of a biomaterial that is not affected by its environment and does not cause inflammatory changes to the surrounding urothelium. In other words, it would be biocompatible, resistant to obstruction, encrustation, bacterial colonization, and cause no irritative voiding symptoms [2, 3]. Also, the secondary procedure that is often required would be eliminated as this increases cost, time, and the potential for morbidity.

Biodegradable ureteral stents have been developed in an attempt to move closer to this ideal stent. The main advantage of a fully degrading stent is foregoing a secondary procedure, thus avoiding the "forgotten stent," which can be a source of significant morbidity [4]. However, this is not the only proposed advantage. Theoretically, the surface of these stents is ever-changing with the degradation process which may help decrease bacterial adhesion, biofilm formation and encrustation [5, 6]. Also, stent design that incorporates early degradation of the bladder coil or progressive softening as the stent degrades may limit lower urinary tract symptoms and VUR during voiding [7, 8]. Although not yet used outside of clinical trials, the future of biodegradable stents is promising.

19.2   Material

Biodegradable polymer use in medicine was first described by Kulkarni *et al.* in 1966 [9]. This group determined that polylactic acid was suitable for use in sutures, vascular grafts, and other surgical implants as it was found to be biocompatible, non-toxic, strong and biodegradable in vivo. Their research opened the door for further experimentation and one year later, Schmitt and Polistina patented polyglycolic acid as another commercially available medical bioabsorbable polymer [10]. Biodegradable materials are now commonly used in medicine and could be considered the standard of care in the world of sutures. Other non-urologic uses include wound dressings, coronary stents, orthopedic bone screws, and dental implants. Metal alloys, such as magnesium and iron, have even been used in degradable coronary stents as they can breakdown into inert materials that do not cause circulatory harm [11].

In urology, biodegradable polymeric materials have been designed for both urethral [12] and ureteral stenting. The development of a clinically useful biodegradable ureteral stent has proved challenging as materials used need to fulfill strict requirements. They need to be biocompatible in order to limit urothelial foreign body reaction; they need to adhere to the basic requirements of stents, namely adequate urinary drainage, ease of deployment and radio-opacity; and they need predictable expansion and degradation rates, which can be influenced by both the type of material and amount used [13]. Breakdown byproducts must be inert, small enough to be eliminated from the urinary tract and not toxic or teratogenic to the host. Even if a biodegradable stent can be developed meeting these standards, they also need to be able to withstand sterilization and storage to be considered for clinical use.

Biodegradable materials used for ureteral stents to date include polylactic acid, polyglycolic acid, polylactic-co-glycolic acid (PLGA), alginate-based materials and chitosan [14–18]. The most recent degradable ureteral stent material, and likely the most promising, is a combination of poly-l-lactic acid, polyglycolic acid and caprolactone (Uriprene™, Poly-Med Inc., Anderson, SC, USA).

19.3   Research

Bergman *et al.* conducted one of the earliest studies of biodegradable material use in the ureter [19]. In a canine model, 4 cm of the mid-ureter in six animals was exchanged for a polylactic acid graft. Eight months post-procedure, four animals demonstrated renal dysfunction secondary to obstructing graft fragments raising concerns about the consequences of unpredictable graft degradation. Another early study with more favorable results utilized a polyglycolic acid tube for stenting a canine following a ureter ureterostomy procedure [20]. The diameter of this stent expanded after insertion to avoid stent migration and it demonstrated comparable flow characteristics to a silastic control stent and degraded by day 7 with no incidence of upper tract obstruction. This study provided in vivo evidence that biodegradable ureteric stents could be safely used while avoiding a secondary procedure for stent removal.

Schlick and Planz conducted the first in vitro work looking at controlling stent degradation based on urinary pH [21, 22]. Stents were composed of experimental plastic biodegradable material designated G100X-15LB and G100X-20LB. In their initial study [21], these stents were placed in artificial urine of varying pH and assessed at periodic time intervals for one month. At pH <7 the stents were stable, but when pH was raised >7 the stents degraded within 48 hours. The second study [22] utilized an experimental ureter model whereby a 30-cm-long plastic biodegradable stent was placed into an infusion set to ensure flow of solution during dissolution. At pH 7.9 all stents dissolved within 20 hours with no evidence of flow obstruction.

The idea that urinary pH may be pharmacologically manipulated to activate stent degradation after desired dwell time is compelling as this may allow one stent design to address a variety of clinical scenarios. However, in practice, stent degradation based on an alkaline urinary pH may prove problematic. Many uropathogens raise urinary pH, which could trigger early degradation. On the other side, pharmacologically raising urinary pH may increase infections for those bacteria known to proliferate in more alkaline urine and may even promote certain types of stone formation (i.e., calcium phosphate, struvite) [23, 24]. It may be for these reasons, and also the difficulty of getting a clinically significant rise in urinary pH pharmacologically, that in vivo studies have not been undertaken.

Polylactic acid stents have been evaluated. Lumiaho *et al.* conducted experiments on a short, expandable, double-helical, self-reinforced biodegradable polylactic acid stent [25–27]. This stent demonstrated favorable drainage characteristics and anti-reflux properties with similar biocompatibility to biostable stents; however, stent degradation was unpredictable with a significant amount of fragments remaining in the ureter at 12 weeks [27]. Polylactic acid stents have also been utilized in canine models of ureteric trauma [28, 29]. In these studies, the stents were designed as simple tubes, and like many biodegradable stents, were designed to expand in diameter by approximately 25% in vivo helping to secure them in place to prevent migration and increase the inner luminal diameter. Urinary flow was preserved, no calcium deposition occurred, and there were no cases of obstruction or stent migration in these studies. There was, however, a trend toward increased inflammatory reaction as well as unpredictable degradation with stent fragments remaining at 120 days post insertion in some cases [28]. Despite this, the biodegradable stent seems effective in treating ureteral injury and may be more advantageous than a biostable stent as there was no need for removal, no encrustation, no reflux of urine in the partial design, and possibly improved symptoms with no coil in the bladder [29].

Multiple authors have conducted studies based on biodegradable ureteral stents made of self-reinforced poly-L-lactic and poly-L-glycolic acid (SR-PLGA). Talja *et al.* assessed a horn-shaped SR-PLGA expandable, biodegradable ureteral stent in a single 37-year-old male with recurrent UPJ obstruction treated by antegrade endopyelotomy [15]. There were no early or late complications, the stent maintained urinary flow while the UPJ healed and at 18 months post stent insertion the UPJ was widely patent. The ability of biodegradable stents to avoid subsequent stent removal and limit complications in a human patient was demonstrated. Around the same time, Olweny *et al.* conducted an endopyelotomy porcine study on the horn-shaped SR-PLGA stent [14]. Favorable radiographic and flow characteristics were once again demonstrated. Unfortunately, these stents induced significant urothelial inflammation raising concerns of biocompatibility. Specifically, three of five animals had stent fragments incorporated into the urothelium and periureteral tissue showing foreign body reaction and inflammation. One animal even had stent fragments eroding into renal parenchyma. These stents were no longer pursued clinically for this reason.

PLGA has also been used in non-horned stent designs. Lumiaho *et al.* evaluated a shortened helical PLGA spiral ureteral stent in a porcine model [30]. This study demonstrated improved drainage and VUR compared to a biostable stent, but biocompatibility was not specifically evaluated. Similar stents have previously been used in the urethra with some success with drainage and compatibility [31] but further efforts are required to determine suitability for upper tract use in the clinical setting. In another study, Zhang *et al.* designed a 4.5 Fr braided thin-walled biodegradable ureteral stent made of a combination of polyglycolic acid and PLGA in a canine model [32]. A thin stent such as this may have applications in the pediatric world where a general anesthetic is often needed for the subsequent stent removal. Strong radial and tensile strength of the biodegradable stent contributed to good flow dynamics and straightforward insertion. All stents degraded by 4 weeks without obstruction or encrustation and histologic tissue reactivity was similar to control biostable stents.

Two groups of biodegradable ureteral stent studies warrant further attention: the Temporary Ureteral Drainage Stent™ (Boston Scientific Corporation, Natick, MA, USA) and the Uriprene™ stent (Poly-Med Inc, Anderson, SC, USA).

19.4 Temporary Ureteral Drainage Stent™

Lingeman *et al.* performed some of the earliest in vivo human trials with an alginate-polymer-based biodegradable ureteral stent known as the Temporary Ureteral Drainage Stent™ (TUDS, Boston Scientific) [16, 33]. This stent was designed as a short-term drainage solution with degradation and spontaneous passage after 48 hours. A pre-clinical swine model of the TUDS demonstrated ease of placement, safety, and similar histopathological changes compared to a commercially available biostable ureteral stent [34].

Phase I trials evaluating durability, patency and safety of the TUDS were conducted in 18 patients post percutaneous nephrolithotomy and looked promising [16]. Day 2 nephrostograms demonstrated ureteral patency in all stented ureters; however, only 11 stents were found to be completely intact at this point indicating premature degradation. All stent material had been removed from the body within 4 weeks with stent migration only occurring in 1 patient on day 2. There were no specific adverse events attributable to the TUDS in this study.

As a follow up to this study, a phase II trial of the TUDS was conducted in 88 patients following uncomplicated ureteroscopy [33]. The TUDS was found to provide adequate drainage for at least 48 hours post-operatively in only 78.2% of patients. Seventeen patients experienced stent extrusion from the upper urinary tract and two others needed active intervention prior to the 48-hour mark. Stents were eliminated at a median of 15 days with 84% of stents completely gone at one month. At 3 months, three patients underwent repeat procedures (shock-wave lithotripsy or ureteroscopy) for retained stent pieces in the renal pelvis.

These studies demonstrate that the TUDS facilitates urinary drainage with favourable tolerability and biocompatibility; however, the real concern about premature stent extrusion resulting in symptoms from obstruction and retained fragments that may serve as a nidus for stone development with need for subsequent and sometimes challenging procedures has limited its clinical use. Even so, these studies are of great value as they have advanced our understanding of biodegradable ureteral stents in the human urinary tract.

19.5 Uriprene^{TM}

Uriprene^{TM} ureteral stents show promise for clinical use (Figure 19.1) [17, 35, 36]. The stent is designed with more coating on the proximal end and less coating on the distal end; therefore, the bladder curl and portion that crosses the ureterovesical junction degrade first, which hypothetically should help avoid ureteral obstruction, may result in less VUR during voiding, decrease bladder infection and improve bladder symptoms.

The first iteration of the Uriprene^{TM} ureteral stent was tested in a pre-clinical porcine study. Stent degradation began at 4 weeks and took between 7 to 10 weeks to fully degrade [35]. This original version provided good drainage with decreased hydronephrosis, predictable degradation in a distal to proximal manner without obstruction. It provided excellent biocompatibility with no stent fragments incorporated into the urothelium and it decreased the incidence of positive urine cultures compared to biostable stents; however, the initial version of the Uriprene lacked axial rigidity making insertion over a regular PTFE wire difficult. It was most easily inserted through a 10Fr ureteral access sheath and preferably over a hydrophilic wire. There were also concerns regarding prolonged degradation time of 7-10 weeks.

The second- and third-generation Uriprene^{TM} stents were developed to maintain the benefits of this biodegradable material but also to degrade faster by altering the percentage of water-soluble polymer in the matrix and to be inserted easier over a regular PTFE wire without an access sheath owing to increased axial rigidity [17, 36]. Once wet, these stents have a very soft durometer, but still maintain their rigidity to provide urinary

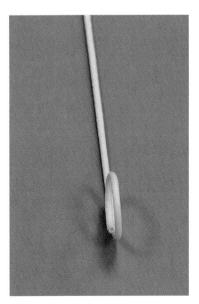
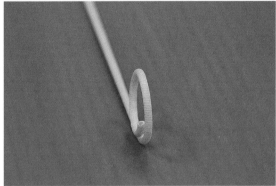

Figure 19.1 Uriprene^{TM} degradable ureteral stent. Source: Poly-Med Inc., Anderson, SC, USA. This stent is composed of three components: an inner coil, an overlaid mesh, and an external coating. Each component is made out of commonly used dissolving suture materials, specifically Glycolide, ε-caprolactone, and trimethylene carbonate. The coating is applied in a gradient fashion with more coating toward the kidney coil and less on the distal end to ensure that it degrades from the bladder end first. Pre-clinical animal studies have shown the stent degrades in 3–4 weeks after implantation. A first-in-human safety study is currently underway.

drainage. These stents were tested in porcine animal models and both generations degraded in a controlled manner without any obstruction from degrading fragments. The second-generation stent degraded by 7 weeks, whereas the third generation stent degraded within 2-4 weeks after implantation. Urinary drainage, determined by intravenous pyelogram, was equally effective compared to control biostable stents and no animal had obstruction from stent degradation. The greatest advantages were that the degradable stents resulted in significantly less inflammation on pathology and much less hydronephrosis compared to ureters stented with biostable stents. A safety pilot study is currently underway at our institution to determine the clinical feasibility of this novel stent.

19.6   Future Directions

Tissue engineered ureteral stents using autologous cells on absorbable scaffolds have been proposed [37, 38]. Conventional stents are recognized by the immune system as non-self and an inflammatory response follows. Stents coated with autologous tissues may bypass this inflammatory response and may be ideal for ureteral replacement/regeneration. This concept was experimentally demonstrated using autologous tissues on engineered biodegradable coronary stents that demonstrated tissue remodeling with collagen and fibroblasts in the stent walls after explantation rather than the typical inflammatory reaction [39]. Autologous chondrocytes and human adipose derived stem cells have been successfully incorporated into biodegradable material suitable for use in the ureter, but to date no human trials have commenced [37, 38].

Drug-eluting and stent-coating technologies have been incorporated on conventional stents, but application has been limited on biodegradable ureteral materials. Heparin, Paclitaxel, Triclosan, and Ketorolac drug-eluting biostable ureteral stents have shown decreased biofilm and stent encrustation, decreased inflammation, antibacterial effects, and a trend toward improved symptom control respectively [40–43]. It is possible that incorporation of these substances into biodegradable materials may prove beneficial, but this has not yet occurred. Preliminary studies investigating the feasibility of biodegradable polymers loaded with biologically active compounds have shown promising results with decreased protein and surface interactions resulting in improved biocompatibility while maintaining biodegradability [44, 45]. Further studies will be forthcoming.

Biodegradable metallic alloys show promise for use in the urinary tract. Lock *et al.* assessed degradation and antibacterial properties of magnesium alloys in artificial urine [46]. Full degradation characteristics are unknown but over a 3-day incubation period magnesium ion concentration in the artificial urine solution increased and as did urine pH. *Escherichia coli* viability and biofilm stent coverage were decreased when compared to biostable stents, which may translate to antimicrobial benefits; however, as other bacteria, such as *Proteus*, that flourish in alkaline environments, further research is warranted before this conclusion can be established.

19.7   Conclusion

Biodegradable stent designs continue to evolve. Benefits of these stents have already been demonstrated including eliminating the secondary procedure for removal, good flow dynamics, decreased stent encrustation, less VUR on those designs with early degradation or elimination of the bladder coil, less bacteruria, and possibly improved comfort. Unfortunately, these benefits have been offset by compatibility issues, unpredictable and inconsistent degradation, retained stent pieces necessitating further intervention, and design flaws making insertion challenging. Further research incorporating new materials, bioactive substances, and designs are needed before a commercially available biodegradable stent comes to market.

References

[1] Dyer RB, Chen MY, Zagoria RJ, Regan JD, Hood CG, Kavanagh PV. Complications of ureteral stent placement. Radiographics : a review publication of the Radiological Society of North America, Inc 2002;22(5):1005–1022. PubMed PMID: 12235330.

[2] Foreman D, Plagakis S, Fuller AT. Should we routinely stent after ureteropyeloscopy? BJU Int 2014;114 Suppl 1:6–8. PubMed PMID: 25070223.

[3] Liatsikos E, Kallidonis P, Stolzenburg JU, Karnabatidis D. Ureteral stents: past, present and future. Expert review of medical devices 2009;6(3):313–324. PubMed PMID: 19419288.

[4] Bhuiyan ZH, Bhuiyan NI, Khan SA, Tawhid MH, Islam MF. Forgotten urological stent. Mymensingh medical journal: MMJ 2011;20(4):632–639. PubMed PMID: 22081182.

[5] Lange D, Bidnur S, Hoag N, Chew BH. Ureteral stent-associated complications--where we are and where we are going. Nature reviews Urology 2015;12(1):17–25. PubMed PMID: 25534997.

[6] Atkins GG BS, LaBerge M, Dooley RL and Shalaby SW. Effect of surface-modified LPPE on bacterial attachment. Trans Soc Biomater 2001;24:507.

[7] El-Nahas AR, El-Assmy AM, Shoma AM, Eraky I, El-Kenawy MR, El-Kappany HA. Self-retaining ureteral stents: analysis of factors responsible for patients' discomfort. Journal of endourology/Endourological Society 2006;20(1):33–37. PubMed PMID: 16426130.

[8] Mosli HA, Farsi HM, al-Zimaity MF, Saleh TR, al-Zamzami MM. Vesicoureteral reflux in patients with double pigtail stents. The Journal of urology 1991;146(4): 966–969. PubMed PMID: 1895452.

[9] Kulkarni RK, Pani KC, Neuman C, Leonard F. Polylactic acid for surgical implants. Archives of surgery 1966;93(5):839–843. PubMed PMID: 5921307.

[10] Schmitt EaP, RA, inventorU.S. Patent 3,297,033. United States, 1967.

[11] Erbel R, Di Mario C, Bartunek J, Bonnier J, de Bruyne B, Eberli FR, *et al.* Temporary scaffolding of coronary arteries with bioabsorbable magnesium stents: a prospective, non-randomised multicentre trial. Lancet 2007;369(9576):1869–1875. PubMed PMID: 17544767.

[12] Kotsar A, Isotalo T, Juuti H, Mikkonen J, Leppiniemi J, Hanninen V, *et al.* Biodegradable braided poly(lactic-co-glycolic acid) urethral stent combined with dutasteride in the treatment of acute urinary retention due to benign prostatic enlargement: a pilot study. BJU Int 2009;103(5):626–629. PubMed PMID: 18990149.

[13] Lange D, Elwood CN, Chew BH. Biomaterials in Urology - Beyond Drug Eluting and Degradable - A Rational Approach to Ureteral Stent Design. In: Pignatello R, ed. Biomaterial - Physics and Chemistry. Rijeka, Croatia: InTech, 2011, pp 459–75.

[14] Olweny EO, Landman J, Andreoni C, Collyer W, Kerbl K, Onciu M, *et al.* Evaluation of the use of a biodegradable ureteral stent after retrograde endopyelotomy in a porcine model. The Journal of urology 2002;167(5):2198–2202. PubMed PMID: 11956478.

[15] Talja M, Multanen M, Valimaa T, Tormala P. Bioabsorbable SR-PLGA horn stent after antegrade endopyelotomy: a case report. Journal of endourology/Endourological Society 2002;16(5):299–302. PubMed PMID: 12184080.

[16] Lingeman JE, Schulsinger DA, Kuo RL. Phase I trial of a temporary ureteral drainage stent. Journal of endourology/Endourological Society 2003;17(3):169–171. PubMed PMID: 12803989.

[17] Chew BH, Lange D, Paterson RF, Hendlin K, Monga M, Clinkscales KW, *et al*. Next generation biodegradable ureteral stent in a yucatan pig model. The Journal of urology 2010;183(2):765–71. PubMed PMID: 20022028.

[18] Venkatesan N, Shroff S, Jayachandran K, Doble M. Polymers as ureteral stents. Journal of endourology/Endourological Society 2010;24(2):191–198. PubMed PMID: 20073560.

[19] Bergman S, Javadpour N, Wade C, Terrill R. Biodegradable ureteral grafts in dogs. Investigative urology 1978;16(1):48–49. PubMed PMID: 689837.

[20] Assimos DG, Smith C, Schaeffer AJ, Carone FA, Grayhack JT. Efficacy of polyglycolic acid (PGA) tubing stents in ureteroureterostomies. Urological research 1984;12(6):291–293. PubMed PMID: 6098061.

[21] Schlick RW, Planz K. Potentially useful materials for biodegradable ureteric stents. British journal of urology 1997;80(6):908–910. PubMed PMID: 9439407.

[22] Schlick RW, Planz K. In vitro results with special plastics for biodegradable endoureteral stents. Journal of endourology/Endourological Society 1998;12(5): 451–455. PubMed PMID: 9847069.

[23] Jones DS, Djokic J, Gorman SP. Characterization and optimization of experimental variables within a reproducible bladder encrustation model and in vitro evaluation of the efficacy of urease inhibitors for the prevention of medical device-related encrustation. Journal of biomedical materials research Part B, Applied biomaterials 2006;76(1):1–7. PubMed PMID: 16206254.

[24] Watterson JD, Cadieux PA, Stickler D, Reid G, Denstedt JD. Swarming of Proteus mirabilis over ureteral stents: a comparative assessment. Journal of endourology/ Endourological Society 2003;17(7):523–527. PubMed PMID: 14565887.

[25] Lumiaho J, Heino A, Tunninen V, Ala-Opas M, Talja M, Valimaa T, *et al*. New bioabsorbable polylactide ureteral stent in the treatment of ureteral lesions: an experimental study. Journal of endourology/Endourological Society 1999;13(2): 107–112. PubMed PMID: 10213104.

[26] Lumiaho J, Heino A, Pietilainen T, Ala-Opas M, Talja M, Valimaa T, *et al*. The morphological, in situ effects of a self-reinforced bioabsorbable polylactide (SR-PLA 96) ureteric stent; an experimental study. The Journal of urology 2000;164(4): 1360–1363. PubMed PMID: 10992415.

[27] Lumiaho J, Heino A, Kauppinen T, Talja M, Alhava E, Valimaa T, *et al*. Drainage and antireflux characteristics of a biodegradable self-reinforced, self-expanding X-ray-positive poly-L,D-lactide spiral partial ureteral stent: an experimental study. Journal of endourology/Endourological Society 2007;21(12):1559–1564. PubMed PMID: 18186698.

[28] Li G, Wang ZX, Fu WJ, Hong BF, Wang XX, Cao L, *et al*. Introduction to biodegradable polylactic acid ureteral stent application for treatment of ureteral war injury. BJU Int 2011;108(6):901–906. PubMed PMID: 21223480.

[29] Fu WJ, Wang ZX, Li G, Cui FZ, Zhang Y, Zhang X. Comparison of a biodegradable ureteral stent versus the traditional double-J stent for the treatment of ureteral injury: an experimental study. Biomedical materials 2012;7(6):065002. PubMed PMID: 23047290.

[30] Lumiaho J, Heino A, Aaltomaa S, Valimaa T, Talja M. A short biodegradable helical spiral ureteric stent provides better antireflux and drainage properties than a double-J stent. Scandinavian journal of urology and nephrology 2011;45(2):129–133. PubMed PMID: 21222571.

[31] Kotsar A, Isotalo T, Mikkonen J, Juuti H, Martikainen PM, Talja M, *et al*. A new biodegradable braided self-expandable PLGA prostatic stent: an experimental study in the rabbit. Journal of endourology/Endourological Society 2008;22(5):1065–1069. PubMed PMID: 18643724.

[32] Zhang MQ, Zou T, Huang YC, Shang YF, Yang GG, Wang WZ, *et al*. Braided thin-walled biodegradable ureteral stent: preliminary evaluation in a canine model. International journal of urology : official journal of the Japanese Urological Association 2014;21(4):401–407. PubMed PMID: 24147536.

[33] Lingeman JE, Preminger GM, Berger Y, Denstedt JD, Goldstone L, Segura JW, *et al*. Use of a temporary ureteral drainage stent after uncomplicated ureteroscopy: results from a phase II clinical trial. The Journal of urology 2003;169(5):1682–1688. PubMed PMID: 12686808.

[34] Auge BK, Ferraro RF, Madenjian AR, Preminger GM. Evaluation of a dissolvable ureteral drainage stent in a Swine model. The Journal of urology 2002;168(2):808–812. PubMed PMID: 12131372.

[35] Hadaschik BA, Paterson RF, Fazli L, Clinkscales KW, Shalaby SW, Chew BH. Investigation of a novel degradable ureteral stent in a porcine model. The Journal of urology 2008;180(3):1161–1166. PubMed PMID: 18639278.

[36] Chew BH, Paterson RF, Clinkscales KW, Levine BS, Shalaby SW, Lange D. In vivo evaluation of the third generation biodegradable stent: a novel approach to avoiding the forgotten stent syndrome. The Journal of urology 2013;189(2):719–725. PubMed PMID: 22982432.

[37] Shi JG, Fu WJ, Wang XX, Xu YD, Li G, Hong BF, *et al*. Tissue engineering of ureteral grafts by seeding urothelial differentiated hADSCs onto biodegradable ureteral scaffolds. Journal of biomedical materials research Part A. 2012;100(10):2612–2622. PubMed PMID: 22615210.

[38] Amiel GE, Yoo JJ, Kim BS, Atala A. Tissue engineered stents created from chondrocytes. The Journal of urology 2001;165(6 Pt 1):2091–2095. PubMed PMID: 11371934.

[39] Nakayama Y, Zhou YM, Ishibashi-Ueda H. Development of in vivo tissue-engineered autologous tissue-covered stents (biocovered stents). Journal of artificial organs : the official journal of the Japanese Society for Artificial Organs 2007;10(3):171–176. PubMed PMID: 17846716.

[40] Krambeck AE, Walsh RS, Denstedt JD, Preminger GM, Li J, Evans JC, *et al*. A novel drug eluting ureteral stent: a prospective, randomized, multicenter clinical trial to evaluate the safety and effectiveness of a ketorolac loaded ureteral stent. The Journal of urology 2010;183(3):1037–1042. PubMed PMID: 20092835.

[41] Chew BH, Cadieux PA, Reid G, Denstedt JD. In-vitro activity of triclosan-eluting ureteral stents against common bacterial uropathogens. Journal of endourology/ Endourological Society 2006;20(11):949–958. PubMed PMID: 17144870.

[42] Cauda F, Cauda V, Fiori C, Onida B, Garrone E. Heparin coating on ureteral Double J stents prevents encrustations: an in vivo case study. Journal of endourology/ Endourological Society 2008;22(3):465–472. PubMed PMID: 18307380.

[43] Liatsikos EN, Karnabatidis D, Kagadis GC, Rokkas K, Constantinides C, Christeas N, *et al*. Application of paclitaxel-eluting metal mesh stents within the pig ureter: an experimental study. European urology 2007;51(1):217–223. PubMed PMID: 16814926.

[44] Brauers A, Thissen H, Pfannschmidt O, Bienert H, Foerster A, Klee D, *et al.* Development of a biodegradable ureteric stent: surface modification and in vitro assessment. Journal of endourology/Endourological Society 1997;11(6):399–403. PubMed PMID: 9440847.

[45] Kotsar A, Nieminen R, Isotalo T, Mikkonen J, Uurto I, Kellomaki M, *et al.* Biocompatibility of new drug-eluting biodegradable urethral stent materials. Urology 2010;75(1):229–234. PubMed PMID: 19647295.

[46] Lock JY, Wyatt E, Upadhyayula S, Whall A, Nunez V, Vullev VI, *et al.* Degradation and antibacterial properties of magnesium alloys in artificial urine for potential resorbable ureteral stent applications. Journal of biomedical materials research Part A 2014;102(3):781–792. PubMed PMID: 23564415.

20

Metallic Ureteric Stents

Ravi Kulkarni

Consultant Urological Surgeon, Ashford and St Peter's Hospitals NHS Foundation Trust, Chertsey, Surrey, UK

20.1 Introduction

The use of metals in surgery dates back to the sixteenth century. The use of gold plates and wires for the repairs of skull fractures was described by Ambroise Pare' in 1546 [1, 2]. Petronius described the use of gold plates for the repair of the cleft palate in 1565. Other metals such as iron, steel, bronze, and subsequently, alloys found their way in surgical practice – mostly in orthopedics. The first use of iron in the fixation of fractures was reported in 1775 [1].

The initial use of metal in the manufacture of stents was in cardiology. A metallic coronary stent was implanted into a patient by Jacques Puel in Toulouse, France on March 28, 1986. They used the term endo-prothèses coronariennes autoexpansives for this device [5]. The natural evolution of this concept has been its adoption in urology for the disobstruction of urethra, prostate, and finally, the ureter.

20.2 Which Metal?

The essential characteristics of any metal to be suitable for the use in human body are its bio-functionality and bio-compatibility [1]. The former refers to the physical properties of the metal that enable it to perform the desired function. The latter relates to the interaction between the metal and the body fluids or tissues. Most metals were found to be unsuitable after the initial enthusiasm.

Ductility, malleability, the ease of molding into suitable shapes, and resistance to compression make metals attractive as stent material. Wider lumen stents created from metals provide better drainage and are likely to stay patent for a longer period of time [3].

However, metallic devices implanted in human body have an important disadvantage. They interact with the tissue fluids and corrode. Corrosion is defined as an interaction between a base metal and its surrounding medium such as liquid or gas. With the exception of the noble metals, this process is inevitable, especially in the urinary tract [1].

Corrosion is rapid when a metal is in contact with an ionic solution. The speed and susceptibility to this process varies between metals – the most noble metals such as gold and platinum show less propensity to corrosion as compared with iron [1].

Ureteric Stenting, First Edition. Edited by Ravi Kulkarni.
© 2017 John Wiley & Sons Ltd. Published 2017 by John Wiley & Sons Ltd.

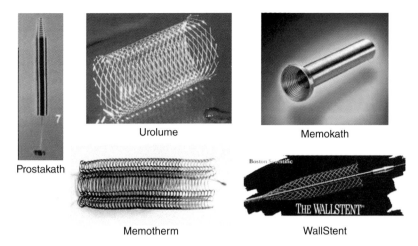

Prostakath

Urolume   Memokath

Memotherm   WallStent

Figure 20.1 Metallic prostatic stents.

The process slows down if the metal is covered with an oxide film [4]. Alloys, as opposed to pure metals, often exhibit different levels of resistance to corrosion. This feature is of considerable significance in urological stents as the human urine is not only ionically rich but also has a variable pH. Both can accelerate corrosion.

Stainless steel was used in the initial versions of urological stents. Fabian's Urological Spiral urethral stent was made from steel [4]. This metal has several disadvantages. Apart from the susceptibility to corrosion and tissue reaction, fragmentation of the material occurred relatively quickly and this reduced its longevity.

Alternative metals such as gold, chromium, and subsequently, alloys were used in the manufacture of urological stents. The Prostakath stent (Figure 20.1) was one of the first such stents which was gold plated [4]. The Urolume prostatic stent made from a complex alloy called Elgiloy, which is a mixture of cobalt, chromium, nickel, molybdenum, iron, and traces of manganese, carbon, silicon phosphorus, sulphur, and berrylium [5].

The next metal selected for the manufacture of stents was titanium. This was followed by newer stents made from its natural successor – NiTinol – the alloy of nickel and titanium [4]. This alloy has many features, which make it unique in the manufacture of urological equipment. Apart from its strength, it is light and can be moulded to fine yet smooth wires. Many devices in the current urological practice such as guidewires and Dormia baskets are made from this alloy.

The initial application of metallic urological stents was in the management of urethral strictures [4]. This concept was extended in the manufacturing of prostatic and subsequently ureteric stents.

The rapid development in the use of metallic stents in the management of coronary and the peripheral vascular disease [4] has been a catalyst in the extension of the concept in urological practice.

The first ureteric stent that entered clinical practice was the Wallstent [6, 7]. Made from stainless steel, the cylindrical segmental stent was designed for insertion in the ureter in both, retrograde as well as an antegrade manner. It was successful in relieving upper tract obstruction caused by malignancy; however, the initial decompression of the obstructed segment was not maintained. Tumor in-growth through the fenestrations of the stent led to re-obstructions in the patients with malignant ureteric obstruction [7, 8]. Removal of these stents proved difficult. However, this stent opened the door to the development of other metallic stents. The principle development was the use of alloys, which have superior bio-compatibility as well as malleability which led to the creation of different designs.

20.3 Other Metallic Ureteric Stents

20.3.1 Memotherm

This NiTinol wire stent was introduced in 1998 by Angiomed (Karlsruhe, Germany). Made from a tightly coiled wire of this alloy, the stent is placed across the narrow segment of the ureter. Its thermal memory is activated to allow expansion to its pre-determined shape. Early experience suggested its efficacy in relieving ureteric obstruction [9–11]. However, these studies were small and had a short-term follow-up. No new studies have been published since the initial experience.

20.3.2 Memokath 051

PNN (formerly Engineers and Doctors, Denmark) developed this stent in 1996. This stent is also made from a variant of the alloy, NiTinol. A special manufacturing process gives the alloy a unique thermal shape memory. If heated to a prespecified temperature, the metal moulds itself into a predesigned shape and becomes hard. It becomes soft when cooled below 10 °C. This property can be utilized to unravel the coiled stent and extract it from the ureter, if necessary.

A wire made from this alloy is tightly coiled into a funnel-shaped stent. The pre-expanded stent is mounted on a catheter. A separate plastic catheter split at its distal end (the lugs) traverses through the lumen of the stent to support its distal end. Its lugs, kept apart by a guidewire, lock the un-expanded stent during the insertion process (Figure 20.2, 20.3, and 20.4).

This stent is inserted into the ureter through a 14 FG introducer sheath. The sheath and its core catheter act as dilator as well as the conduit for the delivery of the un-expanded stent. The stent assembly and the sheath form a set and must be used as a single unit.

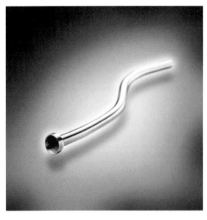

Memokath 051

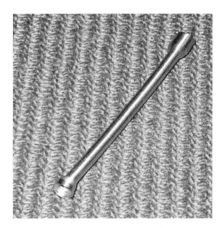

Memokath duel expansion

Figure 20.2 Memokath 051 stents.

The un-expanded stent is inserted into the ureter after the dilatation of the stricture segment. Pre-heated saline or water at 55 °C is injected to induce expansion of the stent to its redetermined shape. It is important to mark the stricture limits with suitable radio-opaque markers placed on the abdominal wall to ensure the placement of the stent in the correct segment of the ureter.

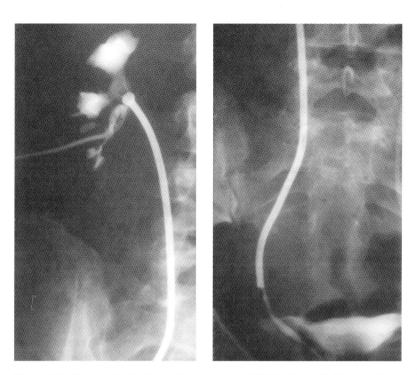

Figure 20.3 Memokath stent in malignant stricture 37 F. Ca Breast. Solitary functioning kidney, total ureteric obstruction. 22 cm Memokath.

(a)   (b)

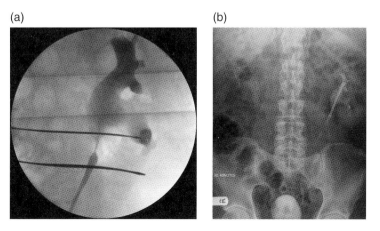

Figure 20.4 Memokath stent in benign stricgture a) Iatrogenic injury at PUJ Solitary kidney b) IVU 1 year after stent insertion.

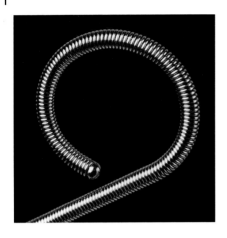

Figure 20.5 Resonance Stent.

Memokath 051 stent is available in fixed lengths: 30, 60, 100, 150, and 200 mm. Longer versions can be manufactured if necessary.

Once expanded, the shaft has a diameter of 10.5FG and the proximal fluted end reaches a width of 21FG.

A duel expansion version has wide ends on either side too is available.

The short- as well as long-term outcomes in the management of malignant and recurrent benign strictures appear to be satisfactory [12–14]. These stents have been effective in the treatment of benign ureteric strictures caused by conditions such as retro-peritoneal fibrosis and renal transplantation [15–17]. They have also found a place in paediatric practice with moderate success [18].

Migration and encrustation can develop and has been reported in 1 to 8% of patients [14, 19, 20]. Prohibitive cost has prevented its widespread use.

20.3.3   Resonance

Introduced in 2007 by Cook (Cook Medical, Bloomington, IN, USA), this solid metal JJ stent is made from an alloy of nickel, cobalt, chromium and molybdenum [21] (Figure 20.5). It has a diameter of 6FG and is available in a variety of lengths from 20 to 30 cm. Introduced in the ureter through a dedicated 8FG access sheath, it curls at both ends when the sheath is withdrawn [21].

This stent has no lumen. It is believed to function on the principle that the urine will flow alongside the stent.

The relief of upper tract obstruction achieved by the Resonance stent is variable. Initial improvement in the drainage in all patients [21] is not sustained. Failure rates from 35-50% have been reported [22, 23]. The results are disappointing in pediatric population [24]. A high failure rate due to migration has been reported in ileal conduits [25].

20.3.4   Allium

This segmental ureteric stent (Allium Medical, Israel) is made from a NiTinol wire, sandwiched between strips of a polymer. This strip of the combined material is moulded into a cylindrical-shaped stent (Figure 20.6). It is available in two diameters of 24 and 26 FG and in the lengths of 100 and 120 mm. Its caudal end is designed to remain in the urinary bladder. It is delivered in to the ureter through a sheath, which has a diameter of 8FG or 10FG. Once in place, the sheath is withdrawn to release and expand the stent.

(a)

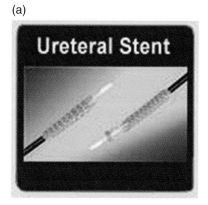

(b)   (c)   (d)

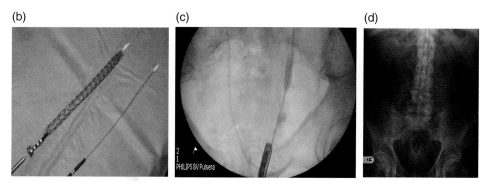

Figure 20.6 a) Allium Stent b) Allium Ureteric Stent c) Ureteric obstruction due to Ca prostate d) Allium stent in-situ for 18 months.

The connections between the composite strips are like a postage stamp and can come apart when the distal end of the stent is pulled. Therefore, the stent, when removed, comes out in the shape of a tape.

This stent too can be inserted in a retrograde as well as an antegrade manner.

Limited published data prevents adequate evaluation of this stent. Satisfactory outcomes have been reported in small series published [26, 27].

20.3.5 Uventa

This stent (Figure 20.7 and 20.8) is manufactured (Taewoong medical, Korea) from NiTinol wire mesh, which is reinforced with a PTFE membrane. The stent is made in three layers: two layers of NiTinol wire mesh are separated by a layer of PTFE. The distal end of the stent has small threads attached to the PTFE coat. These are designed for the extraction of the stent.

The stent is mounted on a delivery system in a compressed form. The two ends of the stent as well as its midpoint are identified with radio opaque markers. Both the central (hollow) metallic support as well as the side port can be used for the injection of saline or contrast. The assembly is locked by a screw mechanism, which needs to be released before deployment.

The stents is available in lengths of 30, 60, 100, and 120 mm. After an initial retrograde pyelogram, the stent is inserted into the ureter over a guidewire. Once the exact position is confirmed, it can be released by withdrawing the external sheath. The stent

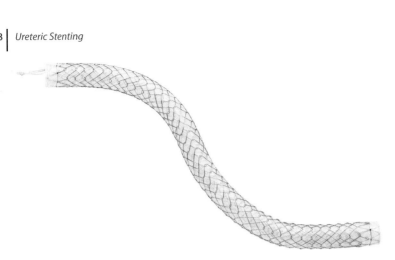

Figure 20.7 Uventa Ureteric Stent.

(a)   (b)   (c)

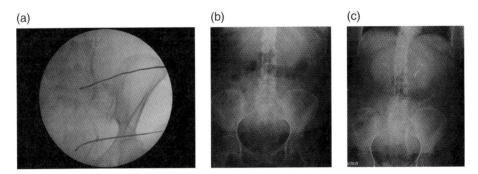

Figure 20.8 Uventa Ureteric Stent a) Left ureteric stricture Recurrent colonic carcinoma b) KUB x ray c) IVU 3 months after stent insertion.

will be released instantly. Multiple stents can be deployed in the same ureter if strictures are located in different areas. An overlap of the stents is suggested. The lumen of the stent opens wide after a period of time.

Published literature suggests good patency rates and ease of insertion. In a series of 54 patients with malignant ureteric obstruction, an overall 81.7% patency rate has been reported [28, 29].

20.3.6 Other Metallic Stents

Another metallic ureteric stent entered transiently during the last decade. The Passager stent (Boston Scientific) had very few published trials. The results were unsatisfactory due to migration of the stent [30–32].

20.4 Results

Segmental metallic stents have been purported to have several advantages over the conventional JJ stents and are also cost effective [3, 29]. The main advantages include longer patency rates and less frequent changes, which leads to cost savings and lack of interruption during other treatments such as radiation or chemotherapy, and so on.

The majority of the stents in this category are segmental. This feature has some advantages. These stents do not traverse the ureteric orifice, and therefore, the patient is spared the bladder irritation – an inevitable consequence of a JJ stent. This improves the quality of life [12–14, 35].

The inherent strength of the metal resists compression, and therefore, patency is unlikely to be compromised. As they provide superior patency rates, early deployment is advantageous [31]. Longer patency rates may reduce the need for frequent stent changes which is translated in cost saving as well as reduction in patient inconvenience [29, 33, 34].

20.4.1 Migration of Metallic Stents

The issue of stent migration is addressed in another section of this book. Metallic stents are not immune from migration. Complete or incomplete, migration leads to recurrence of obstruction. As the segmental stents occupy a part of the ureter, migration can occur in either direction [12]. Even a small degree of movement of the stent can lead to rapid re-occlusion of the ureter. There often is a paucity of symptoms with migration. This can lead to delay in detection and potential loss of renal function.

Retrieval and replacement of migrated metallic stents can be challenging. A full assessment of the renal unit along with its functional status, presence of sepsis and the access to the migrated stents needs to be evaluated before attempts are made to remove such a stent. A proximal access in the form of a nephrostomy tube is advantageous. Stent specific and modified endourological techniques may be needed to remove and replace such stents [36]. This issue is addressed in another chapter of this book.

20.4.2 Encrustation

No stent is immune from encrustation. The potential for encrustation increases with longer indwelling times [37]. This can occur in various forms with metallic stents. The severity can vary from a simple powdery coating of the stent surface to a total occlusion. Detection of encrustation can be difficult and deceptive. Plain x-ray is often unhelpful as the calcification may be masked by the metallic design. Contrast as well as functional imaging with renography is essential. Regular endoscopic evaluation has been suggested in patients with benign disease where the stent may be left in situ for long periods of time.

Removing encrustations or the stent itself can be difficult. Conventional methods such as lithoclast and laser fragmentation can be deployed to remove the calcification prior to the removal of the stent. These may prove difficult. Laser also has the potential of fragmenting the metallic elements of the stent, which can make removal more difficult.

20.4.3 Endothelial Hyperplasia

Tissue reaction is frequently observed at the interface between an indwelling stent and the urothelium. Metallic stents too have been shown to develop this problem, both in animal studies [38] as well as humans [39]. Long-standing ureteric stents have been known to cause secondary occlusion due to such urothelial hyperplasia. The two ends of a metallic stent can induce such reaction to a variable extent. This depends on the material of the stent and the host response.

20.4.4 Impacted Metallic Stents

Occluded and impacted metallic stents present a unique challenge. Such stents are usually indwelling for long periods of time. The presentation is often due to obstruction, infection, or a combination of the two. Deterioration of renal function in a solitary kidney will suggest occlusion.

Removal of such stents needs careful planning. The insertion of a nephrostomy tube at the outset is a useful. This allows the urologist a proximal access for endourological maneuvers. Manufacturers' instructions about the removal need to be heeded as each stent has different mechanical properties. Potential for trauma to the ureteric wall is significant and removal may prove impossible. Alternatives such as a JJ stent through the lumen of the existing device, permanent nephrostomy drainage, or a suitable diversion should be considered.

20.5 Cost

The complexity of design, materials used in the manufacture, the need for additional delivery systems required for the insertion escalates the cost of metallic stents. Although there is variation in the pricing structure of stents from country to country, there is a significant difference between the cost of a JJ stent and a metallic stent. The difference can be between 5 to 20 times.

The longevity of an indwelling metallic stent reduces the need for change and results in cost saving to the healthcare system. This may counter-balance the higher initial cost [39–41].

Improvement of quality of life due to the lack of irritative symptoms can enhance performance and reduce time off work thus resulting in economic and personal gain.

20.6 Current Status

Metallic ureteric stents offer many advantages over the conventional JJ stents. Higher patency rates, longer indwelling times, reduction in stent-related morbidity, and improvement in the quality of life have been reported. However, these need to be balanced against the higher cost, complexity of insertion, and difficulties during removal. Single center experience, small patient numbers, and the lack of randomised multicenter trials preclude adequate evaluation of these devices.

The current literature suggests they are beneficial in the management of malignant ureteric strictures. The role in benign strictures is less well defined. Although the longer periods of patency offer an advantage over the conventional JJ stents, their propensity for encrustation and migration, especially when left indwelling for longer duration, is likely to result in recurrent ureteric obstruction.

They undoubtedly play an important role in the management of ureteric strictures. Natural evolution, such as drug-eluting stents perhaps hold the key to their more definitive role in the future.

References

[1] Gotman I. Characteristics of materials used in implants: metals. In: Stenting the Urinary System, 2 ed, 2004, pp 61–72.

[2] Thurston AJ. Paré and prosthetics: the early history of artificial limbs. ANZ J Surg 2007;77(12):1114–1119.

[3] Hendlin K, Korman E, Monga M. New metallic ureteral stents: improved tensile strength and resistance to extrinsic compression. J Endourol 2012;26(3):271–274.

[4] Mattelaer JJ. History of ureteral and urethral stenting. In: Stenting the Urinary System, 2 ed, 2004, pp 17–24.

[5] Summary of safety and effectiveness data. AMS. March 2014. Available at: www.accessdata.fda.gov/cdrh_docs (accessed 15 October 2016).

[6] Roguin, A. Historical Perspectives in Cardiology. Circulation: Cardiovascular Interventsions 2011;(4):206–209.

[7] Wallsten H. Stenting the Urinary System, 2 ed, 2004, pp 31–38.

[8] Pauer W, Lugmayr H, Urologe A. Self-expanding permanent endoluminal stents in the ureter: 5 years results and critical evaluation. ANZ J Surg 1996;35(6):485–489.

[9] Pandian SS, Hussey JK, McClinton S. Metallic ureteric stents: early experience. Br J Urol 1998;82(6):791–797.

[10] Sibert L, Cherif M, Lauzanne P, Tanneau Y, Caremel R, Grise P. Prospective study of the treatment of localised ureteric strictures by wire mesh stent. Prog Urol 2007;17(2):219–224.

[11] Pauer W, Eckerstorfer GM. Use of self-expanding permanent endoluminal stents for benign ureteral strictures: mid-term results. J Urol 1999;162(2):319–322.

[12] Kulkarni RP, Bellamy EA. A new thermo-expandable shape-memory nickel-titanium alloy stent for the management of ureteric strictures. BJU Int 1999;83(7):755–759.

[13] Kulkarni R, Bellamy E. Nickel-titanium shape memory alloy Memokath 051 ureteral stent for managing long-term ureteral obstruction: 4-year experience. J Urol 2001;166(5):1750–1754.

[14] Agrawal S, Brown CT, Bellamy EA, Kulkarni R. The thermo-expandable metallic ureteric stent: an 11-year follow-up. BJU Int 2009;103(3):372–376.

[15] Bourdoumis A, Kachrilas S, Kapoor S, Zaman F, Papadopoulos G, Buchholz N, Masood J. The use of a thermoexpandable metal alloy stent in the minimally invasive management of retroperitoneal fibrosis: a single center experience from the United kingdom. J Endourol 2014;28(1):96–99.

[16] Bach C, Kabir MN, Goyal A, Malliwal R, Kachrilas S, El Howairis ME, Masood J, Buchholz N, Junaid I. A self-expanding thermolabile nitinol stent as a minimally invasive treatment alternative for ureteral strictures in renal transplant patients. J Endourol. 2013;27(12):1543–1545.

[17] Boyvat F, Aytekin C, Colak T, Firat A, Karakayali H, Haberal M. Memokath metallic stent in the treatment of transplant kidney ureter stenosis or occlusion. Cardiovasc Intervent Radiol 2005;28(3):326–330.

[18] Kamata S, Usui N, Kamiyama M, Yoneda A, Tazuke Y, Ooue T. Application of memory metallic stents to urinary tract disorders in pediatric patients. J Pediatr Surg 2005;40(3):E43–E45.

[19] Klarskov P, Nordling J, Nielsen JB. Experience with Memokath 051 ureteral stent. Scand J Urol Nephrol 2005;39(2):169–172.

[20] Papatsoris AG, Buchholz N. A novel thermo-expandable ureteral metal stent for the minimally invasive management of ureteral strictures. J Endourol 2010;24(3):487–491.

[21] Rao MV, Polcari AJ, Turk TMT. Updates on the use of ureteral stents: focus on the Resonance® stent. Med Devices (Auckl) 2011;4:11–15.

[22] Abbasi A, Wyre HW, Ogan K. Use of full-length metallic stents in malignant ureteral obstruction. J Endourol 2013;27(5):640–645.

[23] Goldsmith ZG, Wang AJ, Bañez LL, Lipkin ME, Ferrandino MN, Preminger GM, Inman BA. Outcomes of metallic stents for malignant ureteral obstruction. J Urol 2012;188(3):851–855.

[24] Gayed BA, Mally AD, Riley J, Ost MC. Resonance metallic stents do not effectively relieve extrinsic ureteral compression in pediatric patients. J Endourol 2013;27(2):154–157.

[25] Garg T, Guralnick ML, Langenstroer P, See WA, Hieb RA, Rilling WS, Sudakoff GS, O'Connor RC. Resonance metallic ureteral stents do not successfully treat ureteroenteric strictures. J Endourol 2009;23(7):1199–1201.

[26] Moskovitz B, Halachmi S, Nativ O. A new self-expanding, large-caliber ureteral stent: results of a multicenter experience. J Endourol 2012;26(11):1523–1527.

[27] Leonardo C, Salvitti M, Franco G, De Nunzio C, Tuderti G, Misuraca L, Sabatini I, De Dominicis C. Allium stent for treatment of ureteral stenosis. Minerva Urol Nefrol 2013;65(4):277–283.

[28] Chung KJ, Park BH, Park B, Lee JH, Kim WJ, Baek M, Han DH. Efficacy and safety of a novel, double-layered, coated, self-expandable metallic mesh stent (Uventa™) in malignant ureteral obstructions. J Endourol 2013;27(7):930–935.

[29] Fiuk J, Bao Y2, Calleary JG3, Schwartz BF1, Denstedt JD. The use of internal stents in chronic ureteral obstruction. J Urol 2015;193(4):1092–1100.

[30] Elsamra SE, Leavitt DA, Motato HA, Friedlander JI, Siev M, Keheila M, Hoenig DM, Smith AD, Okeke Z. Stenting for malignant ureteral obstruction: Tandem, metal or metal-mesh stents. Int J Urol 2015;22(7):629–636.

[31] Kim KH, Cho KS, Ham WS, Hong SJ, Han KS. Early application of permanent metallic mesh stent in substitution for temporary polymeric ureteral stent reduces unnecessary ureteral procedures in patients with malignant ureteral obstruction. Urology 2015;86(3):459–464.

[32] Barbalias GA, Liatsikos EN, Kalogeropoulou C, Karnabatidis D, Zabakis P, Athanasopoulos A, Perimenis P, Siablis D. Externally coated ureteral metallic stents: an unfavorable clinical experience. Eur Urol 2002;42(3):276–280.

[33] Liatsikos EN, Siablis D, Kalogeropoulou C, Karnabatidis D, Triadopoulos A, Varaki L, Zabakis P, Perimenis P, Barbalias GA. Coated v noncoated ureteral metal stents: an experimental model. J Endourol 2001;15(7):747–751.

[34] Baumgarten AS, Hakky TS, Carrion RE, Lockhart JL, Spiess PE. A single-institution experience with metallic ureteral stents: a cost-effective method of managing deficiencies in ureteral drainage. Int Braz J Urol 2014;40(2):225–231.

[35] Joshi HB, Newns N, Stainthorpe A, MacDonagh RP, Keeley FX Jr, Timoney AG. Ureteral stent symptom questionnaire: development and validation of a multidimensional quality of life measure. J Urol 2003;169(3):1060–1064.

[36] Kachroo N, Simpson AD. A novel approach for removing an intra-renal migrated Memokath™ stent. Int J Surg Case Rep 2013;4(10):866–868.

[37] Chew BH, Lange D. Re: ureteral stent encrustation, incrustation, and coloring: morbidity related to indwelling times. J Endourol 2013;27(4):506.

[38] Nishino S, Goya N, Ishikawa N, Tomizawa Y, Toma H. An experimental study of self-expanding ureteric metallic stents: macroscopic and microscopic changes in the canine ureter. BJU Int 2002;90(7):730–735.

[39] Liatsikos EN, Kagadis GC, Barbalias GA, Siablis D. Ureteral metal stents: a tale or a tool? J Endourol 2005;19(8):934–939.

[40] Taylor ER, Benson AD, Schwartz BF. Cost analysis of metallic ureteral stents with 12 months of follow-up. J Endourol 2012;26(7):917–921.

[41] Baumgarten AS, Hakky TS, Carrion RE, Lockhart JL, Spiess PE. A single-institution experience with metallic ureteral stents: a cost-effective method of managing deficiencies inureteral drainage. Int Braz J Urol 2014;40(2):225–231.

21

Removal of Ureteric Stents

Ravi Kulkarni

Consultant Urological Surgeon, Ashford and St Peter's Hospitals NHS Foundation Trust, Chertsey, Surrey, UK

21.1   Introduction

Ureteric stents are inserted for a wide variety of reasons. A definitive plan for the removal or its replacement is usually made after the procedure. This should include the timing and the method of removal. The practice of stent removal varies from country to country and is based on the availability of fiber-optic endoscopes, age of the patient, the type of stent, complexity envisaged, health economics, remuneration and above all, patient preference for topical or general anesthesia.

In the vast majority of patients, stents are deployed for a short-term decompression of the upper urinary tract. The removal of stents in this group of patients is usually decided at the time of insertion. The stent indwelling time is generally under 2 weeks [1]. Patients with recurrent benign ureteric strictures or malignancy are virtually stent-dependent. Removal of stents in these patients can only be considered if a suitable diversion is possible or the renal unit has lost its function when stent will not be necessary (Figure 21.1).

The timing of stent removal depends on many factors. The indication for the stent insertion is probably the most relevant. Stents inserted for the prevention of upper tract obstruction following ureteroscopy can be removed after a few days as the oedema subsides after about 48 hours. A short duration of stenting is generally recommended. Largely determined by local practice and logistics of the facilities for removal, a maximum of 14 days should be considered as adequate [2]. However, this may be prolonged in the presence of sepsis, bleeding, or iatrogenic urothelial trauma. The stent removal in patients with these complicating factors will have to be delayed until these have settled [3].

Conservative management of ureteric trauma usually involves the insertion of a JJ stent. Ureteric injury may heal if the continuity of the urothelium is established. This is encouraged with the placement of a ureteric stent. Stent indwelling time in these situations will vary from a few weeks to several months depending on the severity of trauma and the ancillary procedures undertaken at the time of repair such as suturing of the ureteric wall. Prior radiotherapy, heat damage caused by diathermy or ligasure may necessitate longer period of stenting as healing may be slow.

Ureteric Stenting, First Edition. Edited by Ravi Kulkarni.
© 2017 John Wiley & Sons Ltd. Published 2017 by John Wiley & Sons Ltd.

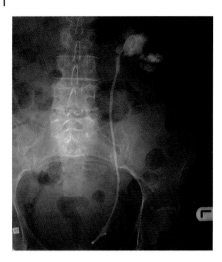

Figure 21.1 Imaging before stent removal. Heavily encrusted stent.

The responsibility of deciding the timing and the technique of stent removal rests in the hands of the urologist (or a radiologist) who inserts it. A plan to undertake the subsequent procedure – either of removal or a change of the stent – needs to be made after insertion. This will help to reduce the un-necessary prolonged periods of stenting and the related morbidity as well as the feared complication of a forgotten stent.

21.2   The Technique of JJ Stent Removal

The standard technique of a JJ stent removal is with the use of a cystoscope. This may be performed under general anesthesia with the use of a rigid cystoscope. The distal end of the stent is held in a biopsy forceps and the stent removed by a gentle pull.

This procedure is more frequently performed under local (topical) anesthesia with the use of a flexible cystoscope. This has many advantages. In addition to the avoidance of a general anaesthesia, it can be performed as a "walk-in-walk-out" procedure (office procedure), which avoids an unnecessary hospital admission. Although cost effective and efficient, this may not be suitable for all patients. Very young or nervous patients are unsuitable and should be offered the choice of a general anesthetic. Previous adverse complications and patient experience too may modify the choice of the technique [4]. Adequate counseling is essential. The use of a ureteroscope to remove stents under local anaesthesia has been described [5].

Imaging in the form of a simple KUB x-ray is advisable prior to removal of a stent that has been placed for a long time. Encrustation may be evident and such stents cannot be removed under local anaesthesia. Failure, patient discomfort, and the need for ancillary procedure can be predicted.

21.3   String on the Stent

Most manufacturers provide JJ stents with pre-attached nylon threads at the distal end. This has several advantages. The stent can be repositioned during insertion if pushed too high. These threads can be left attached to the distal end of the stent and

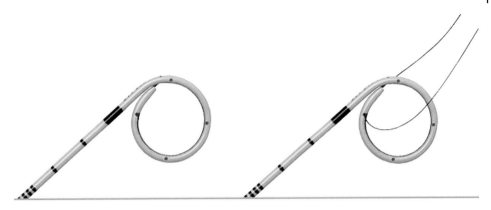

Figure 21.2 Stent on a string.

allowed to protrude through the urethral meatus in both sexes. The patient can be discharged from the hospital with the strings and brought back to the office or the clinic for the removal (Figure 21.2). A gentle pull will unfurl the coils and the stent is removed without resorting to any form of anesthesia. The patient may be instructed to remove the stent, if willing. Satisfactory outcomes with this technique have been described [6, 7].

This technique has many disadvantages. Many patients find this uncomfortable. Pain and anxiety may result in failure of removal. A second procedure may be needed. Patients often experience more pain than anticipated [8]. Snapping of the thread may cause further complications. Case reports where patients have mistaken the broken string for the stent resulting in a retained stent highlights a rare but an important complication of this method [9].

Stent on a string has been used at the end of a PCNL for the drainage of the ureter. A modification of the conventional technique has been described [10]. The stent is placed in an antegrade manner with the strings protruding through the tract in the loin. The stent is removed without anesthesia backward through the PCNL tract after a few days. This technique reduces the need for a separate nephrostomy drainage tube and a cystoscopy for the removal of the stent [11, 12].

21.4 Removal of Segmental and Metallic Stents

Segmental metallic stents need modifications to the conventional endourological techniques. These are often placed inside the ureter and cannot be accessed with a cystoscope. It is essential to familiarize with the recommendations of the manufacturer.

21.4.1 Memokath Stent

These thermo-expandable stents have a unique shape memory. The NiTinol wire used to design this stent softens at temperatures below 10C [13, 14]. Cold saline irrigation will help unravel the stent. The distal end of the stent is grasped in a suitable device, such as a biopsy or dedicated stent removal forceps. The stent can be removed by gentle traction on the wire. The unfurling will only occur if the metal remains below this stipulated

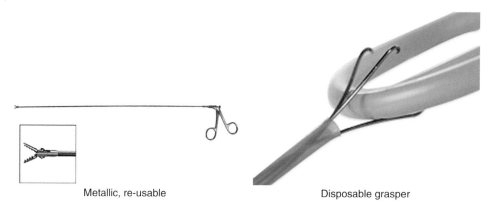

Metallic, re-usable   Disposable grasper

Figure 21.3 Stent removal forceps.

temperature. It is essential to keep the upper end of the stent cooled by continuous infu-sion of cold saline though a ureteric catheter, if necessary. This is important especially in the longer versions of the stent.

Encrusted and migrated Memokath stents are difficult to remove [15]. Clearance of the encrustation may be necessary before stent removal. Proximally migrated stents may require percutaneous removal.

Stents that have become embedded in the urothelium may not be accessible to the jaws of a biopsy forceps (Figures 21.3 and 21.4). Occlusive balloon such as Uromax® can be deployed inside the lumen of the stent (Figure 21.5). The entire assembly is gently dragged down after the expansion of the balloon. Once it is free it from the ureteric wall, it can be removed through a cystoscope.

21.4.2   UVENTA Stent

The distal end of this stent is relatively softer than the main section. This can be held in a suitable forceps. Traction on the stent helps to dislodge the stent from the ureteric wall. It can then be removed through a cystoscope [16, 17]. Stents placed in the ureter can be extracted in a similar manner by grabbing the distal end in a suitable forceps inserted through a ureteroscope.

21.4.3   Allium

This stent is made from a composite of a NiTinol wire sandwiched between two rib-bons of PTFE. This tape is shaped in a cylindrical shape. The two sides of the tape are attached to each other by tiny connections like a postage stamp. These come apart when the most distal end of the strip is pulled. The stent un-ravels and can be removed through the bladder with a cystoscope [18, 19]. There is a paucity of literature on the removal of this stent.

21.4.4   Resonance Stent

This solid metallic stent has curls like a conventional JJ stent on either side. They are designed to unfurl like a JJ stent when stretched. The removal therefore is very similar to that used for a JJ stent provided a suitable grasper is available [20, 21].

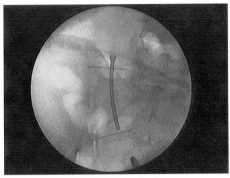

Stent approached
with ureteroscope

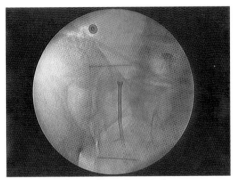

Un-ravelling of stent after
cooling

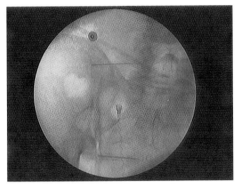

Near complete removal

Figure 21.4 Memokath stent removal.

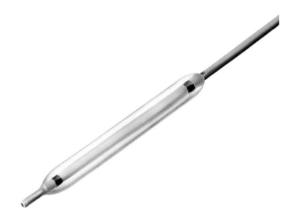

Figure 21.5 Uromax balloon.

Very little published literature gives insight to the technique and difficulties in removal of this stent. As the curves unwind, it can be removed through a cystoscope with the help of a suitable grasper. Modifications to the standard technique have been described [22]. Encrusted Resonance stents will require clearance of the deposits over the stent surface prior to extraction.

21.5   Other Stents

Extraanatomical stents such as Paterson Forrester and Detour stent removal and exchange has been addressed in other chapters. These are complex and need the expertise of an endourologist who has undertaken the insertion of such stents. These patients have difficult urological issues as well as other medical problems.

Careful consideration needs to be given to the choice of anesthesia during exchange of these stents.

Illuminating stents such as Uriglo are used to help identify the ureters during nonurological surgery. These should be removed as JJ stents at the end of the procedure. If ureteric trauma necessitates longer duration of stenting, they should be replaced by conventional JJ stents (Figure 21.6).

21.6   Technical Considerations

Although a straightforward procedure, the technique of stent removal deserves consideration. A JJ stent removed through a rigid cystoscope should be extracted through the sheath of the instrument. The removal of the cystoscope assembly along with the stent as a single unit results in trauma to the urethral epithelium.

The use of topical anesthesia in the form of gel is conventional. One percent lignocaine provides adequate pain relief. However, a 2% gel has been described as superior [23]. However, the merit of this practice has been questioned. Evaluation of pain and patient experience suggests that simple lubricating gel may be just as effective [24, 25]. In fact, some reports suggest more pain with the use of instillagel [26]. However, other studies suggest it is superior to simple lubricating gel or glycerine [27, 28].

Pain during cystoscopic removal of a stent can be variable. The use of more powerful agents such as sedation and inhaled nitrous oxide has been suggested [29, 30].

Adequate volume and contact time are important [31]. Injecting the gel slowly also helps [32]. The temperature of the gel should be given consideration. Pre-cooled gel at temperature below 4C has been shown to be more effective [33]. However, this benefit has been disputed by other studies [34]. Addition of other agents such as DMSO has been reported to be advantageous, especially in males [35]. The use of lignocaine spray

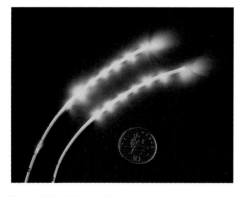
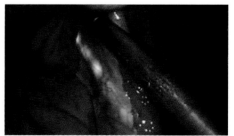

Figure 21.6 Uri-glow Stent.

around the external urethral meatus and the surrounding area in females has been reported to be equally effective [36].

Intra-vesical instillation of local anesthetic such as bupivacaine has been shown to be effective in the management of bladder neoplasms as well as painful bladder syndrome [37–39]. This has been used for stent removal, too.

The type of the grasper for the removal of the stent is based on personal preference. A standard bladder biopsy forceps may not be adequate as the grasp on the stent tip may not be firm. A dedicated stent removal forceps with teeth is superior as it has a better grasp. The use of flat-wire basket, three-pronged grasping forceps and magnets has been described. Various other techniques such as crochet hooks, as well as a snare too have been described [40].

Stents left with a nylon string attached to the distal coil can be removed by a gentle tug on the latter without resorting to the use of a cystoscope [7]. However, snapping of such strings may lead to retention of the stent as the patient may perceive the stent has been removed [41].

The practice of leaving a shorter segment of nylon string to the distal end of the stent helps stent removal as well as correction of malposition [42]. This may also render the stent for removal of alternative devices such as a hook.

Many other ingenious methods of JJ stent removal have been described. The use of a snare suture–shaped like a lasso has the advantage of easy removal with the help of smaller endoscopes especially in children [43].

A modification of the stent-on-the-string principle is a silk tie attached to the lower end of a stent. This serves the same purpose and the use of anesthesia and cystoscopy can be avoided [44].

21.7 Removal of Migrated Ureteric Stents

The issue of stent migration is addressed in another chapter. Removal of migrated stents requires careful planning. A CT IVU should be performed to ascertain the exact position of the stent and the anatomy of the renal unit. Functional assessment with renography is necessary if the stent has been indwelling for a long time. Urinary sepsis should be treated before any intervention. Renal function tests and an overall assessment of the patient including coagulation screening is important as the patient may require insertion of a nephrostomy tube prior to the removal of such stents.

Upper tract drainage with a nephrostomy tube can be a very useful as it will allow decompression, control of sepsis and proximal access if necessary. The tract can be used for a percutaneous removal of the stent especially if it has migrated outside the urinary tract [45].

The application of semi-rigid and flexible ureteroscopes is unavoidable during the removal of migrated, coiled, and knotted stents [46]. A full set of endoscopic equipment including all types of guidewires and graspers is essential [47].

21.8 Removal of Encrusted Stents

Imaging of the urinary tract should not be ignored before removal of a stent. This is especially relevant if the stent has been indwelling for a long period of time. Encrustation and migration is better detected before undertaking the removal.

Encountering such problems after insertion of a cystoscope will lead to failure especially if suitable equipment is not available.

Several options need to be considered for the removal of encrusted ureteric stents. The use of a semi-rigid or a flexible ureteroscope and laser for the fragmentation of encrustation are essential [48]. Heavy encrustation and migration or other complications such as knotting require special considerations [49–51]. Laparoscopic or open procedures too have been described [52].

21.9   Ileal Conduit Stents

There is a significant variation of the type of stents used in the management of uretero-ileal strictures. A single J stent protruding just outside the stoma is the safest option. This technique allows an easy exchange over a guidewire, which can be inserted in the pre-existent stent. The use of JJ stents should be avoided in ileal conduits, as the distal end of these stents will lie within the conduit. Change of these stents will require endoscopic manipulations through the conduit. Loss of access to the upper tracts may result if the stent is pulled out for insertion of a guidewire. Ingenious modifications such as the use of a Foley catheter to inject contrast and gain access have been described [53].

21.10   Antibiotic Prophylaxis

Indwelling ureteric stents get covered with a biofilm and are associated with bacteriuria [54–56]. Over half the patients will harbour bacteria on their stents in 4 weeks. This is not prevented by the use of antibiotics. Urinary tract infection may develop after the removal of a JJ stent [57]. The severity of this may vary [58]. Septicaemia has been reported. Patients with co-existent diabetes, immunosuppression, neutropenia, and other hematological disorders are at a higher risk. A negative urine culture is not entirely reliable [59]. The use of long-term prophylactic antibiotics to prevent septic episodes after a stent removal is not supported by evidence [60].

The use of a prophylactic antibiotic before the removal of a ureteric stent is variable. A single dose of a suitable antibiotic such as an aminoglycoside is recommended [60]. Co-existent infection should be treated prior to the removal of a ureteric stent.

21.11   Other Considerations

The removal of a ureteric stent is a surgical procedure. A formal consent is a standard protocol in most countries. Although local anesthesia is usually adequate, consideration should be given to young patients who often do not tolerate this procedure well. Patient reluctance to a local anesthetic due to apprehension or previous experience should be respected and general anesthesia offered.

Long-term stents often need exchange. So, the removal is only a part of the process. Such procedures need to be taken under a general or regional anesthesia. Local anesthesia can be used in frail patients.

Stent removal is only a part of the patient management. Subsequent steps such as further imaging and follow up plans should be made after stent removal. Healthcare systems vary enormously in the world. The arrangements for re-assessment should be made clear to the patient before discharge.

References

[1] Shigemura K, Yasufuku T, Yamanaka K, Yamahsita M, Arakawa S, Fujisawa M. How long should double J stent be kept in after ureteroscopic lithotripsy? Urol Res 2012;40(4):373–376.

[2] Shigemura K, Yasufuku T, Yamanaka K, Yamahsita M, Arakawa S, Fujisawa M. How long should double J stent be kept in after ureteroscopic lithotripsy? Urol Res. 2012;40(4):373–376.

[3] Brandt AS, von Rundstedt FC, Lazica DA, Roth S. Ureteral reconstruction after ureterorenoscopic injuries. Urologe A 2010;49(7):812–821.

[4] Loh-Doyle JC, Low RK, Monga M, Nguyen MM. Patient experiences and preferences with ureteral stent removal. J Endourol 2015;29(1):35–40.

[5] Söylemez H, Sancaktutar AA, Bozkurt Y, Atar M, Penbegül N, Yildirim K. A cheap minimally painful and widely usable alternative for retrieving ureteral stents. Urol Int 2011;87(2):199–204.

[6] Birch BR, Das G, Wickham JE. Tethered ureteric stents–a clinical assessment. Br J Urol 1988;62(5):409–411.

[7] Barnes KT, Bing MT, Tracy CR. Do ureteric stent extraction strings affect stent-related quality of life or complications after ureteroscopy for urolithiasis: a prospective randomised control trial. BJUI 2014;113(4):605–609.

[8] Nguyen M, Low R, Monga M. Abstract: PD7-08; Session Title: Stone Disease: Therapy I. AUA University, September 2015.

[9] van Diepen S, Grantmyre J. Broken retrieval string leads to failed self-removal of a double-J ureteral stent. Can J Urol 2004;11(1):2139–2140.

[10] Shpall AI, Parekh AR, Bellman GC. Tubeless percutaneous nephrolithotomy with antegrade stent tether: clinical experience. J Endourol 2007;21(9):973–976.

[11] Agrawal MS, Sharma M, Agarwal K. Tubeless percutaneous nephrolithotomy using antegrade tether: a randomized study. J Endourol 2014;28(6):644–648.

[12] Berkman DS, Lee MW, Landman J, Gupta M. Tubeless percutaneous nephrolithotomy (PCNL) with reversed Polaris Loop stent: reduced postoperative pain and narcotic use. J Endourol 2008;22(10):2245–2249.

[13] Kulkarni RP, Bellamy EA. A new thermo-expandable shape-memory nickel-titanium alloy stent for the management of ureteric strictures. BJU Int 1999;83(7):755–759.

[14] Kulkarni R, Bellamy E. Nickel-titanium shape memory alloy Memokath 051 ureteral stent for managing long-term ureteral obstruction: 4-year experience. J Urol 2001;166(5):1750–1754.

[15] Siddique KA, Zammit P, Bafaloukas N, Albanis S, Buchholz NP. Repositioning and removal of an intra-renal migrated ureteric Memokath stent. Urol Int 2006:77(4):297–300.

[16] Chung KJ, Park BH, Park B, Lee JH, Kim WJ, Baek M, Han DH. Efficacy and Safety of a Novel, Double-Layered, Coated, Self-Expandable Metallic Mesh Stent (Uventa™) in Malignant Ureteral Obstructions. J Endourol 2013;27(7):930–935.

[17] Kim JH, Song K, Jo MK, Park JW. Palliative care of malignant ureteral obstruction with polytetrafluoroethylene membrane-covered self-expandable metallic stents: initial experience. Korean J Urol 2012;53(9):625–631.

[18] Moskovitz B, Halachmi S, Nativ O. A new self-expanding, large-caliber ureteral stent: results of a multicenter experience. J Endourol 2012;26(11):1523–1527.

[19] Potretzke AM, Chang H, Kryger JV. Technique for Resonance® stent exchange in patients with extrinsic obstruction: description of a novel approach and literature review. J Pediatr Urol 2012;8(5):557–559. doi: 10.1016/j.jpurol.2012.01.018. Epub 2012 Feb 25.

[20] Nagele U, Kuczyk MA, Horstmann M, Hennenlotter J, Sievert KD, Schilling D, Walcher U, Stenzl A, Anastasiadis AG. Initial clinical experience with full-length metal ureteral stents for obstructive ureteral stenosis. World J Urol 2008;26(3):257–262.

[21] Wang HJ, Lee TY, Luo HL, Chen CH, Shen YC, Chuang YC, Chiang PH. Application of resonance metallic stents for ureteral obstruction. BJU Int 2011;108(3):428–432.

[22] Potretzke AM, Chang H, Kryger JV. Technique for Resonance® stent exchange in patients with extrinsic obstruction: description of a novel approach and literature review. J Pediatr Urol 2012;8(5):557–559.

[23] Dryhurst DJ, Fowler CG. Flexible cystodiathermy can be rendered painless by using 2% lignocaine solution to provide intravesical anaesthesia. BJU Int 2001;88(4):437–438.

[24] Greenstein A, Greenstein I, Senderovich S, Mabjeesh NJ. Is diagnostic cystoscopy painful? Analysis of 1,320 consecutive procedures. Int Braz J Urol 2014;40(4):533–538.

[25] Patel AR, Jones JS, Babineau D. Lidocaine 2% gel versus plain lubricating gel for pain reduction during flexible cystoscopy: a meta-analysis of prospective, randomized, controlled trials. J Urol 2008;179(3):986–990.

[26] Ho KJ, Thompson TJ, O'Brien A, Young MR, McCleane G. Lignocaine gel: does it cause urethral pain rather than prevent it? Eur Urol 2003;43(2):194–196.

[27] Borch M, Scosyrev E, Baron B, Encarnacion J, Smith EM, Messing E. A randomized trial of 2% lidocaine gel versus plain lubricating gel for minimizing pain in men undergoing flexible cystoscopy. Urol Nurs 2013;33(4):187–193.

[28] Goktug HN, Ozturk U, Sener NC, Tuygun C, Bakırtas H, Imamoglu MA. Do lubricants with 2% lidocaine gel have an effect on patient comfort in diagnostic cystoscopy? Adv Clin Exp Med 2014;23(4):585–587.

[29] Kim JH, Park SY, Kim MG, Choi H, Song D, Cho SW, Song YS. Pain and satisfaction during rigid cystoscopic ureteral stent removal: a preliminary study. BMC Urol 2014;14:90.

[30] Young A, Ismail M, Papatsoris AG, Barua JM, Calleary JG, Masood J. Entonox® inhalation to reduce pain in common diagnostic and therapeutic outpatient urological procedures: a review of the evidence. Ann R Coll Surg Engl 2012;94(1):8–11.

[31] Holmes M, Stewart J, Rice M. Flexible cystoscopy: is the volume and content of the urethral gel critical? J Endourol 2001;15(8):855–858.

[32] Khan MA, Beyzade B, Tau W, Virdi JS, Potluri BS. Effect of the rate of delivery of lignocaine gel on patient discomfort perception prior to performing flexible cystoscopy. Urol Int 2002;68(3):164–167.

[33] Goel R, Aron M. Cooled lignocaine gel: does it reduce urethral discomfort during instillation? Int Urol Nephrol 2003;35(3):375–377.

[34] Bhomi KK, Rizal S, Pradhan M, Rijal A, Bhattachan CL. Pain during rigid cystoscopy: a prospective randomized controlled study comparing the benefit of cooled and room temperature lignocaine gel. Nepal Med Coll J 2011;13(1):55–57.

[35] Demir E, Kilciler M, Bedir S, Erken U. Patient tolerance during cystoscopy: a randomized study comparing lidocaine hydrochloride gel and dimethyl sulfoxide with lidocaine. J Endourol 2008;22(5):1027–1029.

[36] Choe JH, Kwak KW, Hong JH, Lee HM. Efficacy of lidocaine spray as topical anesthesia for outpatient rigid cystoscopy in women: a prospective, randomized, double-blind trial. Urology 2008;71(4):561–566.

[37] Taneja R. Intravesical lignocaine in the diagnosis of bladder pain syndrome. Int Urogynecol J 2010;21(3):321–324.

[38] Ahmed M, Acher P, Deane AM. Ureteric bupivicaine infusion for loin pain haematuria syndrome. Ann R Coll Surg Engl 2010;92(2):139–141.

[39] Stravodimos KG, Mitropoulos D, Salvari A, Lampadariou A, Kapetanakis T, Zervas A. Levobupivacaine intravesical injection for superficial bladder tumor resection–possible, effective, and durable. Preliminary clinical data. Int Urol Nephrol 2008;40(3):637–641. Epub 2007 Nov 13.

[40] Kawahara T, Ito H, Terao H, Yamagishi T, Ogawa T, Uemura H, Kubota Y, Matsuzaki J. Ureteral stent retrieval using the crochet hook technique in females. PLoS One 2012;7(1):e29292.

[41] van Diepen S, Grantmyre J. Broken retrieval string leads to failed self-removal of a double-J ureteral stent. Can J Urol 2004;11(1):2139–2140.

[42] Jones JS. Shortened pull-string simplifies office-based ureteral stent removal. Urology 2002;60(6):1095–1097.

[43] Figueroa TE. Retrieval of ureteral stents in children. Tech Urol 1995;1(1):45–47.

[44] Dong J, Lu J, Zu Q, Yang S, Sun S, Cai W, Zhang L, Zhang X. Routine short-term ureteral stent in living donor renal transplantation: introduction of a simple stent removal technique without using anesthesia and cystoscope. Transplant Proc 2011;43(10):3747–3750.

[45] Rhee J, Steele SS, Beiko D. Percutaneous antegrade nephroscopic holmium laser pyelotomy: Novel endourologic technique for removal of extruded ureteral stent. Can Urol Assoc J 2013;7(11,12).

[46] Nettle J, Huang JG, Rao R, Costello AJ. Ureteroscopic holmium laser ablation of a knotted ureteral stent. J Endourol 2012;26(8):968–970.

[47] Lam JS, Gupta M. Tips and tricks for the management of retained ureteral stents. J Endourol 2002;16(10):733–741.

[48] Teichman JM, Lackner JE, Leveillee RJ, Hulbert JC. Total endoscopic management of the encrusted ureteral stent under a single anaesthesia. Can J Urol 1997;4(4):456–459.

[49] Kim MS, Lee HN, Hwang H. Knotted stents: Case report and outcome analysis. Korean J Urol 2015;56(5):405–408.

[50] Bultitude MF, Tiptaft RC, Glass JM, Dasgupta P. Management of encrusted ureteral stents impacted in upper tract. Urology 2003;62(4):622–626.

[51] Shin JH, Yoon HK, Ko GY, Sung KB, Song HY, Choi E, Kim JH, Kim JW, Kim KR, Kwon J. Percutaneous antegrade removal of double J ureteral stents via a 9-F nephrostomy route. J Vasc Interv Radiol 2007;18(9):1156–1161.

[52] Clark C, Bylund J, Paszek M, Lagrange C, Pais VM Jr. Novel approach for removal of heavily encrusted ureteral stent. Can J Urol 2009;16(5):4831–4835.

[53] Wah TM, Kellett MJ. Ureteric catheterization via an ileal conduit: technique and retrieval of a JJ stent. Clin Radiol 2004;59(11):1041–1043.

[54] Stickler DJ, Evans A, Morris N, Hughes G. Strategies for the control of catheter encrustation. Int J Antimicrob Agents 2002;19(6):499–506.

[55] Getliffe K. Managing recurrent urinary catheter encrustation. Br J Community Nurs 2002;7(11):574, 576, 578-580.

[56] Broomfield RJ, Morgan SD, Khan A, Stickler DJ. Crystalline bacterial biofilm formation on urinary catheters by urease-producing urinary tract pathogens: a simple method of control. J Med Microbiol 2009;58(Pt 10):1367–1375.

[57] Nickel JC, Costerton JW. Bacterial biofilms and catheters: A key to understanding bacterial strategies in catheter-associated urinary tract infection. Can J Infect Dis 1992;3(5):261–267.

[58] Riedl CR, Plas E, Hübner WA, Zimmerl H, Ulrich W, Pflüger H. Bacterial colonization of ureteral stents. Eur Urol 1999;36(1):53–59.

[59] Kehinde EO, Rotimi VO, Al-Hunayan A, Abdul-Halim H, Boland F, Al-Awadi KA. Bacteriology of urinary tract infection associated with indwelling J ureteral stents. J Endourol 2004;18(9):891–896.

[60] Moltzahn F, Haeni K, Birkhäuser FD, Roth B, Thalmann GN, Zehnder P. Peri-interventional antibiotic prophylaxis only vs continuous low-dose antibiotic treatment in patients with JJ stents: a prospective randomised trial analysing the effect on urinary tract infections and stent-related symptoms. BJU Int 2013;111(2):289–295.

22

Encrustation of Indwelling Urinary Devices

Justin Chan[1] and Dirk Lange[2]

[1] Department of Urologic sciences, The Stone Centre at Vancouver General Hospital, Jack Bell Research Center, Vancouver, British Columbia, Canada
[2] Director of Basic Science Research, Assistant Professor of Urology The Stone Centre at Vancouver General Hospital, Jack Bell Research Center, Vancouver, British Columbia, Canada

Urinary catheters and stents are common indwelling devices used in the field of urology. While they function to aid the drainage of urine, their long-term use often leads to the development of catheter and stent associated encrustations. Encrustations are minerals that have precipitated, crystallized, and deposited onto urinary implants. The formation of encrustation on catheters and stents are extremely prevalent as up to 50% of all patients that undergo long-term catheterization experience recurrent encrustation formations [1]. In addition to time, other factors that influence indwelling device encrustation are urinary tract infections, type of biomaterial, urine composition, and malignancies [2]. If not addressed, device encrustation will result in significant patient morbidity [1, 3]. Most often, the composition of the encrusting material is the same as that of the original stone, mainly struvite (magnesium ammonium phosphate), calcium phosphate, cystine, uric acid, and calcium oxalate deposits [4]. In this chapter, bacterial and abacterial formation of encrustations, crystalline deposit types, repercussion of encrustation formation, and encrustation prevention will be discussed.

22.1 Bacterial-Associated Encrustation

This type of crystallization is largely due to excessively alkaline urinary conditions [3]. In bacterial-associated encrustation, urea-splitting bacteria are the predominant cause [5]. These bacteria can enter the host by migrating on the urinary implant via the processes of retrograde intraluminal or extra luminal ascent. In retrograde intraluminal ascent, most commonly found with urinary catheters, bacteria originate from collecting bags or from disconnected catheter drainage tube junctions. In contrast, bacteria involved in extra luminal ascent are commonly derived from a colonized urethral meatus [6]. Once the bacteria are in the host, the establishment of a thick bacterial biofilm and the production of urease are important factors in forming encrustation. For a group of bacteria to form a biofilm, the bacteria must fulfill three conditions: 1) the group of microorganisms must attach to one another or adhere to a surface, 2) the

Ureteric Stenting, First Edition. Edited by Ravi Kulkarni.
© 2017 John Wiley & Sons Ltd. Published 2017 by John Wiley & Sons Ltd.

microorganisms must have a change in gene expression that alters their planktonic state phenotype into a biofilm facilitating phenotype and lastly, 3) the biofilm must have an extracellular matrix consisting of host and bacterial products [7]. While not absolutely necessary, the initiation of a biofilm on the surface of indwelling urinary devices is facilitated by the device surface being conditioned. Similar to indwelling medical devices of the circulatory system, urine components become deposited onto the device surface [7]. Once the conditioning film is established, bacterial expressed surface proteins called adhesins recognize their binding partner on the device surface, resulting in a very strong adhesion [5, 8]. In addition to providing sites of attachment for bacteria, the conditioning film also facilitates bacterial adhesion by covering novel anti-adhesive coatings of the indwelling device, thereby rendering them ineffective [9].

If the biofilm-forming uropathogen produces the enzyme urease, the end result is severe device encrustation. Urease is an enzyme that catabolizes urea into ammonia and carbon dioxide, resulting in a significant increase in urine pH and the precipitation of magnesium ammonium phosphate [10]. In general, for precipitation of minerals to occur, the critical urine pH for encrustation formation is 6.8. Urine with pH lower than 6.8 has been shown to produce very small amounts of encrustation [11, 12]. The pH when crystals form in urine is known as the nucleation pH (pHn), which plays a large role in determining the rate of catheter encrustation and blockage [8].

The bacterial species found in the majority of cases of bacterial-derived stent/catheter encrustation is the gram-negative, *Proteus mirabilis* [8, 13, 14]. The prevalence of *P. mirabilis* in cases of urinary implant encrustation can be attributed to its superior colonization ability. Previous studies have shown that if a catheterized urinary tract is infected by equal numbers of *P. mirabilis* and another uropathogenic bacterial species, *P. mirabilis* is capable of out-competing the other bacteria [15]. The superiority of *P. mirabilis* can be attributed to several key virulence factors conveying swarming motility, hemolysin production, uroepithelial cell invasion, the ability to cleave IgA and IgG, lipopolysaccharide and capsular polysaccharide expression, and serum resistance [16]. Furthermore, encrustation due to *P. mirabilis* infection has also been found to be far more severe than with other bacterial species, a characteristic that is likely attributable to the unique isoform of *P. mirabilis* urease, which has been observed to split urea at rates 6 to 25 times faster than ureases produced by other urea-splitting bacteria [17, 18, 19]. Along with *P. mirabilis*, the bacteria *Proteus vulgaris* and *Providencia rettgeri* are also capable of causing encrustation [8], however, in comparison to *P. mirabilis*, *P. vulgaris* and *P. rettgeri* are only isolated in 5-10% of catheter biofilm cases [15].

22.2 Non-Bacterial Causes of Encrustation

Aside from magnesium ammonium phosphate (struvite)-based encrustation, another crystal type that has been found in the presence of bacterial infection is hydroxyapaptite [20, 21, 22, 23]. However, unlike struvite, hydroxyapatite precipitates and crystalizes at a slightly lower pH [24]. Under microscopic examination, hydroxyapatite encrustations are poorly crystallized and appear as microcrystalline aggregates with a globular morphology [8, 24, 25]. These aggregates themselves are not completely pure as they may contain bacteria as well as some carbonate components (that replaces some phosphate ions in apaptite) [4, 8, 23]. This crystalized version of hydroxyapatite is powdery in form and as a result, can cause implant obstruction more easily than larger crystals [24]. Other calcium phosphate crystals that may encrust on catheter and stents are brushite ($CaHPO_4$) and carbonate-apatite ($Ca_{10}(PO_4)_6CO_3$) [4].

22.3   Non-Bacterial Based Indwelling Device Encrustation

In the absence of bacterial infection, the main crystal type to form on stents and catheters are calcium oxalate monohydrate deposits [26, 27]. In order for calcium oxalate monohydrate encrustations to form, they require urine to be in contact with continuous non-renewed and non-protected organic layer. If this condition is met, calcium oxalate monohydrate crystals will be able to start depositing on the catheter and form columnar compact structures [27]. The generation of calcium oxalate crystals is also influenced by the concentration of ions that can complex with either calcium or oxalate. Several of these complexing ions include magnesium and citrate [28]. On top of complexing ions, uric acid has been postulated to play several influential roles in promoting the formation of calcium oxalate crystals. First, some scientists believe that uric acid exerts a direct effect on calcium oxalate crystallization by acting as a heterogeneous nucleant and as an agent that is capable of salting out calcium oxalate from solution [29]. It is also believed that uric acid exerts an indirect influence on the generation of calcium oxalate crystals by acting as an anti-inhibitor. Uric acid is able to reduce the levels of free urinary glycoasminoglycans, which normally act to inhibit calcium oxalate crystallization. With a reduction in free urinary glyocasminglycans, the inhibitory function will be blocked [29]. Unlike the previously mentioned encrusting material, the precipitation of calcium oxalate is not greatly dependent on urinary pH [28].

In addition to being an influential factor for calcium oxalate crystal formation, uric acid is another crystal type that has been identified in catheter and stent encrustations. A previous study investigating catheter and stent encrustations in stone formers has shown uric acid to be a minor component as it only represented 5.2% of the total encrusting material [30]. When uric acid crystals are found in encrustations, they are either in the anhydrous or dihydrate form. Uric acid anhydrous is the predominant form whereas uric acid dehydrate, if present, only accounts for <5% of the encrustation weight [31]. Increased concentrations of urinary uric acid is usually found in individuals with defects in the enzyme xanthine oxidase and unlike other crystal deposits, uric acid crystals tend to form in acidic urinary conditions [28, 31, 32].

The amino acid cystine, in high concentrations, can lead to the formation cystine encrustations on indwelling urinary devices. In normal physiological conditions, humans excrete basal amounts of cystine (0.06-0.17 mmol dm^{-3}), whereas some individuals excrete significantly higher concentrations (1.3-3.3 mmol dm^{-3}) due to genetic defects in tubular reabsorption [28]. Additionally, cystine is an amino acid with rather low solubility [33]. Hence, increased concentration of cystine found in urine can result in tthe precipitation of cystine crystals [28]. Similar to uric acid crystals, cystine crystallization is favored by acidic urinary conditions [34]. Encrustation of indwelling urologic devices represents a major clinical problem in urology. An initial issue with encrustations is that they can cause trauma to the bladder mucosa and urethra. Often encrustations tend to be solid crystalline deposits, and therefore, hard and abrasive [1]. Furthermore, if encrustations are allowed to accumulate, the stent or catheter lumen may become occluded [1, 3]. Blockage of the stent or catheter can result in incontinence due to leakage or urinary retention followed by painful distention of the bladder [1]. Bacteriuria is also commonly associated with encrustations, and thus, the blockage of an urinary implant can lead to retention of bacteria-containing urine, and the resultant vesico-ureteral reflux triggers an ascending infection of the urinary tract, which then, can lead to severe medical conditions such as pyelonephritis, septicemia, and endotoxic shock [35]. If encrustations are present at the time of device removal, extraluminal encrustations may fragment and deposit in the bladder. These fragments may then act as a nucleation centers for bladder stone formation and can lead to further infection [36].

On top of creating complications for patients, encrustations can also cause problems for the attending physician. Catheters or stents that have been encrusted are more difficult to remove [36]. To deal with these encrustations and to remove encrusted catheters or stents, physicians will be required to perform more complex procedures. For stents, if there is minimal encrustation (denoted by minimal linear or bulbous encrustations) and the patient has low stone burden, either ureteroscopy, intracorporeal lithotripsy (with pneumatic lithoclast or laser), or extracorporeal shock wave lithotripsy can be used to aid in encrusted stent removal. For patients with heavily encrusted stents or large stone burdens, percutaneous nephrolithotomy or open surgical removal may be necessary [37]. Likewise for encrusted urinary bladder catheters, extracorporeal shock wave lithotripsy and lithoclast can be used to remove the encrusted catheter. A rigid cystoscope and the creation of suprapubic cystostomy tract can be used to remove the encrusted catheter by crushing the crystal deposits [36].

22.4 Preventing Encrustation of Indwelling Urinary Devices

Since encrustations on urinary indwelling devices represent a common and major problem in urology, much research has been conducted to develop novel methods of preventing encrustation formation. As many encrustations are bacterial-associated, one major area of research is focused on developing biomaterials that are capable of resisting colonization by bacterial biofilms and thus, preventing bacteria-associated encrustations. These biomaterials either have biocides or antibiotic agents incorporated into the polymers of catheters and stents or the biomaterials may be engineered to possess surface properties capable of preventing adherence of bacterial cells [1].

22.5 Stent Coatings

Over the years, several different types of coatings have been used in an attempt to decrease bacterial-associated as well as non-bacterial-associated device encrustation. These include antibiotics, hydrogels, heparin, hyaluronic acid, silver, antimicrobial peptides and biomimetic coatings [38, 39]. While all of these have had varying degrees of success, they have also been fraught with downsides. Historically, stents and catheters have been coated with antibiotics such as ciprofloxacin, gentamicin, norfloxacin, and nitrofurazone. While the use of antibiotic-based coatings showed some success in preventing bacterial colonization and associated encrustation, they only worked over the short term. This phenomenon was likely due to the uncontrolled release of the drugs resulting in initially high enough drug concentrations in the surrounding environment to trigger bacterial killing that decreased significantly with indwelling time as the intensity of drug release decreased [38].

While directly coating urinary stents and catheters with antibiotics have not been fairly successful in preventing bacterial colonization, the use of hydrogel coatings have had some success. A previous study conducted by Desai *et al.* demonstrated that hydrogel coated silicone catheters were capable of preventing bacterial adherence as there was 90% less *Enterococcus faecalis* adhered on coated catheters compared to uncoated catheters [40]. When catheters and stents are coated with hydrogel, hydrogel functions to prevent bacterial colonization by acting as a hydrophilic cross-linked polymer, which absorbs large volumes of liquid [38, 41]. As the hydrogel absorbs liquid, it creates a layer of water on the indwelling device that prevents the deposition of proteins and platelets that may serve as receptors for bacterial adhesion as well as crystal deposition [42]. This in turn can prevent the formation of a conditioning film and potentially subsequent encrustation formation.

Another coating that has shown some promise is the glycosaminoglycan hyaluronic acid, which has been shown to prevent device encrustation by two mechanisms. The first is based on its ability to prevent bacterial-associated encrustation by hindering urinary component deposition and bacterial colonization of the indwelling devices [43]. Secondly, hyaluronic acid is capable of inhibiting the nucleation, growth, and aggregation of certain salts [38]. As such, glycosaminoglycans like hyaluronic acid have been observed to inhibit the growth and aggregation of calcium oxalate crystals by blocking crystal growth sites [43]. While hyaluronic acid seems to be an ideal candidate coating to prevent indwelling device encrustation, all studies performed to date have been in vitro in nature meaning that their efficacy in the clinic remains to be investigated [38].

Similar to hyaluronic acid, heparin is another glycoasminoglycan molecule that has been used to coat urinary indwelling devices. Heparin is a highly sulfated glycosaminoglycan molecule which possesses a very high negative charge density [44]. Its ability to prevent encrustation and bacterial colonization can be attributed its electronegative property, which is believed to repel both gram-positive and gram-negative bacteria from the device surface [39]. While theoretically this makes sense, heparin-coated indwelling devices have had mixed results when tested both in vitro and in vivo. In the in vitro experiments, heparin-coated stents were encrustation-free following 7 days of continuous exposure to artificial urine [45]. In the in vivo experiment, after 120 days of indwelling, heparin-coated stents showed small amounts of deposits on their surface and were not occluded compared to uncoated-stents which were heavily encrusted with some completely obstructed [45]. Conversely, in another in vitro study, heparin-coated stents failed to prevent encrustations from forming. The study showed that heparin-coated stents placed in artificial urine containing urease or had been inoculated with *P. mirabilis* developed a layer of amorphous calcium phosphate [39]. While these results seem to contradict one another, it must be pointed out that both studies utilized encrustation models that yield different types of encrustation. Essentially, what these results show is that no one coating is universally affective at inhibiting crystal nucleation and encrustation in different environments.

Silver is an effective broad-spectrum antimicrobial agent at low concentrations and has been explored as another potential coating to prevent bacterial-based device encrustation [46]. Silver has been exploited in many ways in the research and development of stents as a fully metallic implant, as a coating, or impregnated directly into the device material [38]. Of particular interest to the world of biomaterial design is the fact that prior to implantation the silver coating is inert and has no antimicrobial activity. Upon implantation, however, bodily fluids contact the device surface and activate silver's antimicrobial activity via ionization [38]. When silver is ionized, the silver cations are highly reactive and its ions are capable of modifying bacterial cell walls and membranes and inhibit DNA replication [38]. The silver cations ability to modify different cellular components may be attributed to its ability to displace essential ions such as Ca^{2+} and Zn^+ [47]. The success in preventing bacterial infection has been shown in fully metallic catheter and stents, but success in silver-coated or silver impregnated catheters and stents have been variable [38]. The success of silver coatings is largely questionable as a randomized control clinical study of 1300 patients showed no significant difference in infection rates between silver-coated and uncoated stents [48]. Silver-impregnated catheter and stent showed some success, but also fell short of preventing infection in the long term [1, 49, 50].

Biomimetic coatings have been used on indwelling urinary devices to help them mimic host tissues. Our tissues constantly encounter microbes, but most of the time they remain impervious to bacterial colonization [1]. Mimicry of host tissues on catheters and stents may make these implants less susceptible to bacterial adhesion and encrustation [39]. One biomimetic coating that has been used on these urological devices is phosphorylcholine. Phosphorylcholine is the major polar head group on the outer surface of erythrocytes and can be used on the abiotic surface of catheters and stents to mimic a host cell lipidic membrane [1, 39]. A study conducted by Stickler *et al.* demonstrated mixed results on the ability for phosphorylcholine to decrease stent encrustation. After 12 weeks of implantation in patients, some phosphorylcholine stents were completely free of encrustations, while others were encrusted with their central channels and side-holes completely occluded [1]. Nonetheless, although phosphorylcholine cannot completely eliminate bacterial colonization and/or encrustation, evidence supports its ability to at least reduce their incidence [1].

Most recently, antimicrobial peptides have been pursued as a way to prevent urinary indwelling device biofouling including bacterial-associated encrustation [38]. Currently, there are over 5,000 antimicrobial peptides that have been discovered or synthesized [51]. These unique peptides have been of particular interest in catheter and stent coatings as they confer numerous benefits. For one, they not only have antimicrobial activity but have antiviral, antifungal, antiparasitic, and anti-tumor activity. Antimicrobial peptides also have immune regulatory activity and promote wound healing [52]. The antimicrobial peptides are positively charged and are amphiphilic in nature. These cationic and amphiphilic characteristics allow the peptides to interact with bacterial membranes non-specifically and can cause the disruption of bacterial cell wall and cell membranes [38, 52]. They can also affect DNA or RNA replication, protein synthesis, and other bacterial processes [38]. Their ability to influence numerous processes help reduce the likelihood of bacteria developing resistance [38]. In a recent study conducted by Wang *et al.*, they incorporated an antimicrobial peptide, Bmap-28, into polyurethane membranes (a polymer used in catheters and stents). They showed that polyurethane membranes with Bmap-28 had significantly lower bacterial load after being co-cultured with *P. mirabilis* when compared with control polyurethane membranes. Furthermore, it was observed that the polyurethrane membranes with Bmap-28 incorporated could delay catheter obstruction caused by encrustation [52]. Although antimicrobial peptide coatings are a promising solution, further research has to be conducted to evaluate their suitability for urinary implant usage. Several issues that warrant further research is their potential toxicity to humans, their sensitivity to harsh environmental conditions (susceptibility to proteases and extreme pH), high production costs, folding issues of large antimicrobial peptides, reduced activity when applied as surface coating, and bacterial resistance [51].

Aside from developing coatings to prevent bacterial adherence and encrustations, there is large research focus on constructing urinary stents and catheters with novel materials. In the past, polyethylene was the polymer of choice used to construct ureteral stents, however, its use was fraught with several negative effects including the fact that it was stiff, brittle and had a tendency to fragment [53]. Presently, silicone is one of the materials used in stent construction. Silicone has many desirable characteristics for stent production as currently, it is the polymer that is most resistant to biofilm formation, infection, encrustation, and is one of the lubricious materials [53]. There are, however, several difficulties associated with the use of silicone stents as it is particularly soft and elastic making their use in patients with tight or tortuous ureters difficult [53]. To overcome the issues of both silicone and polyethylene, polyurethrane was developed and is the polymer used in most stents. It was designed to be versatile like silicone yet, strong and rigid like polyethylene [53, 54]. Nevertheless, like other materials, polyurethrane is not free from faults, as it is the cause of significant patient discomfort, ureteral ulceration and erosion, and has poor biodurability [53, 54]. Furthermore, polyurethrane ureteral stents are not free from encrustation, as Singh *et al.* described stent encrustation as one of the most serious complications associated with polyurethrane JJ stents [55].

Currently, research on biodegradable/bioabsorbable compounds for use in ureteral stents is a large area of focus. Like regular urinary implants, biodegradable stents must fulfill all the core characteristics of being biocompatible, have suitable expansion and degradation rates, and guarantee urinary flow for the desired period of time [53]. If all these characteristics are satisfied, the use of these stents may confer various benefits including eliminating the need for a second operation for urinary implant removal and for certain biodegradable stents, even be more resistant to encrustations [56, 57]. One biodegradable material developed by Laaksovirta *et al.* for stent usage is known as SR-PLGA 80/20 (SpiroFlow). This SR-PLGA biodegradable stent is composed of a self-reinforced L-lactide-glycolidic acid co-polymer [57]. Polylactic acid is known for strength, its non-reactivity with tissue and its ability to degrade in vivo. Polyglycolic acid was developed as an alternative to polylactic acid but, is a bioabsorbable polymer [58]. When Laaksovirta *et al.* developed the L-lactide-glycolidic acid co-polymer stent, it was tested in artificial urine. This polymer demonstrated significant resistance to encrustation compared to metallic stents (Prostakath and Memokath 028). At 4 weeks of incubation in artificial urine, no encrustation was noted on the SpiroFlow stents, whereas 8% of the surface area of the Memokath and 1.5% of the Prostakath were encrusted. At 8 weeks, the degree of encrustation increased drastically with 28.4% and 4.1% of the Memokath and Prostakath surface areas, respectively, were encrusted. In contrast, the SpiroFlow stent showed encrustation on only 0.12% of its surface area at 8 weeks and remained stable up till 12 weeks. As is often the case in stent biomaterial design, winning the battle against one stent-associated complications often comes at a price in another area. In the case of biodegradable stents one of the issues that arose due to the significantly different stent material composition was decreased compression strength [57]. As such further research into the ideal stent material is required.

An interesting area to prevent ureteral stent encrustation that has previously been utilized with Foley catheters, is the use of low-energy acoustic waves to prevent biofouling of the device surface. The idea behind their use is that when low-energy acoustic waves are used on indwelling urinary implants, they create a virtual vibrating coat that prevents biofilms and encrustation from forming by inhibiting the adherence of planktonic bacteria or crystals to the device surface [38]. In previous studies, acoustic waves demonstrated to possess broad-spectrum effects as they reduced biofilm burdens caused by different gram-negative and gram-positive bacteria, including the urease positive *P. mirabilis* [59]. A study conducted by Hazan *et al.* demonstrated that acoustics waves kept catheters virtually clean of *Candida albicans*, *P. mirabilis*, and *Escherichia coli* [60]. The difficulty, however, with applying acoustic waves to indwelling devices is that the waves have to be applied continuously on the device surface. Currently, the only way for a patient to receive continuous acoustic wave treatment is to carry a portable actuator, which is not very efficient [38].

Another experimental process to prevent encrustation of urinary catheters is iontophoresis. Iontophoresis is the process where an electrical field is used to prompt diffuse flow of ions in a medium [59]. In an in vivo study conducted by Davis *et al.*, modified catheters that contained platinum electrodes on the catheter tip were implanted in sheep for up to 21 days and underwent iontophoresis process. During the study, bacterial counts in iontophoretic catheterized sheep were found to be 10^3 to 10^4 microbes/mL, whereas control sheep were found to contain 10^7 microbes/mL. In addition, the iontophoretic process was determined to be safe as no significant alterations were found in urine chemistry or the urinary tracts of the sheep [61]. Further research has shown that when the iontophoretic process was used in conjunction with antimicrobial agents, the antimicrobial activity of the antimicrobials were enhanced [59, 62]. Jass *et al.* revealed that when ciprofloxacin, polymyxin B, and piperacillin were used with iontophoresis, the biofilm population of *Pseudomonas aeruginosa* experienced a greater decrease in number than if the biofilm was solely treated by the antibiotics [62]. In an in vitro experiment conducted by Chakravarti *et al.*, electrified iontophoretic catheters with silver electrodes were placed in artificial urine inoculated with *P. mirabillis*. These catheter were shown to be able to reduce bacterial counts via releasing ions with oligodynamic properties that are capable of inhibiting bacterial growth and significantly decrease the encrustation rate of the catheters [63].

Finally, the last way to prevent indwelling device colonization and encrustation is to treat the patient directly and have the afflicted patient take preventative measures. Catheterized patients should have their urine undergo regular bacteriological screening for encrustation causing bacteria. If bacterial species such as *P. mirabillis* are detected, testing for antibiotic susceptibility should be conducted and the patient should start antibiotic treatment immediately [8]. However, caution should be used when treating a patient with antibiotics as antimicrobial treatment can lead to the selection of antibiotic resistant bacteria and to adverse reactions [64]. Aside from antibiotic treatment, a change of diet can help prevent catheter encrustation. The intake of fluids high in citrate such as lemon have been shown to be an effective way of controlling catheter encrustation [65]. Urinary citrate is a natural inhibitor of urinary crystallization [66], including calcium oxalate and calcium phosphate encrustation. Furthermore, citrate has been found to bind to the surface of existing calcium oxalate crystals and prevent crystal development [66].

22.6 Conclusions

Throughout this chapter, both bacterial and abacterial-associated indwelling urinary device encrustation was discussed. Despite much research having gone into the development of methods to prevent it, device encrustation remains a major clinical problem in the field of urology. If untreated, severe medical complications can arise for the afflicted patient and can make the management of the urinary implant increasingly difficult for the attending physician. To mitigate urinary implant encrustation and their associated problems, the research and development of novel coatings and biomaterials for urinary indwelling devices is a constant need.

References

[1] Stickler DJ, Evans A, Morris N, Hughes G. Strategies for the control of catheter encrustation. Int J Antimicrob Agents 2002;19:499–506.

[2] Dakkak Y, Janane A, Ould-Ismail T, Ghadouane M, Ameur A, Abbar M. Management of encrusted ureteral stents. African Journal of Urology 2012;18:131–134.

[3] Getliffe K. Managing recurrent urinary catheter encrustation. British Journal of Community Nursing 2002;7:574–580.

[4] Wilson M, Devine D. Medical Implications of Biofilms. Cambridge University Press, 2003.

[5] Broomfield RJ, Morgan SD, Khan A, Stickler DJ. Crystalline bacterial biofilm formation on urinary catheters by urease-producing urinary tract pathogens: a simple method of control. J Med Microbiol 2009;58:1367–1375.

[6] Nickel JC, Costerton JW. Bacterial biofilms and catheters: A key to understanding bacterial strategies in catheter-associated urinary tract infection. Can J Infect Dis 1992;3:261–267.

[7] Trautner BW, Darouiche RO. Role of biofilm in catheter-associated urinary tract infection. Am J Infect Control 2004;32:177–183.

[8] Stickler DJ, Feneley RCL. The encrustation and blockage of long-term indwelling bladder catheters: a way forward in prevention and control. Spinal Cord 2010;48:784–790.

[9] Gristina AG. Biomaterial-centered infection: microbial adhesion versus tissue integration. Science 1987;237:1588–1595.

[10] Trinchieri A. Urinary calculi and infection. Urologia 2014;81:93–98.

[11] Stickler DJ, Lear JC, Morris NS, Macleod SM, Downer A, Cadd DH, et al. Observations on the adherence of Proteus mirabilis onto polymer surfaces. J Appl Microbiol 2006;100:1028–1033.

[12] Hedelin H, Bratt CG, Eckerdal G, Lincoln K. Relationship between urease-producing bacteria, urinary pH and encrustation on indwelling urinary catheters. Br J Urol 1991;67:527–531.

[13] Burall LS, Harro JM, Li X, Lockatell CV, Himpsl SD, Hebel JR, et al. Proteus mirabilis genes that contribute to pathogenesis of urinary tract infection: identification of 25 signature-tagged mutants attenuated at least 100-fold. Infect Immun 2004;72:2922–2938.

[14] Stickler D, Ganderton L, King J, Nettleton J, Winters C. Proteus mirabilis biofilms and the encrustation of urethral catheters. Urol Res 1993;21:407–411.

[15] Macleod SM, Stickler DJ. Species interactions in mixed-community crystalline biofilms on urinary catheters. J Med Microbiol 2007;56:1549–1557.

[16] Zunino P, Sosa V, Allen AG, Preston A, Schlapp G, Maskell DJ. Proteus mirabilis fimbriae (PMF) are important for both bladder and kidney colonization in mice. Microbiology 2003;149:3231–3237.

[17] Jones BD, Mobley HL. Genetic and biochemical diversity of ureases of Proteus, Providencia, and Morganella species isolated from urinary tract infection. Infect Immun 1987;55:2198–2203.

[18] Waters SL, Heaton K, Siggers JH, Bayston R, Bishop M, Cummings LJ, et al. Ureteric stents: investigating flow and encrustation. Proc Inst Mech Eng H 2008;222:551–561.

[19] Jones DS, Djokic J, Gorman SP. Characterization and optimization of experimental variables within a reproducible bladder encrustation model and in vitro evaluation of the efficacy of urease inhibitors for the prevention of medical device-related encrustation. J Biomed Mater Res B Appl Biomater 2006;76:1–7.

[20] Bichler KH, Eipper E, Naber K, Braun V, Zimmermann R, Lahme S. Urinary infection stones. International Journal of Antimicrobial Agents 2002;19:488–498.

[21] Clapham L, McLean RJC, Nickel JC, Downey J, Costerton JW. The influence of bacteria on struvite crystal habit and its importance in urinary stone formation. Journal of Crystal Growth 1990;104:475–484.

[22] Acton QA. Bacterial Processes—Advances in Research and Application: 2012 Edition. ScholarlyEditions, 2012.

[23] Cox AJC, Hukins DWL, Sutton TM. Infection of catheterised patients: bacterial colonisation of encrusted Foley catheters shown by scanning electron microscopy. Urol Res 1989;17:349–352.

[24] Getliffe KA, Mulhall AB. The Encrustation of Indwelling Catheters. Brit J Urol 1991;67:337–341.

[25] Ron R, Zbaida D, Kafka IZ, Rosentsveig R, Leibovitch I, Tenne R. Attenuation of encrustation by self-assembled inorganic fullerene-like nanoparticles. Nanoscale 2014;6:5251–5259.

[26] Robert M, Boularan AM, El Sandid M, Grasset D. Double-J ureteric stent encrustations: clinical study on crystal formation on polyurethane stents. Urol Int 1997;58:100–104.

[27] Grases F, Sohnel O, Costa-Bauza A, Ramis M, Wang Z. Study on concretions developed around urinary catheters and mechanisms of renal calculi development. Nephron 2001;88:320–328.

[28] Königsberger E, Königsberger L-C. Thermodynamic modeling of crystal deposition in humans. Pure and Applied Chemistry 2001;73:785–797.

[29] Grases F, Sanchis P, Isern B, Perello J, Costa-Bauza A. Uric acid as inducer of calcium oxalate crystal development. Scand J Urol Nephrol 2007;41:26–31.

[30] Bouzidi H, Traxer O, Dore B, Amiel J, Hadjadj H, Conort P, et al. Characteristics of encrustation of ureteric stents in patients with urinary stones. Prog Urol 2008;18:230–237.

[31] Grases F, Costa-Bauza A, Villacampa AI, Sohnel O. Structure of uric acid concretion developed around a catheter. Scand J Urol Nephrol 1997;31:439–443.

[32] Doughty DB. Urinary & Fecal Incontinence: Current Management Concepts. Elsevier Health Sciences, 2012.

[33] Rimer JD, An Z, Zhu Z, Lee MH, Goldfarb DS, Wesson JA, *et al.* Crystal growth inhibitors for the prevention of L-cystine kidney stones through molecular design. Science 2010;330:337–341.

[34] Wagner CA, Mohebbi N. Urinary pH and stone formation. J Nephrol 2010;23 Suppl 16:S165–S169.

[35] Kunin CM. Care of the urinary catheter. Detection, Prevention and Management of Urinary Tract Infections. 4th ed. Philadelphia: Lea and Febiger, 1987. pp. 245–88.

[36] Ho CCK, Khandasamy Y, Singam P, Hong Goh E, Zainuddin ZM. Encrusted and incarcerated urinary bladder catheter: what are the options? The Libyan Journal of Medicine 2010;5:10.3402/ljm.v5i0.5686.

[37] Talati J, Tiselius HG, Albala DM, YE Z. Urolithiasis: Basic Science and Clinical Practice. Springer, London, 2012.

[38] Lo J, Lange D, Chew B. Ureteral stents and Foley catheters-associated urinary tract infections: The role of coatings and materials in infection prevention. Antibiotics 2014;3:87.

[39] Syed T, Tofail SAM, O'Brien P, Chemistry RSo, Craighead H. Biological Interactions with Surface Charge in Biomaterials. RSC Publishing, 2011.

[40] Desai DG, Liao KS, Cevallos ME, Trautner BW. Silver or nitrofurazone impregnation of urinary catheters has a minimal effect on uropathogen adherence. The Journal of Urology 1995;184:2565–2571.

[41] Nakagawa N, Yashiro N, Nakajima Y, Barnhart WH, Wakabayashi M. Hydrogel-coated glide catheter: experimental studies and initial clinical experience. AJR American journal of roentgenology 1994;163:1227–1229.

[42] Noimark S, Dunnill CW, Wilson M, Parkin IP. The role of surfaces in catheter-associated infections. Chemical Society Reviews 2009;38:3435–3448.

[43] Choong SKS, Wood S, Whitfield HN. A model to quantify encrustation on ureteric stents, urethral catheters and polymers intended for urological use. BJU International 2000;86:414–421.

[44] Schierholz J, Beuth J, König D, Nürnberger A, Pulverer G. Antimicrobial substances and effects on sessile bacteria. Zentralblatt für Bakteriologie 1999;289:165–177.

[45] Hildebrandt P, Sayyad M, Rzany A, Schaldach M, Seiter H. Prevention of surface encrustation of urological implants by coating with inhibitors. Biomaterials 2001;22:503–507.

[46] Saint S, Meddings JA, Calfee D, Kowalski CP, Krein SL. Catheter-associated urinary tract infection and the Medicare rule changes. Annals of Internal Medicine 2009;150:877–884.

[47] Schierholz JM, Lucas LJ, Rump A, Pulverer G. Efficacy of silver-coated medical devices. J Hosp Infect 1998;40:257–262.

[48] Riley DK, Classen DC, Stevens LE, Burke JP. A large randomized clinical trial of a silver-impregnated urinary catheter: Lack of efficacy and staphylococcal superinfection. The American Journal of Medicine 1995;98:349–356.

[49] Schierholz JM, Konig DP, Beuth J, Pulverer G. The myth of encrustation inhibiting materials. J Hosp Infect 1999;42:162–163.

[50] Stickler DJ. Biomaterials to prevent nosocomial infections: is silver the gold standard? Curr Opin Infect Dis 2000;13:389–393.

[51] Bahar AA, Ren D. Antimicrobial Peptides. Pharmaceuticals 2013;6:1543–1575.

[52] Wang J, Liu Q, Tian Y, Jian Z, Li H, Wang K. Biodegradable hydrophilic polyurethane PEGU25 loading antimicrobial peptide Bmap-28: a sustained-release membrane able to inhibit bacterial biofilm formation in vitro. Sci Rep 2015;5:8634.

[53] Lange D, Chew BH, Elwood CN. Biomaterials in Urology-Beyond Drug Eluting and Degradable-A Rational Approach to Ureteral Stent Design. INTECH Open Access Publisher, 2011.

[54] Arshad M, Shah SS, Abbasi MH. Applications and complications of polyurethane stenting in urology. J Ayub Med Coll Abbottabad 2006;18:69–72.

[55] Singh I, Gupta NP, Hemal AK, Aron M, Seth A, Dogra PN. Severely encrusted polyurethane ureteral stents: management and analysis of potential risk factors. Urology 2001;58:526–531.

[56] Azuma H, Chancellor MB. Overview of Biodegradable Urethral Stents. Reviews in Urology 2004;6:98–99.

[57] Laaksovirta S, Valimaa T, Isotalo T, Tormala P, Talja M, Tammela TL. Encrustation and strength retention properties of the self-expandable, biodegradable, self-reinforced L-lactide-glycolic acid co-polymer 80:20 spiral urethral stent in vitro. J Urol 2003;170:468–471.

[58] Olweny EO, Landman J, Andreoni C, Collyer W, Kerbl K, Onciu M, *et al.* Evaluation of the Use of a Biodegradable Ureteral Stent After Retrograde Endopyelotomy in a Porcine Model. The Journal of Urology. 2002;167:2198–2202.

[59] Soto SM. Importance of biofilms in urinary tract infections: new therapeutic approaches. Advances in Biology 2014;1–13.

[60] Hazan Z, Zumeris J, Jacob H, Raskin H, Kratysh G, Vishnia M, *et al.* Effective Prevention of Microbial Biofilm Formation on Medical Devices by Low-Energy Surface Acoustic Waves. Antimicrobial Agents and Chemotherapy 2006;50:4144–4152.

[61] Davis CP, Shirtliff ME, Scimeca JM, Hoskins SL, Warren MM. In vivo reduction of bacterial populations in the urinary tract of catheterized sheep by iontophoresis. J Urol 1995;154:1948–1953.

[62] Jass J, Lappin-Scott HM. The efficacy of antibiotics enhanced by electrical currents against Pseudomonas aeruginosa biofilms. Journal of Antimicrobial Chemotherapy 1996;38:987–1000.

[63] Chakravarti A, Gangodawila S, Long MJ, Morris NS, Blacklock ARE, Stickler DJ. An electrified catheter to resist encrustation by *Proteus mirabilis* biofilm. The Journal of Urology 2005;174:1129–1132.

[64] Tenke P, Kovacs B, Bjerklund Johansen TE, Matsumoto T, Tambyah PA, Naber KG. European and Asian guidelines on management and prevention of catheter-associated urinary tract infections. Int J Antimicrob Agents 2008;31 Suppl 1:S68–S678.

[65] Khan A, Housami F, Melotti R, Timoney A, Stickler D. Strategy to Control Catheter Encrustation With Citrated Drinks: A Randomized Crossover Study. The Journal of Urology 183:1390–1394.

[66] Penniston KL, Nakada SY, Holmes RP, Assimos DG. Quantitative Assessment of Citric Acid in Lemon Juice, Lime Juice, and Commercially-Available Fruit Juice Products. Journal of endourology/Endourological Society 2008;22:567–570.

23

Stent Migration

Ravi Kulkarni

Consultant Urological Surgeon, Ashford and St Peter's Hospitals NHS Foundation Trust, Chertsey, Surrey, UK

23.1   Introduction

Ureteric stents are used extensively and for a variety of reasons. The main indications include short- or long-term relief of upper tract obstruction, prevention of pain due to edema after ureteroscopic manipulations, and endo-urological management of ureteric injuries. Stents are also used as splints after ureteric anastomosis, for example, uretero-neo-cystostomy, the formation of an ileal conduit or an orthotopic bladder reconstruction. Ureteric stents play a major role in the management of long-term upper tract obstruction caused by malignancy or recurrent benign strictures.

Ureteric stents are expected to remain in their position and function as effective conduits of urinary drainage. The design of the ureteric stents maintains their desired position. However, stent migration has been observed in 8 to 9.5 % of patients [1–4]. This leads to significant morbidity and also complicates patient management as retrieval or replacement of migrated stents can be complex (Figure 23.1).

23.2   Why Stents Migrate?

There is some debate as to whether stents actually migrate! Incorrect placement during the original procedure if often considered as the main reason for a perceived stent migration. However, true migration can occur due to a variety of reasons.

Distal migration of a JJ stent is related to its shape and the material [5]. A fully coiled stent is less likely to migrate than a J type of curl. A "half turn" coil of a J stent will not be able to overcome the peristaltic activity of the ureter or patient movement and thus will result in its misplacement (Figure 23.2).

Soft stents made from silicone have a higher propensity for migration than those manufactured from stiffer materials like polyurethane.

Iatrogenic migration can occur due to a variety of technical reasons. Premature withdrawal of the guidewire from the stent lumen will lead to incorrect placement of the superior coil of a JJ stent in the upper ureter. Lack of full curling of the upper coil of the stent will also result in the same outcome.

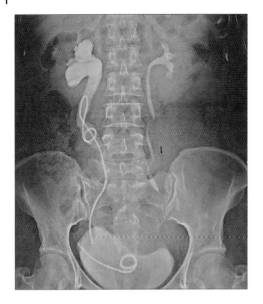

Figure 23.1 Migrated and Fragmented JJ stent.

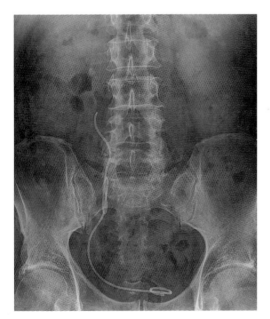
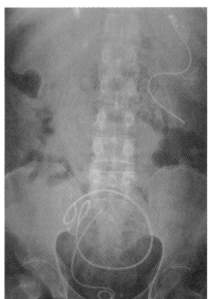

Figure 23.2 Migrated and Fragmented JJ stent.

Proximal migration is associated with the technique of insertion and an incorrect choice of stent length [6, 7]. Inadvertent selection of a short stent may result in the failure of curling of the distal coil, which can lead to an upward migration [8]. The same may result from an over-zealous push during the insertion. Excessive pushing of the distal end of the JJ stent during insertion will lead to the coil to remain in the distal ureter. Proximal migration will result.

Figure 23.3 Misplaced JJ stent. Ante-grade placement of JJ stent in the distal end in vagina. Ureteroscope in distal ureter during re-positioning.

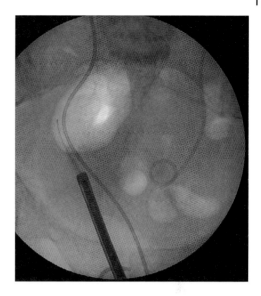

The placement of the proximal coil is also of significance. It should be placed in the renal pelvis and not in the calyx as this would result in proximal migration. Excess of stent length will remain in the in the upper tract and will fall short of the bladder [9].

The reverse can happen during an ante-grade insertion of a JJ stent. It is essential to confirm the position of stent sent after such insertion [10]. Incorrect positioning is more likely as the procedure is often performed under sedation in a radiology suite. There is no access to the bladder in these circumstances and the position of the distal end cannot be visually confirmed. The lower end of the stent may remain in the distal ureter or get misplaced if the guidewire perforates the ureter [11]. (Figure 23.3)

Excessive downward push during an antegrade insertion can lead to distal migration. Retrieval of the distally pushed stent back into the renal pelvis is difficult.

Stents placed in ileal conduits can migrate in either direction.

The use of extra-corporeal shockwave lithotripsy may encourage stent migration [12]. Imaging to assess stone fragmentation will also detect such displacement.

23.3   Where Do Stents Migrate?

Stents can migrate proximally or distally. They may also migrate outside the urinary tract – partially or completely. (Figures 23.4 and 23.5)

Distal migration leading to urinary incontinence due to the extrusion of the distal coil has been reported [13, 14]. Apart from the obvious proximal or distal misplacement, unusual migrations such as extrusion [15], perforation of duodenum [16], intra-peritoneal placement [17], retro-peritoneum [18], vagina, rectum [11], vena cava [19–21], and cardiac chambers [22, 23] have been reported. The lack of fluoroscopy during stent insertion is associated with such unusual placements and migrations. The extraction of such stents requires careful planning and ingenuity. Creative imaging is necessary to detect the exact position and the route taken by the stent.

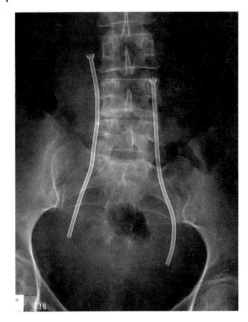
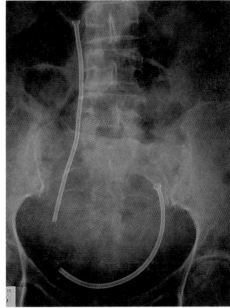

Figure 23.4 Distal migration of Memokath stent a) Bilateral ureteric obstruction due to lymph nodal metastases from carcinoma of anal canal b) Distal migration of left stent 6 months after insertion.

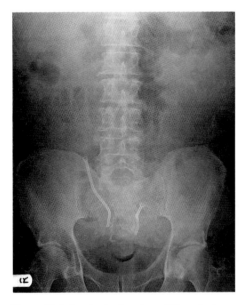
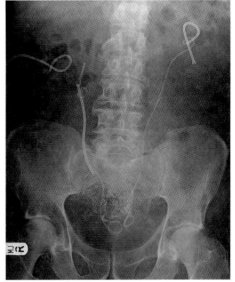

Figure 23.5 Proximal migration of Memokath stents a) Ca rectum. Radiation fibrosis Bilateral Memokath stents b) Migrated stents Bilateral JJ stents and right nephrostomy.

23.4   Stent Length and Migration

Selection of the length of a JJ stent is often arbitrary and based on the judgment of the urologist (or a radiologist) during the insertion. The selection of the stent length is mostly based on the patient's height [24–26]. However, there is little evidence to support this. Direct measurement of the ureter and its perceived length do not correlate well [27]. The accuracy between the exact ureteric length and the patient height is not supported by evidence [27–29]. A direct measurement from a CT scan is more accurate [30].

Various formulae have been described to assess ureteric length [31]. Cadaveric data suggests a lack of correlation between the actual ureteric length and anthropometric measurements [32]. Pediatric surgeons suggest a formula of age in years + 10 as the predictive length of the ureter (in centimeters) in children [33]. The problem of stent migration is observed in about 9% of pediatric procedures such as pyeloplasties [33].

An inappropriately selected stent, which is shorter than the actual length of the ureter will lead to an incorrect placement. The coiled end may remain in the ureter instead of renal pelvis or the bladder. This may create the impression of a migrated stent. The proximal or distal (and sometimes both) may remain in the ureteric lumen due to an error during insertion. The recommended position for the proximal coil is the renal pelvis. Placement of the coils in the upper calyces may result in proximal placement and migration [35].

23.5   Which Stents Migrate?

23.5.1   Stent Diameter, Material and Risk of Migration

As mentioned above, soft stent materials such as silicone are associated with a higher risk of migration compared with the stiffer polyurethane-based stents [34–36].

There is no correlation between stent diameter and migration.

23.5.2   Segmental Stents and Migration

Migration of metallic ureteric stents has been reported [36, 37]. The incidence is variable. Memokath stents have been reported to migrate in 8 to 10% [38, 39].

The incidence of migration of a Resonance stent in ileal conduit is around 90% [40].

23.6   Etiology of Ureteric Stricture and Migration

The recovery of peristalsis of an obstructed ureter after decompression can have a deleterious effect of "milking" the stent in either direction. This will be more likely in benign strictures where the gripping effect of the scar tissue is less firm than malignant tumors. Dilated ureteric lumen too can promote such migration.

Stent design may influence migration. Segmental stents, which are expected to stay only in the ureter, may have a greater propensity to migrate than those, which have a segment in the bladder. Such migrations can be in either direction.

23.7   Detection of Stent Migration

A plain abdominal x-ray is essential after a stent insertion. An incorrectly placed stent can be identified immediately and corrective action taken if the position is less than satisfactory

Stent migration may not cause any symptoms for a prolonged period of time [41]. Such silent migrations present late, with encrustation or sepsis. Imaging undertaken for other reasons may detect a migrated stent. These asymptomatic forgotten stents are usually encrusted and calcified.(Figure 23.6) Proximal migration is more common in this cohort of patients as a distally migrated forgotten stent will encrust and will cause troublesome lower urinary tract symptoms. Asymptomatic distal migration is uncommon.

Patients with other significant comorbidity such as extremes of age, cognitive difficulties, and complex medical issues are more likely to present late with migrated stents.

Persistence of pain, increasing hydronephrosis, failure of improvement (or deterioration) in the renal function in an obstructed system, and inadequate control of sepsis suggest a possibility of migration in the absence of imaging.

23.8   Management of Migrated Stents

Incorrect placement and migration of ureteric stents can pose difficult clinical challenges. Clinical presentation of a migrated stent can vary enormously and often results in delayed detection.

A migrated stent is usually detected by an imaging modality. Removal of such a stent requires a full assessment of the affected renal unit as well as the patient. The exact location, anatomy of the pelvi-calyceal system and renal function in that moity should be

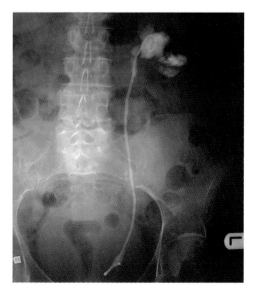

Figure 23.6 Heavily calcified forgotten JJ stent which needed per-cutaneous removal.

evaluated. Coexistent sepsis should be corrected. The degree of encrustation can vary considerably and will have a significant impact on the technique of removal. Fragmentation might have occurred and multiple pieces of a migrated stent may lie in different locations of the urinary system.

Stents that have migrated into the renal pelvis can be removed by endoscopic means with the use of an antegrade or a retrograde technique. The use of a semi-rigid or flexible ureteroscope to retrieve the distal end of the stent is the least invasive method. The use of grasping forceps or a dormia basket to trap the lower end of the stent is usually effective [42]. This can be performed under general or local anesthesia [43]. Ingenious techniques such as the passage of a guidewire to trap and extract the stent have been described [44]. The retrieval of migrated metallic stents is challenging and requires complex endo-urological techniques [45, 46].

Percutaneous removal may be necessary in a small cohort of patients. This approach is necessary when retrograde methods have failed, there is heavy encrustation or complete migration in to the renal pelvis [47]. This is the preferred option in children too [48]. A percutaneous removal can be undertaken with an initial insertion of a nephrostomy tube. This has the advantage of decompression of the system and control of infection. Adequate dilatation of the tract to accommodate a suitable size nephroscope is the preferred method. This also has the advantage of the convenience of deploying laser or lithoclast to fragment the encrustations prior to removal.

A conventional PCNL type of procedure may not be necessary as the mini-PCNL equipment may be able to accept smaller, flexible instruments. This reduces the morbidity of the procedure and the length of stay. The use of laser for the fragmentation of the encrusted stent and a suitable grasping device can be deployed to remove such stents. A fiber-optic ureteroscope can be passed down the ureter if necessary.

Retrograde intra renal surgery too can be used to remove such stents. This, however, can be difficult. The encrustation and fragility of the stent may prevent safe removal in one session. However, this may be the only option if significant comorbidity precludes the use of a percutaneous approach.

23.9   Special Situations

23.9.1   Migrated Memokath Stents

These stents can migrate in either direction. Distal migration is relatively easy to manage. Irrigation with cold saline at a temperature below 10 °C will soften the stent material [49]. The most distal coil of the stent is held in a suitable forceps. The softened stent will unravel if pulled and can be removed through the cystoscope sheath. It is essential to keep the entire stent cooled during removal, as it will harden very quickly due to the body temperature.

Removal of a proximally migrated Memokath stents may need a percutaneous approach. A nephrostomy tube is inserted to decompress the upper tract. Adequate dilatation followed by the insertion of a nephroscope will permit access to the stent. The subsequent steps of removal thereafter are similar to the retrograde procedure. The stent must be removed through the lumen of the sheath of the scope as the partially unravelled stent material can traumatize the renal parenchyma and result in bleeding.

23.9.2 Other Metallic Stents

There is limited published data on the removal of other metallic stents. The technique of removal of such stents needs to be obtained from the manufacturer. Case reports of difficult stent removals and personal communications with a clinician who has the original experience of these stents are often helpful. It may be appropriate to direct such complicated patients to the urologist who has the experience of that specific device.

23.10 Conclusions

Stent migration is the cause of significant morbidity. This complication is preventable in a cohort of patients. Attention to detail, appropriate selection of stent length, use of fluoroscopy, and cystoscopy during insertion will reduce the incidence of incorrect placement. Genuine migration can be detected by early post-insertion imaging. Corrective steps taken quickly will avoid the need for a difficult and invasive extraction at a later date.

References

[1] Leibovici D1, Cooper A, Lindner A, Ostrowsky R, Kleinmann J, Velikanov S, Cipele H, Goren E, Siegel YI. Ureteral stents: morbidity and impact on quality of life. Isr Med Assoc J. 2005 Aug;7(8):491–4.

[2] Ringel A, Richter S, Shalev M, Nissenkorn I. Late complications of ureteral stents. Eur Urol. 2000;38(1):41–44.

[3] Damiano R, Oliva A, Esposito C, De Sio M, Autorino R, D'Armiento M. Early and late complications of double pigtail ureteral stent. Urol Int. 2002;69(2):136–140.

[4] Hao P, Li W, Song C, Yan J, Song B, Li L. Clinical evaluation of double-pigtail stent in patients with upper urinary tract diseases: report of 2685 cases. J Endourol. 2008;22(1):65–70. doi: 10.1089/end.2007.0114.

[5] Saltzman B. Ureteral stents. Indications, variations and complications. Urol Clin North Am.1988;15:481–491.

[6] Breau RH, Norman RW. Optimal prevention and management of proximal ureteral stent migration and remigration. J Urol. 2001;166:890–893.

[7] Slaton JW, Kropp KA. Proximal ureteral stent migration: an avoidable complication? J Urol. 1996;155(1):58–61.

[8] Garrido Abad P, Fernández Arjona M, Fernández González I, Santos Arrontes D, Pereira Sanz I. [Proximal migration of a Double J catheter: case report and review of the literature]. Arch Esp Urol. 2008;61(3):428–431.

[9] Elmalik K, Chowdhury MM, Capps SN. Ureteric stents in pyeloplasty: a help or a hindrance? J Pediatr Urol. 2008;4(4):275–279.

[10] Soh KC, Tay KH, Tan BS, Mm Htoo A, Hg Lo R, Lin SE. Is the routine check nephrostogram following percutaneous antegrade ureteric stent placement necessary? Cardiovasc Intervent Radiol. 2008;31(3):604–609.

[11] Rao AR, Alleemudder A, Mukerji G, Mishra V, Motiwala H, Charig M, Karim OM. Extra-anatomical complications of antegrade double-J insertion. Indian J Urol. 2011;27(1):19–24. doi: 10.4103/0970-1591.78408.

[12] Bregg K, Riehle RA Jr. Morbidity associated with indwelling internal ureteral stents after shock wave lithotripsy. J Urol. 1989;141(3):510–512.

[13] Delasobera BE, Rogers WD. A case of sudden, painless, and persistent urinary incontinence. J Emerg Med. 2013;44(1):e37–e39. doi: 10.1016/j.jemermed.2011.06.123. Epub 2011 Nov 12.

[14] Murtaza B, Niaz WA, Akmal M, Ahmad H, Mahmood A. A rare complication of forgotten ureteral stent. J Coll Physicians Surg Pak. 2011;21(3):190–192.

[15] Shivde SR, Joshi P, Jamkhandikar R. Extrusion of double J stent: a rare complication. Urology 2008;71(5):814–815.

[16] Wall I, Baradarian R, Tangorra M, Badalov N, Iswara K, Li J, Tenner S. Spontaneous perforation of the duodenum by a migrated ureteral stent. Gastrointest Endosc 2008;68(6):1236–1238. doi: 10.1016/j.gie.2008.02.083. Epub 2008 Jun 11.

[17] Wall I, Baradarian R, Tangorra M, Badalov N, Iswara K, Li J, Tenner S. Spontaneous perforation of the duodenum by a migrated ureteral stent. Gastrointest Endosc 2008;68(6):1236–1238.

[18] Abraham G, Das K, George D. Retroperitoneal migration of a Double-J stent: an unusual occurrence. J Endourol 2011;25(2):297–299.

[19] Falahatkar S, Hemmati H, Gholamjani Moghaddam K. Re: Intracaval migration: an uncommon complication of ureteral double-J stent placement. (From: Falahatkar S, Hemmati H, Gholamjani Moghaddam K. J Endourol 2012;26:119-121). J Endourol 2013;27(8):1069–1071.

[20] Ioannou CV, Velegrakis J, Kostas T, Georgakarakos E, Touloupakis E, Anezinis P, Katsamouris AN. Caval migration of a ureteral J-stent after simultaneous ureter and iliac vein perforation during its placement for obstructive pyelonephritis. Int Angiol 2009;28(5):421–424.

[21] Tang Z, Li D, Xiao L, Wan Y, Luo K, Huang L, Zhou J, Huang K. Re: Intracaval migration: an uncommon complication of ureteral double-J stent placement. (From: Endourol 2012;26:119-121). J Endourol. 2012;26(8):1100–1101

[22] Kim TN, Lee CH, Kong do H, Shin DK, Lee JZ. Misplacement or migration? Extremely rare case of cardiac migration of a ureteral j stent. Korean J Urol 2014;55(5):360–362. doi: 10.4111/kju.2014.55.5.360. Epub 2014 May 12.

[23] Hastaoglu IO, Tokoz H, Kavlak E, Bilgen F. Double J ureteral stent displaced through the right ventricle. Interact Cardiovasc Thorac Surg 2014;18(6):853–854. doi: 10.1093/icvts/ivu037. Epub 2014 Mar 14.

[24] Norman RW, Breau RH. Optimal length of ureteric stents. Clin Radiol 2003;58(3):257.

[25] Pilcher JM, Patel U. Choosing the correct length of ureteric stent: a formula based on the patient's height compared with direct ureteric measurement. Clin Radiol 2002;57(1):59–62.

[26] Hruby GW, Ames CD, Yan Y, Monga M, Landman J. Correlation of ureteric length with anthropometric variables of surface body habitus. JU Int 2007;99(5):1119–1122. Epub 2007 Feb 19.

[27] Jeon SS, Choi YS, Hong JH. Determination of ideal stent length for endourologic surgery. J Endourol 2007;21(8):906–910.

[28] Paick SH, Park HK, Byun SS, Oh SJ, Kim HH. Direct ureteric length measurement from intravenous pyelography: does height represent ureteric length? Urol Res. 2005;33(3):199–202. Epub 2005 Feb 25.

[29] Shah J, Kulkarni RP. Height does not predict ureteric length. Clin Radiol 2005;60(7):812–814.

[30] Kawahara T, Ito H, Terao H, Yoshida M, Ogawa T, Uemura H, Kubota Y, Matsuzaki J. Which is the best method to estimate the actual ureteral length in patients undergoing ureteral stent placement? Int J Urol 2012;19(7):634–638.

[31] Shrewsberry AB, Al-Qassab U, Goodman M, Petros JA, Sullivan JW, Ritenour CW, Issa MM. A +20% adjustment in the computed tomography measured ureteral length is an accurate predictor of true ureteral length before ureteral stent placement. J Endourol 2013;27(8):1041–1045.

[32] Novaes HF, Leite PC, Almeida RA, Sorte NC, Barroso U Jr. Analysis of ureteral length in adult cadavers. Int Braz J Urol 2013;39(2):248–256.

[33] Palmer JS, Palmer LS. Determining the proper stent length to use in children: age plus 10. J Urol 2007;178(4 Pt 2):1566–1569.

[34] Hofman R, Hartung R. Ureteric stents and new materials. World Journal of Urology 1989;7:154–157.

[35] Oswalt GC Jr, Bueschen AJ, Lloyd IK. Upward migration of indwelling ureteral stents. J Urol 1979;122(2):249–250.

[36] Chung HH, Kim MD, Won JY, Won JH, Cho SB, Seo TS, Park SW, Kang BC. Multicenter experience of the newly designed covered metallic ureteral stent for malignant ureteral occlusion: comparison with double J stent insertion. Cardiovasc Intervent Radiol 2014;37(2):463–470.

[37] Liatsikos EN, Karnabatidis D, Katsanos K, Kallidonis P, Katsakiori P, Kagadis GC, Christeas N, Papathanassiou Z, Perimenis P, Siablis D. Ureteral metal stents: 10-year experience with malignant ureteral obstruction treatment. J Urol 2009;182(6):2613–2617.

[38] Papadopoulos GI, Middela S, Srirangam SJ, Szczesniak CA, Rao PN. Use of Memokath 051 metallic stent in the management of ureteral strictures: a single-center experience. Urol Int 2010;84(3):286–291.

[39] Agrawal S, Brown CT, Bellamy EA, Kulkarni R. The thermo-expandable metallic ureteric stent: an 11-year follow-up. BJU Int 2009;103(3):372–376.

[40] Garg T, Guralnick ML, Langenstroer P, See WA, Hieb RA, Rilling WS, Sudakoff GS, O'Connor RC. Resonance metallic ureteral stents do not successfully treat ureteroenteric strictures. J Endourol 2009;23(7):1199–1201; discussion 1202.

[41] Cormio L, Piccinni R, Cafarelli A, Callea A, Zizzi V, Traficante A. Asymptomatic spontaneous migration of double pigtail ureteral stent outside the ureter. Int Urol Nephrol 2007;39(1):75–77.

[42] Meeks JJ, Helfand BT, Thaxton CS, Nadler RB. Retrieval of migrated ureteral stents by coaxial cannulation with a flexible ureteroscope and paired helical basket. J Endourol 2008;22(5):927–929.

[43] Livadas KE, Varkarakis IM, Skolarikos A, Karagiotis E, Alivizatos G, Sofras F, Deliveliotis C, Bissas A. Ureteroscopic removal of mildly migrated stents using local anesthesia only. J Urol 2007;178(5):1998–2001.

[44] Fisher JD, Monahan M, Johnston WK 3rd. Improvised method to retrieve a proximally displaced ureteral stent in a remote surgical setting. J Endourol 2013;27(7):922–924.

[45] Potretzke AM, Chang H, Kryger JV. Technique for Resonance® stent exchange in patients with extrinsic obstruction: description of a novel approach and literature review. J Pediatr Urol 2012;8(5):557–559.

[46] Kaplan A, Kolla S, Landman J. Endoscopic Management of Tissue Ingrowth into the Proximal and Distal Components of a Resonance Ureteral Stent. AUA poster, May 7, 2013.

[47] Given MF, Geoghegan T, Lyon SM, McGrath F, Lee MJ. Percutaneous antegrade ureteric stent removal using a rigid alligator forceps. J Med Imaging Radiat Oncol 2008;52(6):576–579.

[48] Lal A, Singhal M, Narasimhan KL, Mahajan JK, Singh JK, Ghai B, Khandelwal N. Percutaneous retrieval of coiled double-J stent from renal pelvis after Anderson-Hynes pyeloplasty: report of two cases. J Pediatr Urol 2012;8(3):e19–e22.

[49] Kulkarni R, Bellamy E. Nickel-titanium shape memory alloy Memokath 051 ureteral stent for managing long-term ureteral obstruction: 4-year experience. J Urol 2001;166(5):1750–1754.

24

Health-Related Quality of Life and Ureteric Stents

Aditya Raja[1] and Hrishi B. Joshi[2]

[1] Research Fellow in Urology, University Hospital of Wales and School of Medicine, Cardiff University, Cardiff, Wales, UK
[2] Consultant Urological Surgeon and Honorary Lecturer, Department of Urology, University Hospital of Wales and School of Medicine, Cardiff University, Wales, UK

24.1 Introduction

Since their introduction, ureteric stents have been known to cause adverse effects. Although much research has focused on attempting to reduce their morbidity in the last 40 years, it still remains the major cause of patient morbidity. Symptoms are known to be both physical and psychosocial and include pain or discomfort (in the loin to groin distribution), lower urinary tract symptoms and sexual dysfunction [1, 2].

Stent technology has evolved since the early days of ureteric stenting. Some of the original ureteric catheters were made out of fabric and coated in varnish [3]. This caused local irritation to the urothelium and caused the stents to become encrusted very quickly. This limited their use and the duration of time they could be left in situ. Later, stents were created out of silicone rubber that impinged on the bladder. Modern stents are composed of a range of hypoallergenic, smooth materials with the view to decrease encrustation rates and stent-related symptoms. Although these devices have continued to evolve, they are still far from perfect and research continues to find ways to reduce patient discomfort.

A review of the early literature shows that following the insertion of a ureteric stent, patients commonly suffer stent-related symptoms such as pain (18-58%), hematuria (34-85%), dysuria (13-72%), frequency of urination (50-85%), and urgency (43-67%) [4]. Less common problems related to ureteric stents include incorrect stent placement and migration. In addition to these symptoms, studies have reported other important HRQoL problems including upper and lower urinary tract sepsis (8-20%), visits to the emergency department, the need to take antibiotics and/or painkillers (66%) [1]. These symptoms may be caused by stent factors (e.g., size, shape or composition) or patient factors (e.g., physical activity, pain caused by reflux) or by some other, currently undiagnosed mechanism. However, these assessments were methodologically weak and unreliable. Subjective HRQoL had not been quantified in an objective way, which made proper evaluation and comparison of HRQoL difficult.

24.2 Development of the Ureteric Stent Symptom Questionnaire (USSQ)

Generic quality of life measures are available such as the SF-36 (and its derivatives and subsequent iterations) and the EuroQol EQ 5-D; however, until recently there had been no intervention-specific measures of HRQoL in patients with in-dwelling ureteric stents [5]. Due to the paucity and heterogeneous nature of these observational studies, it was difficult to come to any objective conclusions. None of the studies investigated used a validated quality of life measure (Figure 24.1).

In 2003, Joshi *et al.* developed the "Ureteric Stent Symptoms Questionnaire" (USSQ). The USSQ is a comprehensive, reliable, and psychometrically valid multidimensional measure that was developed using sound social science methodology,

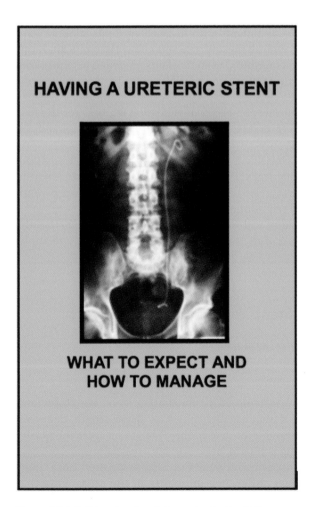

Figure 24.1 Validated patient information leaflet [24].

including qualitative and quantitative research methods, involving both patients and clinicians extensively.

In total, 309 patients helped to develop the USSQ in different phases. During Phase I, nine patients were interviewed after the initial literature review. These, along with studies using existing measures formed the basis of the initial draft of the USSQ. Phase II saw a pilot testing with patients followed by an expert review and then field testing of 40 patients. This produced the final draft, containing 38 items covering six overarching domains. Formal validation was performed in Phase III and reliability, validity, and sensitivity to change were calculated. The measure was found to be internally consistent (Cronbach's alpha >0.7) and test-retest reliability was found to be good (Pearson's coefficient >0.84). Sensitivity to change was good and this was demonstrated by a significant change in score after stent removal. The measure was found to discriminate between those with stents, healthy controls, and patients with urinary stone disease without stents [6].

Results of this work showed that with regard to the morbidity associated with ureteric stents and its effect on HRQoL, 80% of patients with in dwelling stents suffered with difficulty in carrying out activities of daily living and 73% suffered with significant lower urinary tract dysfunction. Patients that required ureteric stents tended to be of working age and 58% of patients reported that their stent-related symptoms had an adverse effect on their work performance.

After the development, USSQ underwent a series of validation studies. For the first time, these studies quantified the symptoms associated with ureteric stents and the effect they have on patients' HRQoL.

Since the original creation of the English version of the USSQ, it has been translated, with linguistic validation in seven languages (French, Italian, Korean, Turkish, Spanish, Mexican Spanish, and Arabic). The Korean version of the USSQ was shown by Park *et al.* in 2012 to be reliable and valid self-administered tool [7].

The USSQ continues to be translated and validated into other languages across the globe. Studies confirm similar impacts of stents on HRQoL across different populations worldwide.

24.3 Data on HRQoL with Stents from Clinical Studies

24.3.1 Studies Involving Different Ureteric Stent Designs – Engineering Methods

24.3.1.1 Stent Designs and Materials

Both industry and researchers have attempted to ameliorate stent symptoms and improve HRQoL by changing stent design attributes such as shape, length, diameter, and stiffness of stents. In total, eight studies have used the USSQ to measure the quality of life of patients with new stent designs [8–15].

Joshi *et al.* compared firm and soft polymer stents in 2005 using the USSQ. They revealed that there was no objective difference in quality of life of patients that had either type of stent [8]. Lingeman *et al.* compared the novel design Boston Scientific Polaris® and Percuflex® stents against control short loop and long tail loop stents. They showed that having less volume of stent material caused less pain (lower USSQ pain domain scores), however this was not shown to be statistically significant [9]. The Bard Inlay® stent showed no change in overall quality of life compared to other stents but patients did report significantly lower USSQ scores in the domain of urinary symptoms. In a similar study in 2011, Davenport *et al.* at did not find any difference in USSQ scores between the Bard Inlay® stent the Polaris® stent [10].

In another study, differing lengths and diameters of stents were compared to assess their impact on quality of life. Studies compared single-length (24 cm) versus multi-length (30 cm), and wider (6Fr) versus thinner (4.8Fr) stent and no significant differences between stents were noted [15].

Two studies compared new stent technology with the older versions with regards to quality of life. The Urovision antirefluxive® stent was tested against a standard Urovision® stent. Patients were found to have less pain on micturition with the antirefluxive stents compared to the controls, however, this was not statistically significant [12].

The PNNMedical Memokath® is a novel, thermo-expandable segmented metallic ureteric stent and can be used in patients with ureteric strictures or malignant extrinsic compression of the ureter. It was compared with a standard ureteric stent and was found to have a statistically positive effect on both light and heavy activity. The Memokath® showed a non-statistically significant decrease in pain and lower urinary tract symptoms compared to the controls [13].

24.4   Studies Comparing Pharmacological Interventions

24.4.1   Pharmacological Agents

The USSQ has been used in 12 clinical trials, testing the efficacy of four drugs to lessen stent-related symptoms (alfuzosin, botulinum type A, tamsulosin, and tolterodine). Gupta *et al.* reported in 2010 that Botulinum type A showed significant reduction in post operative stent-related pain and a decrease in the need for analgesia [16]. Park *et al.* in 2009 compared tolterodine, alfuzosin, and placebo in a randomized controlled trial and found that both drugs had a greater positive effect on HRQoL than the placebo for patients with stents and that there was no significant difference them [17].

A systematic review and meta-analysis by Yakoubi *et al.* in 2011 showed that four studies demonstrated a significant decrease in stent-related discomfort in patients taking alfuzosin and seven studies reported the same with tamsulosin. Both drugs are alpha-1 adrenergic receptor antagonists. Four trials met the inclusion criteria for meta-analysis and included 341 patients, three of these studies examined alfuzosin and one tamsulosin. The analysis showed a significant reduction in urinary symptoms (mean decrease in domain score -6.76, $p = 0.005$) a significant decrease in pain (mean decrease in domain score -3.55, $p = 0.0004$) and significant improvement in general health (mean decrease in domain score -1.90, $p = 0.001$) [18].

24.5   Other Aspects of Ureteric Stents and HRQoL

24.5.1   Position of the Distal End of the Stent and BMI

Giannarini *et al.* used the USSQ to measure ureteric stent-related symptoms compared to position of the stent and BMI. They concluded that the patients were more likely to suffer with symptoms of body pain, decreased work performance, general health, urinary symptoms, and decreased sexual function if the distal loop of the stent crossed the midline. BMI was also found to be related to increased body pain and decreased general health [19].

24.5.2   Other Clinical Scenarios

Patients with renal transplants were found to have lower USSQ scores when the transplant ureter was implanted in the dome of the bladder and that patients suffered with less stent-related symptoms if a transplant ureter was used compared to those with a stent in the native ureter [20].

Barnes *et al.* in 2014 reported that patients with stents with extraction strings attached (for removal without the need of flexible cystoscopy) had no significant difference in HRQoL than those without [21].

In 2015, Abt *et al.* found that intra-vesical stent position on abdominal x-ray did not significantly affect the USSQ scores in their study of 73 patients [22].

24.5.2.1   Patient Information, Counseling, and HRQoL

One aspect of HRQoL and ureteric stenting that has not been fully investigated is the effect of patient education on HRQoL of patients. As early as 2001, the concept of better patient education was investigated and this culminated with the production of an eight-page patient information booklet to give to patients with ureteric stents. This was validated on 30 patients with stents in situ (Figure 24.2). More recently, a study of 74 patients in 2015 showed that patient education on stent-related symptoms before stent insertion led to a significant reduction in the incidence of the stent-related symptoms (Figure 24.3). High-quality patient education is not only advisable from an ethical point of view but could help to reduce the symptoms associated with ureteric stents [23].

24.6   Conclusions

Ureteric stents are an essential part of the armamentarium of an endourologist, however, adverse symptoms associated with ureteric stent use are common and this has a negative affect on the patient's physical and psychosocial well being and overall HRQoL. Symptoms such as pain, lower urinary tract symptoms, as well as sexual dysfunction reduce the HRQoL in over 80% of patients. Patients also describe decreased work performance. The USSQ is a robust, valid, reliable intervention-specific measure to evaluate this morbidity. It has been translated into several languages and this trend endures. It continues to be used to quantify heath-related quality of life in patients with ureteric stents in situ all over the world in both clinical and research settings. Recent, small studies have shown that high-quality patient information leaflets and effective counseling before stent insertion may help to reduce the burden of health-related quality of life effects on stented patients.

URETERIC
STENT SYMPTOMS QUESTIONNAIRE

Questionnaire 1 (*Stent in situ*)

We are interested to know about various aspects of <u>your health, following insertion of the stent</u> and the effect the stent has had on your health.

Please complete the following questionnaire, which has different sections. Please answer all questions in each section.

(We would be grateful if you could complete and post the questionnaire within seven days)

Please complete:

Today's Date: ☐☐ / ☐☐ / ☐☐

Date of Birth: ☐☐ / ☐☐ / ☐☐

Please return to:

Post Code: ☐☐☐☐ ☐☐☐
Hospital Number : ☐☐☐☐☐☐
(for office use)

Figure 24.2 Ureteric stent symptom questionnaire for when stent in situ.

You will see that some questions ask if you have a symptom occasionally, sometimes or most of the time.

Occasionally	=	**less than one third of the time**
Sometimes	=	**between one and two thirds of the time**
Most of the time	=	**more than two thirds of the time**

URINARY SYMPTOMS

Please answer the questions thinking about the urinary symptoms you have experienced <u>following insertion of the stent.</u>

Please put a tick in one box for each question ☑

Please think about your experience since insertion of the stent.

U1. During the day, how often do you pass urine, on average?

Less than hourly ☐ 5   Every 3 hourly ☐ 2

Hourly ☐ 4   Every 4 hours or more ☐ 1

Every 2 hourly ☐ 3

U2. During the night, how many times do you have to get up to pass urine, on average?

None ☐ 1   3 ☐ 4

1 ☐ 2   4 or more ☐ 5

2 ☐ 3

U3. Do you have to rush to the toilet to urinate?

Never ☐ 1   Most of the time ☐ 4
                         (more than two thirds for the time)

Occasionally ☐ 2   All of the time ☐ 5
(less than one third of the time)

Sometimes ☐ 3
(between one and two thirds of the time)

U4. Does urine leak before you can get to the toilet?

Never ☐ 1   Most of the time ☐ 4

Occasionally ☐ 2   All of the time ☐ 5

Sometimes ☐ 3

U5. Do you leak urine without feeling the need to go to the toilet?

Never ☐ 1   Most of the time ☐ 4

Occasionally ☐ 2   All of the time ☐ 5

Sometimes ☐ 3

2

Figure 24.2 (*Continued*)

U6. how often do you feel that your bladder has not emptied properly after you have passed urine?

Never ☐ 1

Occasionally ☐ 2
(less than one third of the time)

Sometimes ☐ 3
(between one and two thirds of the time)

Most of the time ☐ 4
(more than two thirds for the time)

All of the time ☐ 5

U7. Do you have a burning feeling when you pass urine?

Never ☐ 1

Occasionally ☐ 2

Sometimes ☐ 3

Most of the time ☐ 4

All of the time ☐ 5

U8. How often do you blood in your urine?

Never ☐ 1

Occasionally ☐ 2

Sometimes ☐ 3

Most of the time ☐ 4

All of the time ☐ 5

U9. How much blood do you see in your urine?

Do not see any blood ☐ 1

Urine is slightly blood stained ☐ 2

Urine is heavily blood stained ☐ 3

Urine is heavily blood stained and has clot(s) ☐ 4

U10. Overall, how much of a problem are your urinary symptoms to you?

Not at all ☐ 1

A little bit ☐ 2

Moderate ☐ 3

Quite a bit ☐ 4

Extreme ☐ 5

U11. If you were to spend the rest of your life with the urinary symptoms, if any, associated with the stent just the way they are, how would you feel about it?

Delighted ☐ 1

Pleased ☐ 2

Mostly satisfied ☐ 3

Mixed feelings (about equally satisfied and dissatisfied ☐ 4

Mostly dissatisfied ☐ 5

Unhappy ☐ 6

Terrible ☐ 7

Please go to next section --

3

Figure 24.2 (*Continued*)

BODY PAIN (for women):

This section asks about the **body pain or discomfort, which you associate with the stent.**

Please think about your experience **following insertion of the stent.**

P1. Do you experience body pain or discomfort in association with the stent?

      YES ☐₁**, please go to question P2**

      NO ☐₂**, please go to next section on General Health**   (Ignore questions P2 to P9)

P2. Think of the drawings below as the drawings of your body. Please **mark (X) or shade the site(s) where you experience pain or discomfort in association with the stent typically (e.g. during the day to day activities, whenever you pass urine)**

      If you get pain at more than one site, please use a <u>separate mark for each site.</u>

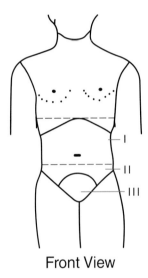
Front View

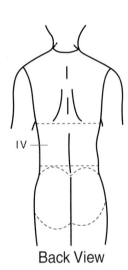
Back View

The numbers I - IV represent following areas for the right and left sides

    I – Kidney front/side area   III – Bladder area

    II - Groin area   IV– Kidney back (loin) area

    Please use O for any other marked area and write the name of the site

P3. Please place a <u>mark (X) to a point on the line below that indicates your pain or discomfort</u> in association with the stent. **Please put a separate mark for each site** if the pain or discomfort is different in severity and write the corresponding number of each site used in the drawing above.

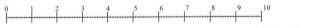

No Pain or discomfort   **Worst Possible Pain**

4

Figure 24.2 *(Continued)*

BODY PAIN (for men):

This section asks about the **body pain or discomfort, which you associate with the stent.**

Please think about your experience **following insertion of the stent.**

P1. Do you experience body pain or discomfort in association with the stent?

YES ☐₁**, please go to question P2**

NO ☐₂**, please go to next section on General Health**   (Ignore questions P2 to P9)

P2. Thinking the drawings below as the drawings of your body, **mark (X) or shade the site(s) where you experience pain or discomfort in association with the stent typically (e.g. during the day to day activities, whenever you pass urine)**

> If you get pain at more than one site, please use a <u>separate mark for each site.</u>

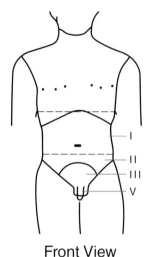
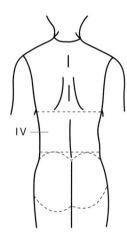

Front View   Back View

The numbers I - V represent following areas for the right and left side.

I – Kidney front/side area	**IV**– Kidney back (loin) area
II - Groin area	**V** – Penis
III – Bladder area	Please use **O** for any other marked site and name that site.

P3. Please place a <u>mark (X) to a point on the line below that indicates your pain or discomfort in</u> association with the stent. **Please put a separate mark for each site** if the pain or discomfort is different in severity and write the corresponding number of each site used in the drawing above.

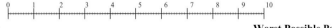

No Pain or discomfort   **Worst Possible Pain**

5

Figure 24.2 *(Continued)*

P4. Which of the following statements best describe your experience regarding <u>physical activities</u> and the pain or discomfort in association with the stent?

I **do not experience any pain** or discomfort during physical activities ☐ 1

I experience pain or discomfort only when I perform **vigorous activities** ☐ 2
(e.g. strenuous sports, lifting heavy objects)

I experience pain when I perform **activities of moderate severity** but not with basic activities ☐ 3
(e.g. walking few hundred yards, driving a car)

I experience pain even when I perform **basic activities** of daily living ☐ 4
(e.g. walking indoors, dressing)

I experience pain while also **being at rest** ☐ 5

P5. Does the pain or discomfort, in association with the stent, interrupt your sleep?

Never ☐ 1   Most of the time ☐ 4

Occasionally ☐ 2   All of the time ☐ 5

Sometimes ☐ 3

P6. Do you experience pain or discomfort, in association with the stent, while passing urine?

Never ☐ 1   Most of the time ☐ 4

Occasionally ☐ 2   All of the time ☐ 5

Sometimes ☐ 3

P7. Do you experience pain or discomfort in the <u>kidney area</u>, while passing urine?

No ☐ 1

Yes ☐ 2

P8. How frequently have you required painkillers to control the pain or discomfort associated with the stent?

Never ☐ 1   Most of the time ☐ 4

Occasionally ☐ 2   All of the time ☐ 5

Sometimes ☐ 3

P9. Overall, how much does the pain or discomfort, in association with the stent, (as distinct from other symptoms) interfere with your life?

Never ☐ 1   Most of the time ☐ 4

Occasionally ☐ 2   All of the time ☐ 5

Sometimes ☐ 3

Please go to next section --

6

Figure 24.2 (*Continued*)

GENERAL HEALTH:

Following insertion of the stent:

G1. Have you had difficulty in performing light physical activities (e.g. walking short distances, driving a car)?

Usually with no difficulty ☐ 1   Usually did not do because of the stent ☐ 4

Usually with some difficulty ☐ 2   All of the time ☐ 0

Usually with much difficulty ☐ 3

G2. Have you had difficulty in performing heavy physical activities (e.g. strenuous sports, lifting heavy objects)?

Usually with no difficulty ☐ 1   Usually did not do because of the stent ☐ 4

Usually with some difficulty ☐ 2   All of the time ☐ 0

Usually with much difficulty ☐ 3

G3. Have you felt tired and worn out?

Never ☐ 1   Most of the time (more than two thirds of the time) ☐ 4

Occasionally (less than one third of the time) ☐ 2   All of the time ☐ 5

Sometimes (between one and two thirds of the time) ☐ 3

G4. Have you felt calm and peaceful?

All of the time ☐ 1   Occasionally (more than two thirds of the time) ☐ 4

Most of the time (less than one third of the time) ☐ 2   Never ☐ 5

Sometimes (between one and two thirds of the time) ☐ 3

G5. Have you enjoyed your social life (going out, meeting friends and so on)?

All of the time ☐ 1   Occasionally ☐ 4

Most of the time ☐ 2   Never ☐ 5

Sometimes ☐ 3

G6. Have you needed extra help from your family members or friends?

Never ☐ 1   Most of the time ☐ 4

Occasionally ☐ 2   All of the time ☐ 5

Sometimes ☐ 3

Please go to next section –

7

Figure 24.2 *(Continued)*

WORK PERFORMANCE:

W1. Regarding your employment status, are you

In full time employment ☐ 1   Student ☐ 4

In part time employment ☐ 2   Unemployed, looking for work ☐ 5

Retired on health ground ☐ 3   Retired for other reason (including age) ☐ 6

Not working for other reason (please specify) ☐ 7 _____

W2. Following insertion of the stent, how many days did the symptoms associated with the stent keep you in bed all or most of the day?

☐☐ Day(s)

W3. Following insertion of the stent, for how many half days or more did you cut down your routine activities because of the symptoms associated with the stent?

☐☐ Half Day(s)

Please answer the questions below (W4 –W7) only if you are in active paid work.
(Otherwise ignore questions W4 – W7).

W4. a) Job title or description of your role: _____

b) Are you an: Employee ☐ 1   Employer ☐ 2   Self employed ☐ 3

Please answer following questions if you have worked after insertion of the stent,

W5. Have you worked for short periods of time or taken frequent rests because of the symptoms associated with the stent?	
Never ☐ 1	Most of the time ☐ 4
Occasionally ☐ 2	All of the time ☐ 5
Sometimes ☐ 3	

W6. Have you worked at your usual job, but with some changes because of the symptoms associated with the stent?	
Never ☐ 1	Most of the time ☐ 4
Occasionally ☐ 2	All of the time ☐ 5
Sometimes ☐ 3	

W7. Have you worked your regular number of hours?	
Never ☐ 1	Most of the time ☐ 4
Occasionally ☐ 2	All of the time ☐ 5
Sometimes ☐ 3	

Please go to next section –

8

Figure 24.2 *(Continued)*

SEXUAL MATTERS:

Please tick one box for each question by thinking about **your experience following insertion of the stent**.

S1. Currently, do you have an active sex life?

No ☐ 1, Please answer question S2 and go to next section (Ignore questions S3 and S4).

Yes ☐ 2, Please go to question S3 (Ignore question S2).

S2. (i) If NO sex life, how long ago did this stop?

After insertion of the stent ☐ 1

Before insertion of the stent ☐ 0

(ii) AND, why did this stop?

Because of the problems associated with the stent ☐ 10

Did not attempt any sexual activity ☐ 0

Some other reason – not to do with the symptoms of the stent ☐ 0

(Ignore questions S3 – S4)

Please answer questions S3 and S4, only if you have answered 'yes' to question S1.

Please think about your experience following insertion of the stent.

S3. Do you have pain when you have sexual intercourse?

Not at all ☐ 1   Severe ☐ 4

Mild ☐ 2   Extreme ☐ 5

Moderate ☐ 3

S4. How satisfied are you with your sex life?

Very satisfied ☐ 1   Dissatisfied ☐ 4

Satisfied ☐ 2   Very dissatisfied ☐ 5

Not sure ☐ 3

Please go to next section ---

9

Figure 24.2 *(Continued)*

ADDITIONAL PROBLEMS:

The following questions ask about your experience following insertion of the stent. Please indicate your experience by ticking the appropriate box.

A1. How many times have you felt you may be suffering from a urinary tract infection (e.g. running temperature, feeling unwell and pain while passing urine)?

Never ☐ 1   Most of the time ☐ 4

Occasionally ☐ 2   All of the time ☐ 5

Sometimes ☐ 3

A2. Have you needed to take antibiotics as a result of insertion of the stent? (Please ignore the course of antibiotics, which may have been given at the time of insertion of the stent.)

Not at all ☐ 1   Two Courses ☐ 3

One Course ☐ 2   Three or more Courses ☐ 4

A3. Have you needed to seek help of a health professional (such as GP, nurse) due to any problem associated with the stent?

Never ☐ 1   Twice ☐ 3

Once ☐ 2   Three or more times ☐ 4

A4. Have you needed to visit the hospital due to any problem associated with the stent?

Never ☐ 1   Twice ☐ 3

Once ☐ 2   Three or more times ☐ 4

GQ In the future, if you were advised to have another stent inserted, how would you feel about it?

Delighted ☐ 1   Mostly dissatisfied ☐ 5

Pleased ☐ 2   Unhappy ☐ 6

Mostly satisfied ☐ 3   Terrible ☐ 7

Mixed feelings (about equally satisfied and dissatisfied) ☐ 4

AQ. If there are any comments you would like to make about the questionnaire or any of your symptoms, please use the space below.

THANK YOU VERY MUCH FOR YOUR HELP

All information will remain confidential

10

Figure 24.2 (*Continued*)

URETERIC
STENT SYMPTOMS QUESTIONNAIRE

Questionnaire 2 (*Post stent*)

We are interested to know about various aspects of <u>your health following removal of the stent</u> and the impact removal of stent has had on your health.

Please complete the following questionnaire, which has different sections. Please answer all questions in each section.

(We would be grateful if you complete and post the questionnaire within seven days)

Please complete,

Today's Date: ☐ / ☐ / ☐

Date of Birth: ☐ / ☐ / ☐

Please return to:

Post Code: ☐☐☐☐ ☐☐☐
Hospital Number: ☐☐☐☐☐☐☐
(for office use)

Figure 24.3 Ureteric stent symptom questionnaire for when stented.

You will see that some questions ask if you have a symptom occasionally, sometimes or most of the time.

Occasionally	=	**less than one third of the time**
Sometimes	=	**between one and two thirds of the time**
Most of the time	=	**more than two thirds of the time**

URINARY SYMPTOMS

Please answer the questions thinking about the urinary symptoms you have experienced <u>following removal of the stent.</u>

Please put a tick in one box for each question   ☑

Please think about your experience since removal of the stent.

U1. During the day, how often do you pass urine, on average?

Less than hourly ☐ 5   Every 3 hourly ☐ 2

Hourly ☐ 4   Every 4 hours or more ☐ 1

Every 2 hourly ☐ 3

U2. During the night, how many times do you have to get up to pass urine, on average?

None ☐ 1   3 ☐ 4

1 ☐ 2   4 or more ☐ 5

2 ☐ 3

U3. Do you have to rush to the toilet to urinate?

Never ☐ 1   Most of the time ☐ 4
(more than two thirds for the time)

Occasionally ☐ 2   All of the time ☐ 5
(less than one third of the time)

Sometimes ☐ 3
(between one and two thirds of the time)

U4. Does urine leak before you can get to the toilet?

Never ☐ 1   Most of the time ☐ 4

Occasionally ☐ 2   All of the time ☐ 5

Sometimes ☐ 3

U5. Do you leak urine without feeling the need to go to the toilet?

Never ☐ 1   Most of the time ☐ 4

Occasionally ☐ 2   All of the time ☐ 5

Sometimes ☐ 3

Figure 24.3 (*Continued*)

U6. How often do you feel that your bladder has not emptied properly after you have passed urine?

Never ☐ ₁   Most of the time (more than two thirds of the time) ☐ ₄

Occasionally (less than one third of the time) ☐ ₂   All of the time ☐ ₅

Sometimes (between one and two thirds of the time) ☐ ₃

U7. Do you have a burning feeling when you pass urine?

Never ☐ ₁   Most of the time ☐ ₄

Occasionally ☐ ₂   All of the time ☐ ₅

Sometimes ☐ ₃

U8. How often do you see blood in your urine?

Never ☐ ₁   Most of the time ☐ ₄

Occasionally ☐ ₂   All of the time ☐ ₅

Sometimes ☐ ₃

U9. How much blood do you see in your urine?

Do not see any blood ☐ ₁   Urine is heavily blood stained ☐ ₄

Urine is slightly blood stained ☐ ₂   Urine is heavily blood stained and has clot(s) ☐ ₅

U10. Overall, how much of a problem are your urinary symptoms to you?

Not at all ☐ ₁   Quite a bit ☐ 1.75

A little bit ☐ 1.25   Extreme ☐ ₂

Moderate ☐ 1.5

U11 If you were to spend the rest of your life with the urinary symptoms, if any, associated with the kidney problem just the way they are, how would you feel about it?

delighted ☐ ₁   Mostly dissatisfied ☐ ₅

pleased ☐ ₂   Unhappy ☐ ₆

Mostly satisfied ☐ ₃   Terrible ☐ ₇

Mixed feelings (about equally satisfied and dissatisfied) ☐ ₄

Please go to next section --

3

Figure 24.3 *(Continued)*

BODY PAIN (for women):

This section asks about the **body pain or discomfort, which you associate with the kidney problem.**

Please think about your experience **following removal of the stent.**

P1. Do you experience body pain or discomfort in relation to your kidney problem?

YES ☐₁, **please go to question P2**

NO ☐₂, **please go to next section on General Health**   (Ignore questions P2 to P9)

P2. Think of the drawings below as the drawings of your body. Please **mark (X) or shade the site(s) where you experience pain or discomfort in relation to your kidney problem typically (e.g. during the day to day activities, whenever you pass urine)**
If you get pain at more than one site, please use a <u>separate mark for each site.</u>

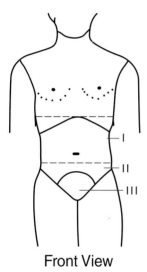

Front View

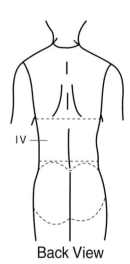

Back View

The numbers I - IV represent following areas for the right and left sides

I – Kidney front/side area   III – Bladder area
II - Groin area   IV– Kidney back (loin) area
Please use O for any other marked area and write the name of the site

P3. Please place a <u>mark (X) to a point on the line below that indicates pain or discomfort</u> in relation to your kidney problem. **Please put a separate mark for each site** if the pain or discomfort is different in severity and write the corresponding number of each site used in the drawing above.

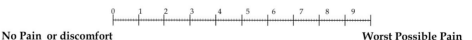

No Pain or discomfort   **Worst Possible Pain**

4

Figure 24.3 (*Continued*)

BODY PAIN (for men):

This section asks about the **body pain or discomfort, which you associate with your kidney problem.**

Please think about your experience **following removal of the stent.**

P1. Do you experience body pain or discomfort in relation to your kidney problem?

YES☐₁, **please go to question P2**

NO ☐₂, **please go to next section on General Health**   (Ignore questions P2 to P9)

P2. Think of the drawings below as the drawings of your body. Please **mark (X) or shade the site(s) where you experience pain or discomfort in relation to your kidney problem typically (e.g. during day to day activities, whenever you pass urine)**

If you get pain at more than one site, please use a <u>separate mark for each site.</u>

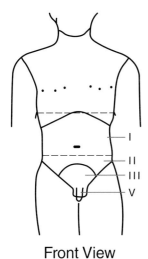

Front View

Back View

The numbers I - V represent following areas for the right and left sides

I – Kidney front/side area   **IV**– Kidney back (loin) area
II - Groin area   **V - Penis**
III – Bladder area   **Please use O**   for any other marked area and write the name of the site

P3. Please place a <u>mark (X) to a point on the line below that indicates your pain or discomfort in</u> relation to your kidney problem. **Please put a separate mark for each site** of the pain or discomfort is different in severity and write the corresponding number of each site used in the drawing above.

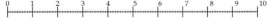

No Pain or discomfort   **Worst Possible Pain**

5

Figure 24.3 (*Continued*)

P4. Which of the following statements best describe your experience regarding <u>physical activities</u> and the pain or discomfort in relation to your kidney problem?

I **do not experience any pain** or discomfort during physical activities ☐ 1

I experience pain or discomfort only when I perform **vigorous activities** ☐ 2
(e.g. strenuous sports, lifting heavy objects)

I experience pain when I perform **activities of moderate severity** but not with basic activities ☐ 3
(e.g. walking few hundred yards, driving a car)

I experience pain even when I perform **basic activities** of daily living ☐ 4
(e.g. walking indoors, dressing)

I experience pain while also **being at rest** ☐ 5

P5. Does the pain or discomfort, in relation to your kidney problem, interrupt your sleep?

Never ☐ 1   Most of the time ☐ 4

Occasionally ☐ 2   All of the time ☐ 5

Sometimes ☐ 3

P6. Do you experience pain or discomfort, in relation to your kidney problem, while passing urine?

Never ☐ 1   Most of the time ☐ 4

Occasionally ☐ 2   All of the time ☐ 5

Sometimes ☐ 3

P7. Do you experience pain or discomfort in the <u>kidney area</u>, while passing urine?

No ☐ 1

Yes ☐ 2

P8. How frequently have you required painkillers to control the pain or discomfort associated with the kidney problem?

Never ☐ 1   Most of the time ☐ 4

Occasionally ☐ 2   All of the time ☐ 5

Sometimes ☐ 3

P9. Overall, how much does the pain or discomfort, in relation to your kidney problem, (as distinct from other symptoms) interfere with your life?

Not at all ☐ 1   Quite a bit ☐ 4

A little bit ☐ 2   Extremely ☐ 5

Moderately ☐ 3

Please go to next section --

6

Figure 24.3 (*Continued*)

GENERAL HEALTH:

Following removal of the stent:

G1. Have you had difficulty in performing light physical activities (e.g. walking short distances, driving a car)?

Usually with no difficulty ☐ 1   Usually did not do because of the stent ☐ 4

Usually with some difficulty ☐ 2   Usually did not do for other reasons ☐ 0

Usually with much difficulty ☐ 3

G2. Have you had difficulty in performing heavy physical activities (e.g. strenuous sports, lifting heavy objects)?

Usually with no difficulty ☐ 1   Usually did not do because of the stent ☐ 4

Usually with some difficulty ☐ 2   Usually did not do for other reasons ☐ 0

Usually with much difficulty ☐ 3

G3. Have you felt tired and worn out?

Never ☐ 1   Most of the time (more than two thirds of the time) ☐ 4

Occasionally (less than one third of the time) ☐ 2   All of the time ☐ 5

Sometimes (between one and two thirds of the time) ☐ 3

G4. Have you felt calm and peaceful?

All of the time ☐ 1   Occasionally ☐ 4

Most of the time ☐ 2   Never ☐ 5

Sometimes ☐ 3

G5. Have you enjoyed your social life (going out, meeting friends and so on)?

All of the time ☐ 1   Occasionally ☐ 4

Most of the time ☐ 2   Never ☐ 5

Sometimes ☐ 3

G6. Have you needed extra help from your family members or friends?

Never ☐ 1   Most of the time ☐ 4

Occasionally ☐ 2   All of the time ☐ 5

Sometimes ☐ 3

Please go to next section ---

7

Figure 24.3 (*Continued*)

WORK PERFORMANCE:

W1. Regarding your employment status, are you

In full time employment ☐ 1   Student ☐ 4

In part time employment ☐ 2   Unemployed, looking for work ☐ 5

Retired on health ground ☐ 3   Retired for other reason (including age) ☐ 6

Not working for other reason (please specify) ☐ 7 _____

W2. Following removal of the stent, how many days did the symptoms associated with the kidney problem keep you in bed all or most of the day or result in the loss of a full day's work?

☐☐ Day(s)

W3. Following removal of the stent, for how many <u>half days</u> did you cut down your routine activities (including work) because of the symptoms associated with the kidney problem?

☐☐ Half Day(s)

Please answer the questions below (W4 –W7) only if you are in active paid work.

(Otherwise ignore questions W4 – W7).

W4. a) Job title or description of your role: _____

b) Are you an: Employee ☐ 1   Employer ☐ 2   Self employed ☐ 3

<u>**Please answer following questions if you have worked after removal of the stent,**</u>

W5. Have you worked for short periods of time or taken frequent rests because of the symptoms associated with the kidney problem?
Never ☐ 1   Most of the time ☐ 4
Occasionally ☐ 2   All of the time ☐ 5
Sometimes ☐ 3

W6. Have you worked at your usual job, but with some changes because of the symptoms associated with the kidney problem?
Never ☐ 1   Most of the time ☐ 4
Occasionally ☐ 2   All of the time ☐ 5
Sometimes ☐ 3

W7. Have you worked your regular number of hours?
Never ☐ 5   Most of the time ☐ 2
Occasionally ☐ 4   All of the time ☐ 1
Sometimes ☐ 3

Please go to next section --

8

Figure 24.3 (*Continued*)

SEXUAL MATTERS:

Please tick one box for each question by thinking about **your experience following removal of the stent**.

S1. Currently, do you have an active sex life?

No ☐ 1,   Please **answer question S2 and go to the last question GQ.**

Yes ☐ 2,   Please **go to question S3 (Ignore question S2).**

S2. (i) If NO sex life, how long ago did this stop?

After insertion of the stent ☐ 1

Before insertion of the stent ☐ 0

(ii)AND, why did this stop?

Because of the kidney problem ☐ 10

Did not attempt any sexual activity ☐ 0

Some other reason – not to do with the kidney problem ☐ 0

(**Ignore questions S3 – S4)**

Please answer questions S3 and S4, only if you have answered 'yes' to question S1.
Please think about your experience following removal of the stent.

S3. Do you have pain when you have sexual intercourse?

Not at all ☐ 1   Severe ☐ 4

Mild ☐ 2   Extreme ☐ 5

Moderate ☐ 3

S4. How satisfied are you with your sex life?

Very satisfied ☐ 1   Dissatisfied ☐ 4

Satisfied ☐ 2   Very dissatisfied ☐ 5

Not sure ☐ 3

GQ In the future, if you were advised to have another stent inserted, how would you feel about it?

Delighted ☐ 1   Mostly dissatisfied ☐ 5

Pleased ☐ 2   Unhappy ☐ 6

Mostly satisfied ☐ 3   Terrible ☐ 7

Mixed feelings (about equally satisfied and dissatisfied) ☐ 4

AQ. If there are any comments you would like to make about the questionnaire or any of your symptoms, please use the space below.

THANK YOU VERY MUCH FOR YOUR HELP
(Please complete the enclosed questionnaires)

9

Figure 24.3 *(Continued)*

References

[1] Joshi HB, Stainthorpe A, Keeley FX, Jr., MacDonagh R, Timoney AG. Indwelling ureteral stents: evaluation of quality of life to aid outcome analysis. J Endourol 2001;15(2):151–154.

[2] Bregg K, Riehle RA, Jr. Morbidity associated with indwelling internal ureteral stents after shock wave lithotripsy. J Urol 1989;141(3):510–512.

[3] Yachia, D, editor. Stenting the urinary system. 2nd ed. Oxford: ISIS Medical Media; 2004.

[4] Joshi HB, Okeke A, Newns N, Keeley FX, Jr., Timoney AG. Characterization of urinary symptoms in patients with ureteral stents. Urology 2002;59(4):511–516.

[5] Dellis A, Joshi HB, Timoney AG, Keeley FX, Jr. Relief of stent related symptoms: review of engineering and pharmacological solutions. J Urol 2010;184(4):1267–1272.

[6] Joshi HB, Newns N, Stainthorpe A, MacDonagh RP, Keeley FX, Jr., Timoney AG. Ureteral stent symptom questionnaire: development and validation of a multidimensional quality of life measure. J Urol 2003;169(3):1060–1064.

[7] Park J, Shin DW, You C, Chung KJ, Han DH, Joshi HB, *et al.* Cross-cultural application of the Korean version of Ureteral Stent Symptoms Questionnaire. J Endourol 2012;26(11):1518–1522.

[8] Joshi HB, Chitale SV, Nagarajan M, Irving SO, Browning AJ, Biyani CS, *et al.* A prospective randomized single-blind comparison of ureteral stents composed of firm and soft polymer. J Urol 2005;174(6):2303–2306.

[9] Lingeman JE, Preminger GM, Goldfischer ER, Krambeck AE. Assessing the impact of ureteral stent design on patient comfort. J Urol 2009;181(6):2581–2587.

[10] Davenport K, Kumar V, Collins J, Melotti R, Timoney AG, Keeley FX, Jr. New ureteral stent design does not improve patient quality of life: a randomized, controlled trial. J Urol 2011;185(1):175–178.

[11] Calvert RC, Wong KY, Chitale SV, Irving SO, Nagarajan M, Biyani CS, *et al.* Multi-length or 24 cm ureteric stent? A multicentre randomised comparison of stent-related symptoms using a validated questionnaire. BJU Int 2013;111(7):1099–1104.

[12] Ritter M, Krombach P, Knoll T, Michel MS, Haecker A. Initial experience with a newly developed antirefluxive ureter stent. Urol Res 2012;40(4):349–353.

[13] Maan Z, Patel D, Moraitis K, El-Husseiny T, Papatsoris AG, Buchholz NP, *et al.* Comparison of stent-related symptoms between conventional Double-J stents and a new-generation thermoexpandable segmental metallic stent: a validated-questionnaire-based study. J Endourol 2010;24(4):589–593.

[14] Lee C, Kuskowski M, Premoli J, Skemp N, Monga M. Randomized evaluation of Ureteral Stents using validated Symptom Questionnaire. J Endourol 2005;19(8):990–993.

[15] Damiano R, Autorino R, De Sio M, Cantiello F, Quarto G, Perdona S, *et al.* Does the size of ureteral stent impact urinary symptoms and quality of life? A prospective randomized study. Eur Urol 2005;48(4):673–678.

[16] Gupta M, Patel T, Xavier K, Maruffo F, Lehman D, Walsh R, *et al.* Prospective randomized evaluation of periureteral botulinum toxin type A injection for ureteral stent pain reduction. J Urol 2010;183(2):598–602.

[17] Park SC, Jung SW, Lee JW, Rim JS. The effects of tolterodine extended release and alfuzosin for the treatment of double-j stent-related symptoms. J Endourol 2009;23(11):1913–1917.

[18] Yakoubi R, Lemdani M, Monga M, Villers A, Koenig P. Is there a role for alpha-blockers in ureteral stent related symptoms? A systematic review and meta-analysis. J Urol 2011;186(3):928–934.

[19] Giannarini G, Keeley FX, Jr., Valent F, Manassero F, Mogorovich A, Autorino R, *et al.* Predictors of morbidity in patients with indwelling ureteric stents: results of a prospective study using the validated Ureteric Stent Symptoms Questionnaire. BJU Int 2011;107(4):648–654.

[20] Regan SM, Sethi AS, Powelson JA, Goggins WC, Milgrom ML, Sundaram CP. Symptoms related to ureteral stents in renal transplants compared with stents placed for other indications. J Endourol 2009;23(12):2047–2050.

[21] Barnes KT, Bing MT, Tracy CR. Do ureteric stent extraction strings affect stent-related quality of life or complications after ureteroscopy for urolithiasis: a prospective randomised control trial. BJU Int 2014;113(4):605–609.

[22] Abt D, Mordasini L, Warzinek E, Schmid HP, Haile SR, Engeler DS, *et al.* Is intravesical stent position a predictor of associated morbidity? Korean J Urol 2015;56(5):370–378.

[23] Abt D, Warzinek E, Schmid HP, Haile SR, Engeler DS. Influence of patient education on morbidity caused by ureteral stents. Int J Urol 2015;22(7):679–683.

[24] Joshi HB, Newns N, Stainthorpe A, MacDonagh RP, Keeley FX, Jr., Timoney AG. The development and validation of a patient-information booklet on ureteric stents. BJU Int 2001;88(4):329–334.

25

Evidence Base for Stenting

Rami Elias[1] and Edward D. Matsumoto[2]

[1] Laparoscopy and Endourology Fellow, Division of Urology, McMaster University, Hamilton, Ontario, Canada
[2] Professor of Urology, Division of Urology, Department of Surgery, DeGroote School of Medicine, McMaster University, Hamilton, Ontario, Canada

25.1 Contemporary Use of Ureteric Stents in Endourology

The ureteric stent, although simple, is a vital instrument for the modern day urologist. The ureteric stent serves an important role in endourological procedures from its role as an adjunctive device to being used as a primary tool. The breadth of use in current procedures are numerous and will be detailed in the other chapters of this textbook. We will focus on the most commonly contended scenarios where stents may or may not be utilized. This chapter will critically appraise the medical literature surrounding these scenarios and will provide an examination of the supporting evidence behind their management.

25.2 Evidence-Based Medicine Primer

Evidence-based medicine (EBM) is the approach to medicine, which is based upon the best scientific data available in the literature. EBM provides a conceptual framework, which healthcare providers can use during problem solving. This involves gathering the information in the literature, processing it, and putting into practice the information that is most relevant to the question. One must be able to effectively critically appraise the information gathered before putting it into practice. In the scientific literature, studies exist on a continuum of quality and scale. Pooled studies or large randomized controlled trials (RCTs) occupy one extreme and tend to replicate results that are more reliable and valid, or closer to the "truth." On the other end of the spectrum, expert opinion and small case series data may drastically differ on the spectrum of validity and therefore must be judged as such when critically appraising the literature. The use of evidence-based data allows practitioners to provide the highest quality of care when compared to subjective and often unreliable data derived from other sources (Table 25.1).

Ureteric Stenting, First Edition. Edited by Ravi Kulkarni.
© 2017 John Wiley & Sons Ltd. Published 2017 by John Wiley & Sons Ltd.

Table 25.1 Oxford Center for Evidence-Based Medicine.

Level of Evidence	Description
1a	Systematic Review (with homogeneity) of RCTs*
1b	Individual RCT (with narrow Confidence Interval)
1c	All or none
2a	Systematic Review (with homogeneity) of cohort studies
2b	Individual cohort study (including low quality RCT)
2c	"Outcomes" Research; Ecological studies
3a	Systematic Review (with homogeneity) of case-control studies
3b	Individual Case-Control Study
4	Case-series Poor quality cohort studies Poor quality case-control studies
5	Expert opinion without explicit critical appraisal, or based on physiology, bench research or "first principles"

* RCT, randomized control trial.

25.3 Randomized Controlled Trials

Randomized controlled trials (RCTs) are considered the gold standard when evaluating the effects of novel treatments. They are often used to measure both efficacy and effectiveness of a medical intervention. *Efficacy* measures the degree of treatment effect under ideal circumstances where *effectiveness* measures results under "real-world" clinical settings [1]. A RCT can be formulated to measure either property depending on the populations used, eligibility criteria, health outcomes measured, and follow-up duration. RCTs can also be classified by the manner with which participants are exposed to an intervention (Table 25.2). The most common trial design would be a *parallel group trial* where participants are randomized to one of the intervention arms.

Table 25.2 Types of randomized control trials.

Type of RCT	Definition
Parallel Group Trial	Participants are randomized to one of the intervention groups
Crossover Trial	Participants are exposed to each intervention in a random sequence
Cluster Trial	Cluster or groups of participants are randomly allocated to different study arms
Factorial Trial	Participants are randomized to individual interventions or a combination of interventions
Split Body Trial	Separate body parts within each participant is randomized

Source: [20].

Multiple validated tools exist for assessing the reporting and quality of various study designs. Clinicians should use these during their appraisal of the literature, dependent on the type of study being evaluated (Table 25.3).

The guideline is presented in the form of an itemized checklist and divides a scientific report into its five major components (Table 25.4). The first step when assessing a trial for quality is identifying the author(s) research question and the trial design. The title should contain these major components using the widely recognized PICOT format

Table 25.3 Reporting guidelines and quality assessment statements for across study designs.

Study Type	Reporting Guideline	
Meta-Analysis	PRISMA	Preferred Reporting Items for Systematic Reviews and Meta-Analyses
Systematic Review	PRISMA	Preferred Reporting Items for Systematic Reviews and Meta-Analyses
Randomized Control Trial	CONSORT	Consolidated Standards of Reporting Trials
Diagnostic/Prognostic Study	STARD	Standards for Reporting of Diagnostic Accuracy
Observational Study	STROBE	Strengthening the Reporting of Observational Studies in Epidemiology
Qualitative Research	SRQR	Standards for Reporting Qualitative Research
Case Report	CARE	CAse REport Guidelines

Table 25.4 The essential components of the CONSORT.

Section	Essential Components
Introduction	Title Abstract
Methods	Trial Design Participants Interventions Outcomes Sample Size Randomization Allocation Concealment Blinding Statistical Methods
Results	Outcomes Baseline Data Participant Flow Ancillary Analyses
Discussion	Generalizability Interpretation Limitations
Other	Registration Protocol Funding

Table 25.5 The PICOT framework.

Component	Explanation
Population	The study group examined including age group, gender, and disease status where applicable
Intervention	The type of intervention that is examined
Comparator	The alternative treatment that is used in comparison
Outcome	The desired effect or outcome measured
Time-frame	The specific duration of data collection and follow-up

(Population/patients, Intervention, Comparison/control, Outcome, Time) (Table 25.5). The report's abstract should have a clear depiction of the research question. Explicit objectives and the overall hypothesis should be outlined in the introduction of the study.

25.4   Meta-Analysis and Systematic Reviews

A meta-analysis is a statistical technique used for combining results from multiple independent studies. The goal is to provide an estimate of a treatment effect based on pooled analysis of similarly designed studies. The robustness of a meta-analysis is dependent on the ability to identify these trials, evaluate their quality, and include the properly conducted trials for grouped analysis. The Preferred Reporting Items for Systematic Reviews and Meta-Analyses (PRISMA) Statement is a standardized reporting system for meta-analyses that aides in the quality assessment.

25.5   The Evidence for Treatment of Acute Infectious Obstruction

Management of an infected and obstructed urinary collecting system is a common clinical scenario seen in urology practice. Frequently, the offending cause of the acute obstruction is related to a ureteral stone, but other etiologies have been well-documented in the literature. This section will focus primarily on ureteral calculi-related obstruction and resultant infected hydronephrosis. The need for immediate recognition of urosepsis and subsequent decompression is of paramount importance to reduce morbidity and mortality. We will provide references to and describe the results of critically appraised literature in order to support diagnostic and treatment measures for acute infectious obstruction.

From a urological perspective, optimal urosepsis management requires early-goal directed therapy in addition to antimicrobial exposure to both blood and urinary tract [2]. Urosepsis is defined as the response to a systemic infection originating from the genitourinary system and is recognized by the clinical parameters of the systemic inflammatory response (Table 25.6). Other tenets of management include blood pressure stabilization via volume expansion and adequate tissue oxygenation. Of particular importance in septic stone management is control of complicating

Table 25.6 Systemic inflammatory response syndrome criteria.

Criteria	Upper Limit	Lower Limit
Body Temperature	>38°C	<36°c
Heart Rate	>90/minute	———
Respiratory Rate	>20/minute	———
PaCO2	<32 mmHg	———
White Blood Cell Count	>12x10^9/L	<4 x10^9/L

factors in the urinary system, primarily the obstructed collecting system. Both ureteral stenting and percutaneous nephrostomies have been well-documented management options for immediate genitourinary decompression with advantages and disadvantages for each.

Proponents of percutaneous drainage via nephrostomy advocate this technique to avoid unnecessary stone manipulation, potential ureteral perforation, and exacerbation of the urosepsis episode. An additional advantage is the avoidance of a general anesthetic for insertion. If necessary, sedation can be used to augment the procedure for patient comfort. Disadvantages would include injury to adjacent organ(s), such as the liver, spleen, and/or colon, pleural transgression, and/or significant vascular injury at time of insertion. Ipsilateral renal loss would be the most devastating sequelae. The major complication rate of this procedure ranges in the literature but is approximately less than 4%, but can range from <1% up to 15% [3]. Other benefits include insertion by either an interventional radiologist or trained urologist; however, some centers may have limited access to this approach. The rate of successful insertion of a percutaneous nephrostomy approaches 99% in skilled hands; however, this number decreases in patients with a non-dilated collecting system or complex stone disease such as a stag horn stone [3]. The most important contraindication to this method would be uncorrected coagulopathy.

Comparatively, the risk profile for retrograde stent insertion is more favorable with no documented renal loss or severe hemorrhagic complication. Besides the safety record, the lack of external appliances decreases the risk of further procedures from secondary accidental dislodgement. Other advantages include the ability to perform the procedure regardless of coagulopathy profile and easy access for delayed stone intervention. Retained ureteral stents is a unique complication that has been well reported. Encrustation, migration, fragmentation, obstruction, and ensuing renal failure can occur [4]. Unfortunately, the rate of success of retrograde ureteric stent insertion is not fully described in the literature and is limited by the quality of studies reporting this number.

Ultimately, the decision between these two techniques would be made after considering patient clinical factors, in addition to the availability of an interventional radiologist, operating suite, and anesthetic support.

Certainly, regional practice patterns can influence decision making, as is evident in the United Kingdom. Lynch and colleagues performed a formal postal questionnaire to all members of the British Association of Urological Surgeons, The British Society of Interventional Radiologists, and the British Society of Urogenital Radiology (Quality: Level 5). The preferred technique for renal de-obstruction in the clinically septic patient was percutaneous nephrostomy with rates of 78% and 88% for radiologists and urologists

respectively. The primary limitation of this cross- sectional survey was a poor respond-
ent rate (19%), making extrapolation very limited. Nonetheless, regarding specialist
preference, this has been the only study polling urologists' and radiologists' direct opin-
ions [5]. Practice patterns in North America and elsewhere have not yet been reported
in the literature.

There have been a limited number of studies directly comparing percutaneous
nephrostomy and retrograde ureteral stents for acutely infectious, obstructed hydronephrosis related to stones. The quality of the literature is variable but consists of mainly
small, properly formed, RCTs, with the exception of one case series (Table 25.7).

The first study was performed by Pearle and colleagues. This meticulously performed
RCT (Quality: Level 1b) compared percutaneous nephrostomy and retrograde ureteral
stents in 42 consecutive patients with normalization of either a white blood cell count
or temperature as the primary outcome. Sample size and power calculations were performed prior to study initiation. Explicit inclusion criteria were used to narrow the subject pool. The primary outcome, time to normalization, or white blood cell count or
temperature, was clearly stated, in addition to the secondary outcome measures.

This RCT was more methodical than the other studies that addressed this comparison. Patient parameters between the two equal groups of 21 were compared and found
to be similar with respect to age, gender, and stone size. Time to normalization of the
primary outcomes was found to be non-statistically significant between the two groups.
This trial did identify a shorter procedural and fluoroscopic time favoring retrograde
catheterization (32.7 minutes and 5.1 minutes respectively) compared to percutaneous
nephrostomy (49.2 and 7.7 minutes). The only treatment failure occurred in the percutaneous group and was salvaged via an endoscopic approach. Although length of stay
was a secondary outcome and was influenced by other medical comorbidities, it did not
significantly differ between groups, having a duration of five or fewer days. Cost analysis was performed based on average disposable use and included radiologist, anesthetic,
and urologist fees. The total cost of retrograde stent insertion was $2,401.33 U.S. dollars
compared to $1,137.01 for the percutaneous approach. The former price was not sig-
nificantly altered when sedation was used versus general anesthetic. Fiscal calculations
are limited in their extrapolation to other healthcare systems. The authors ultimately
concluded that was no difference in clinical efficacy between the two methods, however, cost favored percutaneous nephrostomy by nearly a factor of two.

A second RCT, performed by Mokhmalji *et al.*, [6] observed 40 consecutive cases
of stone-related, infected, hydronephrosis that were randomized equally to either

Table 25.7 Trials comparing acute decompression techniques retrograde stent versus percutaneous
nephrostomy tube insertion.

Author, Year of Publication	Type of Study	Outcome	Number of Events	Level of Evidence
Pearle *et al.*, 1998 [21]	Randomized Control Trial	Time to normalization of white count or temperature	42	1b
Mokhmalji *et al.*, 2001 [6]	Randomized Control Trial	Relief of symptoms	40	1b
Yoshimura *et al.*, 2005 [22]	Outcomes Research	Risk factors for drainage	53	2c

percutaneous or endoscopic decompression (Quality: Level 1b). The main exclusion criteria that precluded randomization included end stage hydronephrosis or conditions that necessitate one type of diversion over the other (pediatric cases, conduits, poor coagulation or solitary kidney). Clinical parameters related to the course of the procedure (success, analgesic use, x-ray exposure), subsequent progress (administration of IV antibiotics), and quality of life were all measured. The latter was assessed via two validated quality of life questionnaires, immediately after the procedure and two to four weeks later.

Although this was a RCT, there were some methodological issues identified with this trial. The primary outcome measurement was not clearly identified. Additionally, sample size calculations were not included in the report; thus, whether the study was adequately powered is questionable. Interestingly, 20% of individuals randomized to ureteral stent insertion failed, requiring conversion to a percutaneous approach. The converse was not the case, with all of nephrostomies successfully inserted. Whether Intention-to-Treat analysis was completed is unclear as this was not stated. The x-ray exposure, administration of analgesics, and time on IV antibiotics all favored nephrostomy insertion but did not reach statistical significance. Duration of diversion was longer in the ureteral stent group than the nephrostomy group with 56% and 20% respectively at four weeks. Lastly, the quality of life results tended to favor nephrostomy insertion particularly when looking at a prolonged dwell time; however, it was found not to be statistically significant. Although the authors suggested that the percutaneous approach was more favorable, based on the evidence, these conclusions could not be drawn.

The final paper found in the literature regarding surgical decompression in an emergent setting is a retrospective, cohort study by Yoshimura and colleagues (Quality: Level 2b). The primary goal of the study was to examine the characteristics of patients with urosepsis associated with upper urinary tract calculi requiring emergency drainage. The authors identified 59 emergency drainage procedures for urosepsis with 35 ureteral stent insertions and 24 percutaneous nephrostomies. The authors also followed clinical parameters during the hospital stay and compared them to a cohort of individuals who did not require emergent treatment. They noted that patients undergoing ureteral stenting had more rapid progression of inflammatory markers and more severe thrombocytopenia. However, these patients were younger and more likely to have an earlier recovery. These results should be taken cautiously as their event rate was low compared to the number of variables compared. The main drawback behind this study is its cohort design. Being a retrospective and observational one could not prove causation with any of the outcomes that were measured. The primary purpose is to describing the characteristics of patient presentations, type and frequency of drainage, in addition to several other clinical parameters. Unfortunately, no conclusions can be drawn between the comparison of nephrostomy tube usage and ureteric stents and thus has limited usefulness for decision making.

Overall, it is clear that the mainstay of treatment for stone-related obstruction and urosepsis is emergent decompression. There is obvious evidence necessitating immediate identification and action to prevent patient morbidity. Major European and North American consensus clearly state that either method of decompression is sufficient in their respective guidelines. Based on the literature, controversy still remains. The two RCTs were limited in their sample size and had differing conclusions. Depending on the clinical scenario, percutaneous nephrostomy insertion may have a higher procedural success rate and improved patient perceived quality of life with the trade off a higher risk profile. Conversely, ureteral stent insertion has been shown to be equally as efficacious but with a potential for higher cost.

25.6   Ureteroscopy and Post-Procedure Stent Insertion

Ureteric stents have long been seen as a necessary adjunctive device in the armamentarium of the modern day urologist. Ureteral stenting after endoscopic lithotripsy is thought to prevent ureteral obstruction and renal colic that may develop secondary to stone manipulation [7]. It has also been suggested that improved healing and reduced stricture formation are added benefits [8]. Opponents describe an increased procedural cost, significant stent-associated lower urinary tract symptoms and the need for delayed cystoscopic removal. This section will examine the use of ureteral stenting in the setting of an uncomplicated, ureteroscopic stone lithotripsy. The term uncomplicated has been defined as a procedure with minimal or no ureteral trauma, minimal or no dilation, and minimal or no residual burden [9]. There have been several large pooled analyses of RCTs to aid urologists in the decision making for ureteral stent utilization.

The first meta-analysis was performed by Makarov *et al.* [10] after pooling 10 RCTs comparing the use of ureteral stents post-ureteroscopy for stones versus no use of ureteral stents post-ureteroscopy (Quality: Level 1a). The primary outcome was urologic complication and was predefined as a secondary procedure, emergency department evaluation, and/or hospital admission. The search strategy and data extraction method was thorough and clearly outlined, however, the number of trial found compared to the number ultimately included was not described. The reasons behind exclusions of certain trials were unclear and thus, a source of bias. Additionally, an individual quality assessment of the RCTs was not completed. After a total of 891 subjects were analyzed, there was a 4% lower rate of urologic complications in patients who underwent ureteral stenting. Although the results did initially achieve statistical significance, there was a substantial degree of heterogeneity, $I^2 = 86.2\%$. To address this, a random-effects model, a statistical analysis used to address a large, measurable degree of difference between the studies, was used. Ultimately, the confidence intervals were too wide (CI -10.1%, 1.8%) to support a conclusion with statistical significance. An attempt to analyze for publication bias was performed in the form of a funnel plot and statistical analysis, subsequently showing none present. The authors did make an attempt to explain the amount of heterogeneity between the trials and cited factors such as use of ureteral dilation, multiple types of lithotripsy, and variable size of scope as reasons for the observed differences. Despite the lack of evidence from the pooled data, there was a discordant conclusion with the support of omitting a ureteral stent post-ureteroscopy. Based on the evidence, this is not the case and the question remains unanswered.

The second meta-analysis was published by Pengfei *et al.* [11] and included 16 trials with a total of 1573 patients (Quality: Level 1a). The search strategy was clear, systematic and involved multiple investigators. The exclusion criteria were more explicit in this study, choosing individuals who lacked any type of complicating feature such as solitary kidney, renal failure, pregnant status or concomitant ureteral stricture. Their reasoning for choosing an "index stone patient" was to reduce the potential amount of variability observed. A particular strength of this study was their individual assessment of quality for each study included using the Cochrane Collaboration Reviewers'

Handbook and the other published guidelines [12]. The reasons behind study exclusion was also clearly explaining in the methods section. In this study, multiple outcome measures were extracted including stone-free rate, operative time, lower urinary tract symptoms, urinary tract infection, pain, unplanned medical visits, and late complications. The authors then pooled the data and compared the outcomes using the only the RCTs with the available data. The conclusions were that the unstented group had a shorter operative time and reduced lower urinary tract symptoms including hematuria. Both these conclusions, although statistically significant, was accompanied by a significant level of heterogeneity despite using a random-effects model, $I^2 = 77\%$ and 69% respectively. In fact, with the exclusion of urinary frequency or urgency, heterogeneity was substantial and significant across all outcomes, I^2 between 69%–88%. There was analysis showing no difference in unplanned medical visits, admissions to the hospital or late complications between the groups, however, the type of analysis is unclear and a forest plot of the data was not included. Another questionable feature was the lack of heterogeneity analysis for these outcomes, making the ability to draw conclusions questionable. One answer that can be extracted from this pooled data is whether there is increased lower urinary tract symptoms, frequency or urgency, with stented versus non-stented. There was a significant finding based on pooled data of homogenous trials with an almost nil level of variance. Although this finding seems overtly obvious, it is supported by the current evidence. Ultimately, it is clear that it is unsuitable to pool the data across these RCTs because of the inherit level of variability between studies. Thus, the recommendation against routine stenting is unsubstantiated when critically evaluating the evidence.

Lastly, Nabi *et al.* [13] also completed a meta-analysis combining trials examining stenting use after uncomplicated ureteroscopy. The systematic review was properly conducted with a clear research question and impetus for the analyses in addition to an explicit search strategy. Nine trials reporting on 831 participants were identified for pooled analysis. Each trial was individually analyzed for design differences to account for variability including a quality assessment. A flow diagram of studies was present in the paper outlining the exact reasons for exclusions. After combining the available results, the authors identified an increased rate of lower urinary tract symptoms (frequency/urgency and dysuria). Similar to the aforementioned meta-analyses, the level of heterogeneity was quite substantial for all pooled calculations with an $I^2 > 70\%$, making the ability to validate the results questionable. Again we see a properly constructed systematic review combining studies that are not overtly suitable for pooled analysis. The only valid pooled analysis was across culture proven urinary tract infections showing no difference between groups. The authors did identify several key limitations behind the primary data to help them interpret their conclusions. One factor that affected the variability was the lack of clear definition of an uncomplicated ureteroscopy. They also identified the lack of standardized outcome measures across the trials making pooled analysis difficult. The authors also identified that the poor quality of trials and inconsistent reporting of outcomes limit the validity in observed conclusions.

The current ureteral guidelines for the management of ureteral calculi endorsed by the AUA and EUA groups state the use of ureteral stenting after ureteroscopy for stone management is an optional adjunctive procedure [14]. Conversely, the use of routine stent insertion for extra-corporal shock wave lithotripsy is not recommended.

It is not surprising that the results of the aforementioned studies are concordant with each other since they included many of the same randomized control trials. A summary of the available meta-analyses in the literature is provided (Table 25.8). However, it is clear that a large degree of heterogeneity exists across the primary RCTs in the current literature for this research question. This variability limits the usefulness of pooled data and thus the conclusions that can be drawn. The main pitfalls with the data are the small sample sizes, the quality of individual studies and the quality of reporting of these studies. Sources of variability across the different RCTs have been identified to help with the interpretation of the data (Table 25.9). These discrepancies may account for the large amount of heterogeneity of the data.

Table 25.8 Meta-analyses comparing ureteral stents versus no ureteral stents post ureteroscopy.

Author, Year of Publication	Type of Study	Outcomes	Number of Trials & Patients	Level of Evidence
Nabi *et al.*, 2007 [13]	Meta-Analysis	Complications Operative Time	9/831	1a
Makarov *et al.*, 2008 [10]	Meta-Analysis	Urologic Complications	10/891	1a
Pengfei *et al.*, 2011 [11]	Meta-Analysis	Stone-Free Rates Complications	16/1573	1a

Table 25.9 Randomized control trials comparing outcomes for stented versus non-stented group.

Author, Year of Publication	Outcome Measured	Number of Renal Units	Sources of Heterogeneity
Denstedt *et al.*, 2001 [7]	Symptoms, UTI, Complications	58	Intra-operative dilatation patients excluded Stents removed at first visit (variable)
Netto *et al.*, 2001 [23]	Symptoms, Success, Complications, Cost	295	Antibiotics post-op Ultrasonic fragmentation Population from Brazil
Borboroglu *et al.*, 2001 [24]	Symptoms, Analgesia Use, Complications	113	Variable scope size Six patients removed from study without analysis
Byrne *et al.*, 2002 [25]	Operative Time, Symptoms, UTI, Complications	60	Blinding not described Upper tract urothelial cancers included
Chen *et al.*, 2002 [26]	Symptoms, Analgesia, Complications, Stone Free Rate	60	Blinding not described Patients admitted post-op Population from Taiwan
Cheung *et al.*, 2003 [27]	Operative Time, Symptoms, Intra- Operative Parameters, Complication, Stone Free Rate	58	Blinding not described Intra-operative ureteral edema formally evaluated
Srivastava *et al.*, 2003 [28]	Pain, Success Rate, Stent Symptoms, Stricture Formation	48	Blinding not described 8.5F semi-rigid scope
Damiano *et al.*, 2004 [29]	Operative Time, Symptoms, Complications	104	Pneumatic lithotripsy Stone size >1cm included Intra-operative ureteral edema formally evaluated Antibiotics post-op

(Continued)

Table 25.9 *(Continued)*

Author, Year of Publication	Outcome Measured	Number of Renal Units	Sources of Heterogeneity
Jeong *et al.*, 2004 [30]	Symptoms, Operative Time, Hospital Stay	45	Blinding not described Patients admitted post-op Population from Korea
Grossi *et al.*, 2006 [31]	Symptoms, Hydronephrosis, Residual Fragments	56	Pneumatic lithotripsy Up to 8.5F scope Screening US post-op
Hussein *et al.*, 2006 [32]	Symptoms, Hydronephrosis	56	Bilharzial lesions Variable spinal anesthetic Balloon dilatation Egyptian population
Ibrahim *et al.*, 2008 [33]	Symptoms, Stone Free Rate, Complications, Stone Recurrence	220	Variable balloon dilatation Up to 10.5F scope Antibiotics post-op
Isen *et al.*, 2008 [34]	Symptoms, Complication, Stricture Formation	43	Up to 9.8F scope Endoscopic forceps used Antibiotics post-op
Xu *et al.*, 2009 [35]	Operative Time, Symptoms, Complication, Stone Free Rate	110	Stone size up to 2cm Laser lithotripsy Chinese population
Cevik *et al.*, 2010 [36]	Operative Time, Symptoms, Hospital Stay, Complications, Stone Free Rate	60	Weak allocation concealment Pneumatic lithotripsy Screening IVP post-op

25.7 Tubeless Percutaneous Nephrolithotomy

Percutaneous nephrolithotomy (PCNL) has a well established role in urology for treatment of large and complex stones in the kidney after it was first described by Scandinavian authors Fernström *et al.* in 1976 [15]. The traditional technique mandated the insertion of a nephrostomy tube after the procedure was completed. The benefits of this was to maintain drainage of the collecting system, tamponade the recently made tract and allow for second look procedures [16]. Since its inception, alterations have been proposed to minimize patient morbidity including the "mini-perc" [17], small caliber nephrostomy and "tubeless" PCNLs. The proponents of the latter advocated reduced pain, decreased hospital stay and morbidity.

For the purposes of this section, the evidence for the use of ureteric stents during a PCNL will be examined. *Tubeless PCNL* will be defined as the ancillary use of ureteric stents after a PCNL without the concomitant use of a nephrostomy tube. The first description of a tubeless PCNL was published by Bellman *et al.* in 1997 [18]. At the end of the procedure, the author placed a Double J ureteric catheter in the ureter with visual and fluoroscopic guidance. The first 30 patients had a temporary percutaneous council tip catheter inserted and removed in the recovery unit. This was then modified and the ureteric catheter was the sole method of drainage for the remaining 20 patients. This trial identified low a complication rate and ultimately the feasibility of this technique. Randomized control trials were formed following the advent of tubeless PCNL. These trials often had either a ureteric stent or ureteric catheter cannulated along the entire ureter into the bladder. Standard PCNL was often compared to tubeless PCNL (with ureteric decompression) or to small bore nephrostomy tubes.

Borges *et al.* [19] performed a systematic review and identified ten randomized control trials to include in a meta-analysis. The research questions clearly outlined with a meticulous search strategy. A summary of study selection process was included. Although limited, a quality assessment was reported and identified the risk of bias for most of the included RCTs. The details behind the surgical techniques for each study was outlined and described to account for potential study differences. When comparing stone-free rates between tubeless (stented) and conventional PCNL, there was no difference between the two groups. The pooled analyses showed no degree of heterogeneity for this outcome. Hematocrit drop did not differ either while reduced length of stay and prolonged urinary leakage did favor the tubeless group. Again, the measure of variability across the RCTs for those outcomes were nil as well. Of note, if an outcome analysis had a considerable degree of heterogeneity (>50%), the authors did try to provide explanation. They accounted for the large degree of heterogeneity for the operative time ($I^2 = 55\%$) outcome by identifying that different types of stent and insertion techniques were used. A lengthy discussion was included that described the limitation of each analyses. The implications for practice were discussed as well as potential future research questions.

Based on these studies and their incorporated randomized trials, there is evidence that tubeless PCNL is a reasonable option in a select group of individuals. The RCTs for this research question appear to be more suitable for pool analysis, making interpretation and conclusions from this data more valid. Reduced hospital stay may be a primary benefit with no identifiable increase in complication rate. Whether this translate to a lower cost has yet to be determined.

25.8   Conclusion

For the contemporary urologist, it is essential to stay current with the literature in order to provide patients with evolving surgical techniques. In order to do so, the ability to critically appraise a scientific study is a skill that is necessary in the armamentarium of a modern day clinician. This chapter has helped construct a framework on how to dissect a trial to evaluate the validity of the results and the potential usefulness for application. We have outlined the necessary components of a meta-analysis and randomized control trial, however, this chapter only serves as a primer to the subject of evidence based medicine. An example of its application has been conducted by the evaluation of urologic literature in endourology. The primary pitfalls with the studies present in this subject area are the small sample sizes, variable degree of reporting, and a high level of heterogeneity between studies. Nonetheless, future research should focus on larger samples with a more stringent methodological process to answer the aforementioned research questions.

References

[1] Godwin M, Ruhland L, Casson I, *et al.* Pragmatic controlled clinical trials in primary care: the struggle between external and internal validity. BMC Med Res Methodol 2003;3:28.

[2] Wagenlehner FM, Weidner W, Naber KG. Optimal management of urosepsis from the urological perspective. Int J Antimicrob Agents 2007;30:390–397.

[3] Ramchandani P, Cardella JF, Grassi CJ, *et al.* Quality improvement guidelines for percutaneous nephrostomy. J Vasc Interv Radiol 2003;14:S277–81.

[4] Aron M, Ansari MS, Singh I, *et al.* Forgotten ureteral stents causing renal failure: multimodal endourologic treatment. J Endourol 2006;20:423–428.

[5] Lynch MF, Anson KM, Patel U. Current opinion amongst radiologists and urologists in the UK on percutaneous nephrostomy and ureteric stent insertion for acute renal unobstruction: Results of a postal survey. BJU Int 2006;98:1143–1144.

[6] Mokhmalji H, Braun PM, Martinez Portillo FJ, Siegsmund M, Alken P, Köhrmann KU. Percutaneous nephrostomy versus ureteral stents for diversion of hydronephrosis caused by stones: a prospective, randomized clinical trial. J Urol 2001;165:1088–1092.

[7] Denstedt JD, Wollin TA, Sofer M, Nott L, Weir M, D'A Honey RJ. A prospective randomized controlled trial comparing nonstented versus stented ureteroscopic lithotripsy. J Urol 2001;165:1419–1422.

[8] Harmon WJ, Sershon PD, Blute ML, Patterson DE, Segura JW. Ureteroscopy: current practice and long-term complications. J Urol 1997;157:28–32.

[9] Haleblian G, Kijvikai K, de la Rosette J, Preminger G. Ureteral stenting and urinary stone management: a systematic review. J Urol 2008;179:424–430.

[10] Makarov DV, Trock BJ, Allaf ME, Matlaga BR. The effect of ureteral stent placement on post-ureteroscopy complications: a meta-analysis. Urology 2008;71:796–800.

[11] Pengfei S, Yutao L, Jie Y, *et al.* The results of ureteral stenting after ureteroscopic lithotripsy for ureteral calculi: a systematic review and meta-analysis. J Urol 2011;186:1904–1909.

[12] Cochrane Handbook for Systematic Reviews of Interventions. The Cochrane Colloboration, 2011.

[13] Nabi G, Cook J, N'Dow J, McClinton S. Outcomes of stenting after uncomplicated ureteroscopy: systematic review and meta-analysis. BMJ 2007;334:572.

[14] Preminger GM, Tiselius HG, Assimos DG, *et al.* 2007 guideline for the management of ureteral calculi. J Urol 2007;178:2418–2434.

[15] Fernström I, Johansson B. Percutaneous pyelolithotomy. A new extraction technique. Scand J Urol Nephrol 1976;10:257–259.

[16] Srinivasan AK, Herati A, Okeke Z, Smith AD. Renal drainage after percutaneous nephrolithotomy. J Endourol 2009;23:1743–1749.

[17] Jackman SV, Docimo SG, Cadeddu JA, Bishoff JT, Kavoussi LR, Jarrett TW. The "mini-perc" technique: a less invasive alternative to percutaneous nephrolithotomy. World J Urol 1998;16:371–374.

[18] Bellman GC, Davidoff R, Candela J, Gerspach J, Kurtz S, Stout L. Tubeless percutaneous renal surgery. J Urol 1997;157:1578–1582.

[19] Borges CF, Fregonesi A, Silva DC, Sasse AD. Systematic review and meta-analysis of nephrostomy placement versus tubeless percutaneous nephrolithotomy. J Endourol 2010; 24(11).

[20] Chan AW, Altman DG. Epidemiology and reporting of randomised trials published in PubMed journals. Lancet 2005;365:1159–1162.

[21] Pearle MS, Pierce HL, Miller GL, *et al.* Optimal method of urgent decompression of the collecting system for obstruction and infection due to ureteral calculi. J Urol 1998;160:1260–1264.

[22] Yoshimura K, Utsunomiya N, Ichioka K, Ueda N, Matsui Y, Terai A. Emergency drainage for urosepsis associated with upper urinary tract calculi. J Urol 2005;173:458–462.

[23] Netto NR, Ikonomidis J, Zillo C. Routine ureteral stenting after ureteroscopy for ureteral lithiasis: is it really necessary. J Urol 2001;166:1252–1254.

[24] Borboroglu PG, Amling CL, Schenkman NS, *et al.* Ureteral stenting after ureteroscopy for distal ureteral calculi: a multi-institutional prospective randomized controlled study assessing pain, outcomes and complications. J Urol 2001;166:1651–1657.

[25] Byrne RR, Auge BK, Kourambas J, Munver R, Delvecchio F, Preminger GM. Routine ureteral stenting is not necessary after ureteroscopy and ureteropyeloscopy: a randomized trial. J Endourol 2002;16:9–13.

[26] Chen YT, Chen J, Wong WY, Yang SS, Hsieh CH, Wang CC. Is ureteral stenting necessary after uncomplicated ureteroscopic lithotripsy? A prospective, randomized controlled trial. J Urol 2002;167:1977–1980.

[27] Cheung MC, Lee F, Leung YL, Wong BB, Tam PC. A prospective randomized controlled trial on ureteral stenting after ureteroscopic holmium laser lithotripsy. J Urol 2003;169:1257–1260.

[28] Srivastava A, Gupta R, Kumar A, Kapoor R, Mandhani A. Routine stenting after ureteroscopy for distal ureteral calculi is unnecessary: results of a randomized controlled trial. J Endourol 2003;17:871–874.

[29] Damiano R, Autorino R, Esposito C, *et al.* Stent positioning after ureteroscopy for urinary calculi: the question is still open. Eur Urol 2004;46:381–387; discussion 387.

[30] Jeong H, Kwak C, Lee SE. Ureteric stenting after ureteroscopy for ureteric stones: a prospective randomized study assessing symptoms and complications. BJU Int 2004;93:1032–1034; discussion 1034.

[31] Grossi FS, Ferretti S, Di Lena S, Crispino M. A prospective randomized multicentric study comparing stented vs non-stented ureteroscopic lithotripsy. Arch Ital Urol Androl 2006;78:53–56.

[32] Hussein A, Rifaat E, Zaki A, Abol-Nasr M. Stenting versus non-stenting after non-complicated ureteroscopic manipulation of stones in bilharzial ureters. Int J Urol 2006;13:886–890.

[33] Ibrahim HM, Al-Kandari AM, Shaaban HS, Elshebini YH, Shokeir AA. Role of ureteral stenting after uncomplicated ureteroscopy for distal ureteral stones: a randomized, controlled trial. J Urol 2008;180:961–965.

[34] Isen K, Kenan I, Bogatekin S *et al.* Is routine ureteral stenting necessary after uncomplicated ureteroscopic lithotripsy for lower ureteral stones larger than 1 cm. Urol Res 2008;36:115–119.

[35] Xu Y, Wei Q, Liu LR. A prospective randomized trial comparing non-stented versus routine stented ureteroscopic holmium laser lithotripsy. Saudi Med J 2009;30:1276–1280.

[36] Cevik I, Dillioglugil O, Akdas A, Siegel Y. Is stent placement necessary after uncomplicated ureteroscopy for removal of impacted ureteral stones. J Endourol 2010;24:1263–1267.

26

Robotic Ureteric Reconstruction

Helena Gresty[1], Navroop Johal[1] and Pardeep Kumar[2]

[1] Department of Academic Surgery, The Royal Marsden NHS Foundation Trust, London, UK
[2] Consultant Urological Surgeon, Department of Academic Surgery, The Royal Marsden NHS Foundation Trust, London, UK

26.1   Introduction

The da Vinci robotic platform has facilitated a marked increase in minimally invasive reconstruction of the urinary tract. Three-dimensional vision combined with adjustable magnification allows for improved depth perception and identification of peri-ureteric structures. Optimal ergonomics, tremor filtration, as well use of instruments with seven degrees of motion, provide the precision of movement required to perform fine dissection and suturing. Newer incarnations of the robotic platform incorporate increased reach, multi-quadrant access, and the ability to alter patient position during surgery – all of which facilitate surgery on the entire ureter. Urologists are thus taking advantage of these technical advances and embarking on a relatively shorter learning curve compared to laparoscopic surgery [1].

While the reported experience of robotic ureteric surgery in the literature is certainly less than that of robotic prostatectomy, cystectomy, or partial nephrectomy there has been a surge of case reports and series that show the robotic approach to the ureter to be feasible, safe, and with encouraging outcomes.

26.2   General Considerations

The majority of patients, particularly those with multiple comorbidities, benefit from minimally invasive surgical techniques. Despite this the surgeon must consider that certain patients are not suitable for this approach. Severe cardiopulmonary disease may make pneumo-peritoneum hazardous. Patient positioning in Trendelenberg can present additional anesthetic demands. Multiple previous abdominal surgeries may result in difficulties with adhesions.

A particular issue with the ureter is the discrepancy between pre-operative investigation and intra-operative findings. Pre-operative assessment of the diseased/obstructed ureter is covered in detail elsewhere in this text. Often multiple techniques are utilized including CT urogram, antegrade nephrostogram, retrograde urography, MAG3 renogram, and direct visualization with ureteroscopy. It is the author's experience that these modalities may underestimate the extent of pathology, particularly in cases of retroperitoneal fibrosis or iatrogenic ureteric strictures. In these cases, often more of the ureter requires replacement than was initially suspected in order to effect optimal outcomes. In robotic surgery, this may require extra port placement, change in patient position, or conversion to open surgery.

Indications for ureteric reconstruction include iatrogenic injury, stricture and obstruction, reconstruction of congenital defects, particularly in the pediatric population, and excision of urothelial tumors in highly selected cases. Decisions on operative approach are analogous to open surgery. Etiology, location, length of ureteric abnormality, suitability of the bladder for flap formation, and low-pressure drainage should all be considered.

Particular to robotic surgery are the following issues:

- *Port placement* – Port placement is generally more cranial than that for a robotic prostatectomy. This facilitates access to the mid-ureter allowing for adequate mobilization. Extra ports when required during the case should be placed – morbidity from port placement under vision and pneumoperitoneum is minimal.
- *Handling of the ureter* – Haptic feedback is absent in robotics. Experienced robotic surgeons compensate for this with a heightened awareness of tissue dynamics with movement, using this as a surrogate for touch. Unfortunately even the grasping forceps designed for handling bowel will cause damage to the ureteric adventitia. A key component of robotic ureteric surgery is adopting a "no-touch" technique. This utilizes vessel loops to facilitate ureteric mobilization as well as Weck Hem-o-lok clips or similar to act as a site for holding the ureter safely. In non-cancer cases the redundant ureter to be excised is used as a handle to manipulate the ureter after distal division and only excised at the last moment to minimize handling of the healthy ureter.
- *Suture choice* – Bladder closure is most efficiently achieved using a barbed suture. In the author's opinion, this suture type is not suitable for ureteric suturing.
- *Stent placement* – Flexibility is required as no two cases undergoing reconstruction are the same. Access to the bladder is facilitated by bringing the robotic cart in from the side (so called "side docking"). This allows ureteric stent placement cystoscopically. If this is unavailable or unfeasible, then standard guide wires can be passed through any laparoscopic port. Again, placement of a dedicated suprapubic 3 or 5 mm port to facilitate stent placement is recommended if this provides the optimal angle with which to pass the stent. Guidewires can even go down a 14G vascular access cannula passed through the abdominal wall.
- *Watertight* – It is the author's standard practice to test reconstruction by filling the bladder. This is generally carried out via the urethral catheter with a bag of saline at around 100 cm above the patient. An extra suture can be easily placed during the case when required.

A number of established open techniques have been adapted for a minimally invasive approach over the last two decades. These include the ureteroneocystostomy, psoas hitch, Boari flap, and uretero-ureterostomy.

26.3 Ureteroneocystostomy

Ureteroneocystostomy (UNC) refers to the re-implantation of the ureter into the bladder following excision of a diseased segment. It is the procedure of choice for ureteric pathology in close proximity to the bladder up to 5 cm in length. Iatrogenic injuries to the ureter are most likely at this level, this being the most common indication for UNC in the adult population. Other indications include distal ureteric cancers as well as ureteric obstruction secondary to other pelvic tumors and/or their treatment (e.g., radiotherapy for cervical cancer). The technique is also used in the pediatric population to treat high-grade or refractory vesico-ureteric reflux.

26.3.1 Patient Positioning and Port Placement

The patient should be in lithotomy with a moderate or steep Trendelenberg. Intermittent pneumatic calf compression is essential for deep vein thrombosis prophylaxis and the patient should receive a broad-spectrum antibiotic at induction of anesthesia. A urethral catheter is placed at the beginning of the case. The authors use an intravenous giving set connected to this catheter to facilitate simple filling and emptying of the bladder by the circulating nursing team during the case.

Port placement is similar to that for a radical cystectomy. This facilitates access to the ureter above the common iliac artery as well as mobilization of the large bowel where required. The initial 8-mm camera is placed just above the umbilicus. A 30-degree telescope is used for the procedure. Two 8-mm trocars are placed lateral to the rectus muscle on either side near the anterior axillary line and just below the level of the umbilicus. An additional 8-mm trocar is placed three finger breadths above the iliac crest for the fourth robotic arm on the contralateral side to the ureter of interest. This facilitates medial retraction of bowel and bladder when required. A 12-mm assistant port is required on the side of the ureter to be operated on for suction and suture needle delivery. On occasion an addition 5-mm port in the mid trans-pyloric plane is used.

26.3.2 Procedure

The surgeon may wish to perform prior or simultaneous cystoscopy. If the latter is planned a "side dock" of the robotic cart will be required to facilitate access to the perineum. Dependent on the pathology, placement of a ureteric stent or catheter can be carried out. An alternative is to carry out intravesical mobilization of the ureteric orifice by bladder cuff excision with a Collins knife.

A trans-peritoneal approach is favored by the authors, although extra-peritoneal surgery is feasible in very short distal strictures. After port placement and robot docking the retroperitoneum on the side of interest is exposed by incising the peritoneum and medializing the large bowel along the line of Toldt. Careful mobilization of the ureter at the level of the common down to the uretero-vesical junction is carried out. The adventitial layer of the ureter is preserved to avoid de-vascularization. This is achieved by medial and lateral ureteric dissection until a window is made behind the ureter. A vessel loop is then placed around the ureter and secured as a loop with a Weck Hem-o-lok clip. This facilitates a "no-touch" technique – the aim is to never actually grip the healthy ureter with the robotic instruments.

The affected distal ureter is excised down to the bladder with robotic scissors and placed in a nubert bag or similar for later retrieval. In the context of ureteric resection for cancer, tumor spillage is avoided with the use of Weck Hem-o-lok clips on either side of the remaining ureter. In cases of distal ureteric tumor resection an ipsilateral lymph node dissection is carried out prior to ureteric reconstruction. This also allows time for any intra-operative ureteric margin frozen sections to be reported.

Attention is then turned to the bladder dividing the urachus and mobilizing it in a similar fashion to trans-peritoneal robotic prostatectomy. The bladder is filled and emptied using the urethral catheter to ensure adequate mobilization has been achieved. The Weck Hem-o-lok clip used to occlude the upper ureter is grasped and the ureter "offered up" to the bladder to ascertain the optimal site of re-implantation. Division of the contralateral bladder pedicle may be required to mobilize the bladder and ensure a tension-free anastamosis. Alternative forms of reconstruction in the form of a psoas hitch or Boari flap should be considered if there is insufficient ureteric length to form a tension free anastomosis.

The detrusor is divided with cautery in the line of re-implantation. This is best achieved with the bladder filled. The bipolar instrument (either robotic fenestrated bipolar or robotic Maryland dissecting forceps) is ideal for this task. It may be necessary to switch this instrument to the side of the ureter being operated on to ensure that an adequate detrusor tunnel is formed. At the site of implantation the dissection is continued through to the urothelium and a cystostomy formed, again in the line of re-implantation. A 4/0 coated polyglactin suture is then placed at the apex of this cystostomy.

The ureter is spatulated, care being taken that the magnification in robotic surgery may overestimate the size of the spatulation. The previously placed 4/0 suture allows the back wall of the anastamosis to be sutured. A stent is placed as previously described and the anastmosis completed. The detrusor tunnel is closed over the ureter as an anti-reflux mechanism with a similar 3/0 suture.

At the end of the reconstruction the bladder is filled to ensure suture lines are watertight. A non-suction drain is left at the operative site utilizing one of the trocar placement sites.

In the authors practice the urethral catheter is removed at a week following a satisfactory cystogram and stent removed at 4–6 weeks.

26.3.3 Literature

Yohannes *et al.* [2] were the first to publish the technique of robotic UNC for a distal ureteric stricture in a man with failed endoscopic treatment and recurrent stone disease. They reported an operative time of 210 minutes with less than 50 ml blood loss and no intra-operative or post-operative complications. A number of authors have since published relatively small case series of UNC, often alongside a variety of robotic ureteric procedures and in combination with a psoas hitch or Boari flap [3–7].

Musch and colleagues [8] recently published a series of 16 patients who underwent robotic distal ureteric surgery for various pathologies. Three patients underwent extravesical anti-refluxing re-implantation without a psoas hitch or Boari flap, two for strictures, and one for persistent vesiculoureteric reflux. Two patients underwent intravesical reimplants following inadvertent bilateral ectopic ureteric transection during robotic radical prostatectomy and resection of megaureter. The operative duration ranged from 153–460 minutes with a hospital stay ranging from 6–22 days. Of these five patients, all were asymptomatic at follow-up and had no hydronephrosis on follow-up imaging.

26.4 Psoas Hitch

In circumstances where ureteric length is insufficient for direct tension-free bladder reimplantation in the form of a UTC, additional length may be gained from a psoas hitch. Although practice varies, this technique is usually adopted for excised ureteric length between 5 cm to 10 cm. A Boari flap may be adopted, often in conjunction with a psoas hitch, when further ureter is excised or if the bladder is insufficiently mobile [9].

26.4.1 Patient Positioning and Port Placement

This is similar to robotic UNC. The only adjustment is that the ipsilateral 12 mm trocar for the patient-side surgeon is placed higher to facilitate access to the psoas tendon for stabilization of the reconstruction.

26.4.2 Procedure

The ureter should be mobilized and the area of interest excised as described for UNC. The space of Retzius is developed, the bladder filled with normal saline, and the degree of bladder and ureteric mobility assessed. If a psoas hitch is required the contra-lateral superior vesicle pedicle is divided unless the bladder is very large. Using a no-touch technique, by grasping the occluding Weck Hem-o-lok clip, the proximal ureter is placed over the anterior aspect of the bladder. In contrast to a ureteroneocystostomy, a full-thickness incision is made in a line *perpendicular* to the line of the ureter to be re-implanted. An 8- to 10-cm incision is required as a minimum. Again, this is best achieved with the bladder filled via the urethral catheter. This facilitates an increase in length of available bladder to bridge the ureteric defect. The psoas tendon is exposed and two sutures at least 2 cm apart anchor the bladder to the tendon. This is carried out to provide stability to the reconstruction and facilitate re-implantation. The ureter is anastamosed to the apex of the cystostomy with similar sutures as for UNC. A ureteric stent is placed and the bladder defect closed. The authors prefer a barbed 2/0 sture for this purpose. The reconstruction is tested as watertight with subsequent management as per UNC.

26.4.3 Literature

De Naeyer *et al.* [10] were the first group to report a single case of robotic psoas hitch in the literature. Patil and colleagues [11] later published a series of twelve patients in a multi-institutional review of robotic UTC with psoas hitch between 2004 and 2006. The indications were stricture disease and uretero-vaginal fistula. They reported no intra-operative or postoperative complications and reported a mean blood loss of 48 mls (45–100 ml range) and mean operative time of 208 minutes (80 to 360 min range). They used intravenous urography and MAG3 to assess postoperative outcomes and reported normal findings in 10 patients and mild residual hydronephrosis in 2 patients. Interestingly, the group also retrospectively compared their robotic data to that of open and laparoscopic approaches to psoas hitch and found the robotic technique to be associated with shorter hospital stay and lower blood loss.

26.5 Boari Flap

The Boari flap is a well-established technique for mid and upper ureteric reconstruction. It provides a tunneled extension of the bladder to bridge a ureteric lesion of 10–15 cm in length [9]. It is often combined with a psoas hitch that acts as an anchor and facilitates tension free re-implantation of the ureter.

26.5.1 Patient Positioning and Port Placement

This is similar to the robotic psoas hitch. It is useful to tilt the operating table laterally away from the ureter of interest as well as place the patient in Trendelenberg to facilitate upper ureteric dissection.

26.5.2 Procedure

A similar approach to the dissection of the distal ureter and mobilization of the bladder is performed as described for UTC and psoas hitch. The bladder should be filled and a vesical flap dissected using electrocautery along the anterior surface of the bladder, at least 2 cm from the bladder neck. Some authors have described the use of a triangle shaped flap but the authors prefer a "U" shape. In order to avoid flap ischemia it is of crucial importance that the ratio of flap base to length should not exceed 3:1. Several surgeons also use an anchoring suture on the psoas tendon at this point. The ureter is spatulated as previously described. The posterior surface of the anastomosis is formed first using interrupted sutures. A ureteric stent is then placed. The bladder defect is then closed using a 2/0 barbed suture starting at the inferior aspect. Suturing continues cranially and the flap is tubularized. Finally the superior and anterior aspect of the tube is used to complete the anterior ureterovesical anastamosis. Interrupted sutures are then used to complete the two-layer closure of the bladder. The visceral peritoneum overlying the bladder is closed over the suture line to further reinforce the reconstruction.

26.5.3 Literature

Casati and Boari [12] first described the use of a bladder flap to repair ureteric defects over 100 years ago. Although the open Boari flap is well described and often utilized by urologists, there is relative paucity of laparoscopic data [13, 14]. Since Schimpf and Wagner [7] published two cases of robotic Boari flap among a series of 11 robotic distal ureteric reconstructions in 2009, a number of groups have gone on to confirm the feasibility of the robotic approach [8, 15, 16].

Do *et al.* [17] published their group's experience of eight cases in 2014 and also provided an excellent summary of the current literature within the field. Their cohort of patients had stricture disease caused by a variety of pathologies including iatrogenic injury and previous pelvic malignancy. They detail a mean operative time of 171.9 min (range 115–240) and a blood loss of 161.3 ml (50–250 ml range). There were no conversions to open and no intraoperative complications although one patient had a prolonged anastomotic leak, which was managed with catheterization alone.

In a detailed series by Musch and colleagues [8], robotic Boari flap was performed in five patients, including two patients with distal ureteric transitional cell carcinoma. Their operative time ranged from 230 to 320 minutes with the oncological resections taking the longest time. They reported one prolonged anastomotic leak and one case of urine leak causing a chemical peritonitis.

In contrast to robotic psoas hitch, no group have yet compared their robotic outcomes to that of laparoscopic or open techniques and comparative studies would certainly be highly valued in the field.

26.6   Ureteroureterostomy

A short ureteric defect in the upper or mid ureter may be repaired by direct ureteric anastamosis. Although it may be technically feasible to perform in the distal ureter, UTC with or without psoas hitch or Boari flap is favored so as to minimize the risk of ischemic stricture formation.

26.6.1   Patient Positioning and Port Placement

This is similar to the robotic Boari flap.

26.6.2   Procedure

The area of interest in the mid- or upper ureter should be dissected and mobilized as described in UTC proximally. Concurrent ureterenoscopy to visualize the precise target area may be helpful and requires a double sterile field and side docking of the robotic cart. Buffi *et al.* [18] used this technique to manage coexisting ureteric stones during the procedure. The diseased segment should be excised and managed as previously described to expose two healthy ends of ureter. Care should be taken to assess for ureteric length to ensure tension free anastamosis. The ends should be spatulated using robotic Pott's scissors in opposite orientations and re-anastamosed over a ureteric stent. The authors favor the formation of a watertight anastamosis with two continuous 4-0 absorbable sutures run from each apex. The anastamosis is ideally encased with redundant omentum or mobilized parietal peritoneum.

26.6.3   Literature

Several authors have published the outcomes of robotic ureteroureterostomy as isolated case reports or small series [4, 18–21].

Hemal and colleagues [4] as part of their large case series of 44 patients undergoing robotic ureteric reconstruction report 11 cases of ureteroureterostomy. Indications were proximal ureteric stricture in 7 cases and a retrocaval ureter in 4 patients. Operative time was less than that seen in distal ureteric reconstruction ranging from 75–140 min with a mean length of stay of 3 days. All cases were relieved of symptoms and had no strictures on radionuclide scintigraphy. The only complication reported was one post-operative infection with *C. difficil* managed with antibiotics. No cases in their whole series were converted to open and similarly there were no urine leaks.

Lee *et al.* [21] describe successful re-anastomosis in three carefully selected patients with short ureteric lesions just proximal to the iliac vessels. One patient was taken back to theatre at day one post op when urine was noted in the periureteric drain. When the JJ stent was removed it was found to be kinked and was likely crushed by the robotic instruments. The stent was exchanged and drainage settled without any manipulation of the anastomosis. Follow-up IV urogram or retrogram pyelgraphy showed good patency of repair in all patients. All patients were pain free and two patients had improved drainage and split function at follow-up. Guazzoni's group [18] published a series of five similar cases in *European Urology* in 2011. They highlight the particular advantage of concurrent flexible ureterorenoscopy, which was essential in locating the site of stricture in three of five patients.

26.7   Conclusion

Robotic ureteric reimplantation is feasible, safe, and can deal with the majority of mid and lower ureteric strictures. Reconstruction of upper ureteric strictures remains a challenge when stricture length is long.

References

[1] Passerotti CC, Passerotti AM, Dall'Oglio MF, Leite KR, Nunes RL, Srougi M, Retik AB, Nguyen HT. Comparing the quality of the suture anastamosis and the learning curves associated with performing open, freehand and robotic-assisted laparoscopic pyeloplasty in a swine animal model. J Am Coll Surg 2009;208(4): 576–586.

[2] Yohannes P, Chiou RK, Pelinkovic D. Rapid communication: pure robot-assisted laparoscopic ureteral reimplantation for ureteral stricture disease: case report. J Endourol 2003;17(10):891–893.

[3] Williams SK, Leveillee RJ. Expanding the horizons: robot-assisted reconstructive surgery of the distal ureter. J Endourol 2009;23(3):457–461.

[4] Hemal AK, Nayyar R, Gupta NP, Dorairajan LN. Experience with robot assisted laparoscopic surgery for upper and lower benign and malignant ureteral pathologies. Urology 2010;76(6):1387–1393.

[5] Pugh J, Farkas A, Su LM. Robotic distal ureterectomy with psoas hitch and ureteroneocystostomy: surgical technique and outcomes. Asian Journal of Urology 2015;2(2):123–127.

[6] Glinianski M, Guru KA, Zimmerman G, Mohler J, Kim HL. Robot-assisted ureterectomy and ureteral reconstruction for urothelial carcinoma. J Endourol 2009;23(1):97–100.

[7] Schimpf MO, Wagner JR. Robot-assisted laparoscopic distal ureteral surgery. JSLS 2009;13(1):44–49.

[8] Musch M, Hohenhorst L, Pailliart A, Loewen H, Davoudi Y, Kroepfl D. Robot-assisted reconstructive surgery of the distal ureter: single institution experience in 16 patients. BJU Int 2013;111(5):773–783.

[9] Nakada SY, Hsu THS. Management of upper urinary tract obstruction. In: Wein AJ, Kavoussi LR, Novick AC, Partin AW, Peters CA, eds. *Campbell-Walsh Urology* 10th Edition, Vol II, Chapt. 41. Philadelphia, PA: Saunders 2012, pp. 1122–1168.

[10] De Naeyer G, Van Migem P, Schatteman P, Carpentier P, Fonteyne E, Mottrie AM. Case report: pure robot-assisted psoas hitch ureteral reimplantation for distal-ureteral stenosis. J Endourol 2007;21(6):618–620.

[11] Patil NN, Mottrie A, Sundaram B, Patel VR. Robotic-assisted laparoscopic ureteral reimplantation with psoas hitch: a multi-institutional, multinational evaluation. Urology 2008;72(1):47–50.

[12] Casati E, Boari A. Contributo sperimentale alla plastica dell'urretere. Atti Acad Med Natl 1894;14:149.

[13] Seideman CA, Huckabay C, Smith KD, Permpongkosol S, Nadjafi-Semnani M, Lee BR, Richstone L, Kavoussi LR. Laparoscopic ureteral reimplantation: technique and outcomes. J Urol 2009;181(4):1742–1746.

[14] Castilloa OA, Travassos J, Escobar JF, Lopez-Fontanaa G. Laparoscopic ureteral replacement by Boari flap: multi-institutional experience in 30 cases. Actas Urol Esp 2013;37(10):658–662.

[15] Yang C, Jones L, Rivera ME, Varlee GT, Deane LA. Robotic-assisted ureteral reimplantation with Boari flap and psoas hitch: a single-institution experience. J Laparoendosc Adv Surg Tech A 2011;21(9):829–833.

[16] Kozinn SI, Canes D, Sorcini A, Moinzadeh A. Robotic versus open distal ureteral reconstruction and reimplantation for benign stricture disease. J Endourol 2012;26(2):147–151.

[17] Do M, Kallidonis P, Qazi H, Liatsikos E, Ho Thi P, Dietel A, Stolzenburg JU. Robot-assisted technique for boari flap ureteral reimplantation: is robot assistance beneficial? J Endourol 2014;28(6):679–685.

[18] Buffi N, Cestari A, Lughezzani G, Bellinzoni P, Sangalli M, Scapaticci E, Zanoni M, Annino F, Larcher A, Lazzeri M, Rigatti P, Guazzoni G. Robot- assisted uretero-ureterostomy for iatrogenic lumbar and iliac ureteral stricture: technical details and preliminary clinical results. Eur Urol 2011;60(6):1221–1225.

[19] Mufarrij PW, Shah OD, Berger AD, Stifelman MD. Robotic reconstruction of the upper urinary tract. J Urol 2007;178(5):2002–2005.

[20] Passerotti CC, Diamond DA, Borer JG, Eisner BH, Barrisford G, Nguyen HT. Robot-assisted laparoscopic ureteroureterostomy: description of technique. J Endourol 2008;22(4):581–586.

[21] Lee DI, Schwab CW, Harris A. Robot-assisted ureteroureterostomy in the adult: initial case series. Urology 2010;75(3):570–573.

27

Indwelling Ureteric Stents – Health Economics Considerations

Dominic A. Teichmann[1] and Hrishi B. Joshi[2]

[1] Specialist Registrar in Urology, University Hospital of Wales and School of Medicine, Cardiff University, Wales, UK
[2] Consultant Urological Surgeon and Honorary Lecturer, Department of Urology, University Hospital of Wales and School of Medicine, Cardiff University, Wales, UK

27.1   Introduction

Indwelling ureteric stents have multiple applications with the aim of either preventing or relieving obstruction and facilitating renal drainage. Their uses are widely described in the acute setting to relieve infected obstruction in the presence of a ureteric stone, especially associated with infection, to prevent scarring and allow drainage in transplanted kidneys, to mitigate compression in malignancy or fibrosis encompassing the ureter and after an ureteroscopy.

Although useful, they have implications for patients' health-related quality of life as well as significant impact on resources [1]. Controversies also surround the use of stents in many of these situations when service and patient impact are taken into account.

Relatively little attention has been paid to performing detailed outcomes assessments of stent usage and evaluating associated health economic considerations.

27.2   Health Economic Evaluations

Health economic evaluations reflect efficacy or can demonstrate effectiveness statistically by modeling. Comparative health economic analyses can be classified according to the type of comparison regarding the costs and consequences. Depending on the type of analysis, the assessment of outcome ranges from "non-assessment" through to assessment in non-monetary, naturalistic units to monetary assessment. These can be classified in the following categories [2].

| | Measurement | | |
Method of analysis	Assessment of costs	Assessment of outcome	Cost-outcome comparison
Cost-minimization analysis (CMA)	Monetary	None	None
Cost-effectiveness analysis (CEA)	Monetary	Natural units	Costs per outcome unit
Cost-utility analysis (CUA)	Monetary	Utility values	Costs per QALY
Cost-benefit analysis (CBA)	Monetary	Monetary	Net costs

In recent work by Joshi *et al.*, the mean EuroQol utility values, which indicate patient satisfaction with treatment, were significantly reduced following stent insertion. Stents are associated with negative functional capacity and reduced utility values. (Indwelling ureteral stents: evaluation of symptoms, quality of life, and utility) [3]. These might have significant influence on indirect costs considerations. Data for health economic analyses of stents remain limited, having been derived from diverse sources (e.g., pooled data sets, meta-analyses, unverifiable assumptions) and are affected by uncertainties. Most of the available data is related to the cost-benefit analyses that involve direct costs only and might not apply to different healthcare systems.

We have considered the evidence in three common settings in which ureteric stents are utilized. The context of their clinical application is fundamental to the subsequent outcome and health economic assessments.

27.3   Short-Term Application

This is the most common use of the ureteric stents made of polymeric materials. Most of the health economic data relates to the peri-intervention insertion of stents. Post-ureteroscopy stenting: This has remained a topic of some contention with the argument based upon to what degree the antecedent procedure was "complicated" or "uncomplicated."

The use of ureteral stents in these circumstances has been the topic of several studies and systematic reviews.

Direct costs are impacted by the use of the stent, variably longer operating time due to their insertion and repeat admission for removal of the stent (if the attached strings are not left ex-corporis). Indirect costs also play a factor in relation to stent related symptoms, conceivably requiring time off work and loss of QoL and slower return to normal physical activities.

Liang Tange *et al.*'s paper in 2011 [4] made some efforts to delineate and a multitude of different outcome measures pertaining to the use and non-use of stents post uncomplicated ureteroscopy.

In the 14 trials examined, only two evaluated return to normal activities where no significant difference was found between the stent and non-stent groups. In one study, however, which included the use of the validated Ureteric Stent Symptom questionnaire (USSQ) found that the QoL was significantly worse in the stented group. Notably, two-thirds of patients in Srivastava's study [5] would opt for a non-stented option in future if given the choice for the same procedure.

Five studies reported that stenting increased cost overall, whereas 10 studies reported significantly increased operating time, a key cost-driver, in the stented group.

Unplanned medical visits and readmission rates in 11 studies, comprising 1103 patients, showed a higher all-cause readmission rate in the non-stented group, although this did not reach statistical significance. Examining the sub-groups of the uretero-scopic intervention undertaken, be it holmium laser or pneumatic lithotripsy showed no significant difference in re-admission rates and thus they were analyzed as a homog-enous group.

Dysuria, frequency, and hematuria were the only remaining factors, which were sig-nificantly higher in the stented group that could conceivably impact on quality of life, but would not be likely to be a de facto component of a direct or indirect cost increase.

A meta-analysis in the British Medical Journal by Nabi *et al.* [6] in 2007 of nine RCTs comprising 831 patients reported similar findings to the Chinese group. Their sub-group analysis of cost, once again, found the methodology with which this was analyzed inconsistent. Among the studies, however, operation time and overall cost were once again found to be higher in the stented patient group.

In conclusion, it seems more work needs to be done in defining the terminology of "uncomplicated ureteroscopy" so as to undertake further studies with more standardized outcome measures, trial design, QoL outcome measures and cost-effectiveness data.

The conception of a validated costing model would greatly improve the methodology with which cost analyses are undertaken and would allow more accurate and reliable comparison between healthcare institutions on a national scale, and healthcare systems internationally.

At present, evidence suggests benefit with the avoidance of stenting following uncom-plicated ureteroscopy on the basis of shorter operating time, fewer direct material and stent-removal costs, and improved quality of life outcomes measures in relation to indirect costs. However, this must be balanced against the higher likelihood of post-procedural re-admission risk and the associated financial implications.

27.4 Medium- to Long-Term Application: Chronic Obstructive Uropathy

Here the cost analyses have hinged upon the repeated use of polymeric stents in com-parison with long-term metallic stents.

In a 2011 review of practice by Gonzalez *et al.* [7] comparing standard PTFE stents against a nickel-titanium prosthesis "Memokath" in Spain found the metal, thermo-expandable stent to be of high initial cost (€4865 per treatment) in comparison to PTFE stent usage (€1275) in a day-case setting. This results in €3589 cost excess with the use of the Memokath. They did, however, report that this cost excess was recovered after the third change of the PTFE stent.

These results carry limitations as the cost analysis was hypothetical, thus potentially missing re-admissions and complications associated with the procedure in a real-world setting. Furthermore, there was not mention of the intended length of use of the memokath stent. Their decision tree analysis was based on an 80% likelihood of collateral adverse effects with use of PTFE stents and a 0% likelihood of the same with the metallic stent. The absence of patient reported complications in the use of metallic stents, although different from PTFE stents, is not absent in the majority of published literature.

Lopez-Huertas *et al.* [8] examined use of metallic stents in specifically benign upper tract obstruction in a small patient group. They examined actual cost per patient in comparison with PTFE stent usage, individualized the number of stent changes in a year for each patient, and based their result on the mean cost. They found that the annual cost for polymer stent maintenance was $10,362, representing a 43% reduction in cost per patient, per year. Three out of the thirteen patients had metallic stents discontinued prematurely due to irritative voiding symptoms and gross hematuria, only one of these resolved with subsequent placement of PTFE stent.

Despite the robust methodology, the low patient number, incomplete follow-up, and non-generalizability of cost remain an issue with this study. It does, however, seem to suggest a trend toward metallic stents being a feasible alternative to frequent PTFE stent changes in chronic disease management, with the cost equilibrium being met by the lesser change frequency.

These findings seemed to be corroborated by Taylor *et al.* [9] in 2012 in a cohort of 21 patients whose all-cause obstructive pathology cost of stent placement and exchange (PTFE versus metal) within an American private healthcare system. They demonstrated a saving of between 48%–74% on an annual basis, with the variability dependent on frequency of exchange.

Similarly Baumgarten *et al.* [10] examined a series of 97 metallic stent placements in 50 patients for malignancy and chronic ureteric compromise due to ureterostomy or ileal conduit formation. They have the largest case series examining this intervention and drew similar conclusions to Lopez-Huertas' paper as pertaining to cost-effectiveness due to lesser frequency of stent exchange. The cost analysis, however, was somewhat presumptive as some costs were extrapolated and costs associated with clinical failure of the stent were not reported.

These studies would benefit significantly from a cohesive and unified cost analysis methodology allowing for comparison between studies and evaluation of different management strategies.

In conclusion, most of the published literature seems to suggest that in terms of cost, irrespective of country or healthcare system, changeable metallic ureteral stents confer a cost-benefit in all-cause ureteral obstruction on the basis of decreased replacement-frequency requirement.

This stands to reason, as long as their use is judiciously applied in a chronic patient population where multiple stent exchanges are envisaged to justify the initially high material outlay costs.

27.5 Comparator Assessment: Nephrostomy and Stenting

Two modes of management of obstructed system exist consisting of a percutaneous nephrostomy with or without a subsequent anterograde stent, or a cystoscopically placed retrograde stent. A number of factors influence the decision regarding the above treatment modality with both patient and "institution" factors playing a role. Clinical circumstances and resource limitations often influence type of drainage used.

A recent study undertaken by Chitale *et al.* [11] in Norwich examined the cost implications of a single-stage nephrostomy and anterograde stent placement versus a "traditional" interval two-stage approach in upper urinary tract obstruction due to all-cause ureteric drainage compromise.

This group found there would be a significant cost saving in the procedural and length of stay-related costs of the one-stage procedure. They found the difference in hospital length of stay for all-cause pathological upper tract obstruction to be in the region of fewer 10 days, signifying a saving of approx £2,500 in their institution, with a procedural cost reduction of £665 to £376 (43%). The procedure was also found to be safe, with a similar analgesic and antibiotic regimen utilized in the two protocols.

There were some relative and absolute contra-indications to its use with hemorrhage, urosepsis, and untreated acute renal failure, respectively, being conditions precluding the use of the single stage procedure. Irrespective of the above, this study indicates that in a suitable group of patients a single-stage diversion could be a cost-effective and safe solution to achieve renal drainage.

27.6 Other/Miscellaneous Considerations

The forgotten stent: Complications associated with the prolonged use of stents are well documented and troublesome to manage, resulting in unnecessary morbidity for the patient and stress for the responsible surgeon.

Monga *et al.* [12] found that stents "forgotten" >6 months resulted in 68% being calcified, 45% fragmented with 52% subsequently requiring ureteroscopy, 32% ESWL, and 26% PCNL to ensure safe removal. This is clearly an important problem.

Utilizing and maintaining a reliable system to monitor stent insertion and prompt removal is an important facet of their use.

Only few papers have examined the fiscal argument behind the imperative to maintain an effective stent register. Lynch *et al.* [13] looked at average costs of follow-up procedures required to manage the forgotten stent within an NHS model. A simple non-elective cystoscopy cost £430, with ESWL costing £1499 and ureteroscopic or open procedures incurring a cost in the region of £2815–£6610.

Boboroglu and Kane [14] found that patients with forgotten stents required between two to six procedures to render them stent free, with the implied cost, therefore, being considerable.

Sancaktutar *et al.* [15] undertook a more thorough study in a cohort of 26 patients where stents had been retained for a period of greater than 12 months from point of insertion. Management and costs of the individuals were retrospectively analyzed. In their cohort, the mean cost of management was 6.9-fold higher than in the event of timely removal. The mean indwelling time of the forgotten stents was 31.2 months with a significant range of 14 to 120 months. The long retention period of several stents often meant a multimodal and complex treatment approach was required. The average excess cost for the management of these patients with the above modalities was calculated to be $1,225 USD, including hospitalization and procedure costs. A notable consideration is that financial burden increased in line with duration of the stent retention.

With the common usage of intra-ureteric stents in urological practice and no unified approach regarding their follow-up and retrieval despite the existence of a stent register, there is a significant patient and financial benefit to be sought from engendering the use of a robust system.

27.6.1 Methods of Ureteric Stent Extraction, Post-Procedural Considerations and Cost

The practice of allowing ureteral stent strings to protrude from the ureter allowing for either patient or physician removal without further invasive procedure as seemingly obvious benefits. However, its practice is by no means widespread and respective sequelae little documented.

Although no explicit cost analysis was performed one can gain an impression of the relevant clinical and cost issues surrounding stent removal from recent work done by a group at the University of Iowa, comprising a retrospective review by Bockholt *et al.* [16] and a subsequent small randomized prospective series by Barnes *et al.* [17].

Bockholt *et al.* performed a retrospective analysis of 181 unilateral ureteroscopic procedures undertaken for stones receiving ureteral stents. Despite the disproportionately low number of patients receiving a stent with extraction strings left in situ (23%) they suggested that there was no significant difference in post-procedure related events (PREs) between those with and those without extraction strings, regardless of gender. This review served as a useful scoping exercise to inform the primary end-points of the subsequent randomized series of 68 patients receiving ureteric stents following routine URS for stones disease. Their primary outcome measures consisted of "urinary symptoms" and "general health" domains of the validated USSQ (Ureteric Stent Symptom Questionnaire), which was completed at 1d, 6d, and 6w post-operatively. They showed no difference in post-operative pain, urinary symptoms, general health, or work-performance scores between the groups.

Furthermore, no difference in UTI or unscheduled health consultations were demonstrated. Fifteen percent of the string group had inadvertent stent removal, none of which required replacement or had clinically significant sequelae.

No explicit cost-analysis was performed, which is clearly a significant limitation in this context, however, the cogent implication was that no clinically deleterious consequences associated with ureteric stent strings and patient removal were identified and thus this method provides a cost-effective alternative to cystoscopic stent removal. Work has only been done in relation to stone disease and given the potential for inadvertent extraction, one should be cautious where infection, ureteral perforation, or endo-pyelotomy are features of the clinical case.

Explicit cost analyses in a sufficiently powered randomized study such as this would add credibility to the reasonable conclusions drawn and may widen judicious use of ureteral stent extraction strings in procedures where ureteric stent is deemed clinically necessary.

Regarding the future for development of a management strategy for patients with ureteric obstruction Gershman *et al.* [18] undertook some work examining an efficacy and cost-comparison between "office-based" procedures and those undertaken with a daycare surgical admission. Procedures examined included retrograde pyelography, upper tract BCG instillation and ureteric stent insertion and exchange.

They found that in a multitude of clinical scenarios including malignancy and primary stent insertion, procedures undertaken in a office setting by an experienced practitioner with the availability of radiological screening were a safe and cost-effective alternative to daycare surgical admission and general anesthesia.

Given the appropriate case selection this strategy would appear to be a cost-efficient alternative to hospital-based procedures and ought to be a region if interest in terms of service development.

27.6.2 Renal Transplant

Routine stenting of the transplanted ureter in renal transplant recipients has been common practice for some time. Most recently, the associated increased incidence of infective and symptomatic complications associated with the use of the ureteric stent has warranted its re-evaluation. The cost implications of routine stenting and subsequent removal need to be balanced with the risk of anastomotic disruption and consequent healthcare costs.

Wilson *et al.* [19] had recently advocated the continued use of ureteric stents in this scenario for the prevention of urological complications, however, quality of life (QoL) and economic issues had yet to be evaluated.

Tavakoli *et al.* [20] examined the urological complications and healthcare expenditure in renal transplant patients in a series of 201 adult patients over 3 years who were randomized into "stented" and "non-stented" groups following surgery. In their study significantly more patients in the non-stented group received a living donor kidney and acute rejection was more frequent in the stented group, although this did not reach statistical significance. There were no deaths and no significant difference in graft failure between the groups.

Of the no-stent group, 7.7% suffered from urinary tract obstruction compared with none in the stented group ($p < 0.004$) and similarly, significantly more patients in the non-stent group suffered from urinary leakage (8.9% versus 0.9%, $p < 0.008$). Nine patients required re-implantation in the non-stented group as opposed to one in the stented group.

Cost analysis revealed the mean cost per patient in the stented group to be £755 in comparison with £906 in the non-stented group. Furthermore, the total number of hospital days for the stented group was 68 with primarily urinary infective complications in comparison to 126 in the non-stented group, with the majority due to urological mechanical complications.

Their findings agreed with Wilson's [21] paper, concluding that in the 3-month period examined, stenting significantly decreased the incidence of urological complications.

There was an increased incidence of post-operative urinary tract infection, especially beyond 4 weeks of insertion, although this was rarely associated with long-term adverse outcome in terms of graft function or survival.

Furthermore, stenting was found to be cost effective. Stent removal costs were the single largest expenditure in the stented group, however, this was still lower on average than dealing with the cost of complications in the non-stented group, with the average being £2,718.

This makes a compelling case for stenting both on a surgical outcome, and cost basis in this scenario. Quality of life and stent symptoms were not assessed in this study.

Similar studies examining the pediatric transplant population, despite not using cost as a primary endpoint did not reach the same conclusions.

Excess costs were seen in respect to stent removal and need for general anesthesia but without the associated mechanical obstructive complications seen in their adult counterpart. More work is required in this domain, but, as is usual, the management of adults and children cannot be considered equivalent in the respect of ureteric stents in renal transplant recipients.

27.7 Conclusion

Ureteric stents are a simple urological adjunct, which creates complex urological and healthcare–related problems, least of all in terms of cost.

Indications for their use are multiple and the evidence base for their use is changing in the many domains of their utility. This creates problems for clinicians who are keen to achieve the best possible outcomes for patients while avoiding the stent-related complications discussed above and their implications on cost.

Health economic considerations have not necessarily always been at the forefront of the clinician's mind when choosing a treatment course for their patients, however, it is becoming a more focal topic. This can be seen as an opportunity rather than a regrettable circumstance, as making robust health-economic evaluations also constitute a valid platform for evidence-based medicine and achieving the most effective utilization of resources.

The assessment of cost in healthcare is a divisive subject but one that needs to become as axiomatic of a consideration regarding the implementation of any clinical intervention as the examination of outcomes and efficacy. The methodology for assessing cost as detailed in the studies in this chapter has been diverse, and would benefit from standardization, especially within a nationally funded healthcare model with a centralized recommendations and policy.

It might be difficult to firmly recommend a specific strategy in using a stent, or stent type in a given clinical situation based on the current evidence alone. However, it would be advisable to only employ their use carefully after thorough patient counseling, ensuring it is a fully informed decision.

References

[1] Joshi HB. Ureteric stents: overview of current practices and problems. British Journal of Medical and Surgical Urology 2012;5(Suppl):S3–S10.

[2] Walter E, Zehetmayr S. Guidelines on Health Economic Evaluation Consensus paper. April 2006, IPF Institute.

[3] Joshi HB, Stainthorpe A, MacDonagh RP, Keeley FX Jr, Timoney AG, Barry MJ. Indwelling ureteral stents: evaluation of symptoms, quality of life and utility. J Urol 2003;169(3):1065–1069.

[4] Tang L, Gao X, Xu B Jianguo Hou Zhenshe, JH. Placement of ureteral stent after uncomplicated ureteroscopy: Do we really need it? Urology 2011;78(60):1248–1256.

[5] Srivastava A, Gupta R, Kumar A, Kapoor R, Mandhani A. Routine stenting after ureteroscopy for distal ureteral calculi is unnecessary: results of a randomized controlled trial. J Endourol 2003;17(10):871–874.

[6] Nabi G, Cook J, N'Dow J, McClinton S. Outcomes of stenting after uncomplicated ureteroscopy: systematic review and meta-analysis. BMJ. 2007;334(7593):572. Epub 2007 Feb 20.

[7] Luis Llanes González, *et al.* Decision analysis for the economic evaluation of the management of chronic obstructive uropathy. General Urology Arch Esp Urol 2011;64(9):875–881.

[8] López-Huertas HL, Polcari AJ, Acosta-Miranda A, Turk TM. Metallic ureteral stents: a cost-effective method of managing benign upper tract obstruction. J Endourol 2010;24(3):483–485. doi: 10.1089/end.2009.0192.

[9] Taylor ER, Benson AD, Schwartz BF. Cost analysis of metallic ureteral stents with 12 months of follow-up. J Endourol 2012;26(7):917–921. doi: 10.1089/end.2011.0481. Epub 2012 Apr 17.

[10] Baumgarten AS, Hakky TS, Carrion RE, Lockhart JL, Spiess PE. A single-institution experience with metallic ureteral stents: a cost-effective method of managing deficiencies in ureteral drainage. Int Braz J Urol 2014;40(2):225–231. doi: 10.1590/S1677-5538.IBJU.2014.02.13.

[11] Chitale S1, Raja V, Hussain N, Saada J, Girling S, Irving S, Cockburn JF. One-stage tubeless antegrade ureteric stenting: a safe and cost-effective option? Ann R Coll Surg Engl 2010;92(3):218–224. doi: 10.1308/003588410X12518836439128. Epub 2009 Dec 7.

[12] Monga M1, Klein E, Castañeda-Zúñiga WR, Thomas R. The forgotten indwelling ureteral stent: a urological dilemma. J Urol 1995;153(6):1817–1819.

[13] Lynch MF, Ghani KR, Frost I, Anson KM. Preventing the forgotten ureteric stent: results from the implementation of an electronic stent register. BJU Int 2007;99:245–246.

[14] Borboroglu PG, Kane CJ. Current management of severely encrusted ureteral stents with a large associated stone burden. J Urol 2000;164(3 Pt 1):648–650.

[15] Sancaktutar AA, Söylemez H, Bozkurt Y, Penbegül N, Atar M. Treatment of forgotten ureteral stents: how much does it really cost? A cost-effectiveness study in 27 patients. Urol Res 2012;40(4):317–325. doi: 10.1007/s00240-011-0409-3. Epub 2011 Aug 11.

[16] Bockholt NA, Wild TT, Gupta A, Tracy CR. Ureteric stent placement with extraction string: no strings attached? BJU Int 2012;110(11 Pt C):E1069-E1073. doi: 10.1111/j.1464-410X.2012.11219.x. Epub 2012 May 11.

[17] Barnes KT, Bing MT, Tracy CR. Do ureteric stent extraction strings affect stent-related quality of life or complications after ureteroscopy for urolithiasis: a prospective randomised control trial. BJU Int 2014;113(4):605–609. doi: 10.1111/bju.12541.

[18] Gershman B, Eisner BH, Sheth S, Sacco DE. Ureteral stenting and retrograde pyelography in the office: clinical outcomes, cost effectiveness, and time savings. J Endourol 2013;27(5):662–666. doi: 10.1089/end.2012.0644.

[19] Wilson CH, Rix DA, Manas DM, editorial group: Cochrane Kidney and Transplant Group. Routine intraoperative ureteric stenting for kidney transplant recipients. JRNL 2013;6:CD004925. DOI: 10.1002/14651858.CD004925.pub3

[20] Tavakoli A, Surange RS, Pearson RC, Parrott NR, Augustine T, Riad HN. Impact of stents on urological complications and health care expenditure in renal transplant recipients: results of a prospective, randomized clinical trial. J Urol 2007;177(6): 2260–2264; discussion 2264.

[21] Wilson CH, Bhatti AA, Rix DA, Manas DM. Routine intraoperative stenting for renal transplant recipients. Transplantation 2005;80(7):877–882.

28

Ureteric Stents: The Future

Ravi Kulkarni

Consultant Urological Surgeon, Ashford and St Peter's Hospitals NHS Foundation Trust, Chertsey, Surrey, UK

Ureteric stenting is a common urological procedure. Mundane it may seem, it is an integral part of every urologist's workload. It helps to relieve upper tract obstruction. Improvement in renal function and relief of pain are attractive benefits from this small device though it comes at a price. Every patient needs to appreciate the inevitable morbidity associated with ureteric stenting.

Attempts to improve the stents in order to minimize the associated complications have never stopped. Their size, shape, curls, materials, and coating have evolved since the original stent was used in clinical practice. However, the reduction in the morbidity associated with JJ stents is minimal. The relief of upper urinary tract obstruction, too, cannot be taken for granted. Failure of stent function and complications, such as migration, often lead to complex clinical scenarios, which are difficult to manage. Encrustation remains the most intractable of all the problems associated with stents.

Segmental and metallic stents have improved the longevity of the indwelling time and the durability of upper tract decompression. The reduction in lower urinary tract irritation associated with some of these stents is a welcome improvement. However, the complexity of insertion as well as removal of these devices needs to be taken into account as these issues necessitate involvement of specialist teams with expertise.

Cost is a major consideration in healthcare around the globe. Although JJ stents are relatively inexpensive, repeated stent changes add up to the cost of the overall patient care in the long run. Metallic stents offer superior durability and reduce the frequent need for stent changes. However, this benefit is blunted by their cost, complexity of insertion, and removal.

There are other considerations. Forgotten stents result in significant morbidity and associated grief to the patient as well as the healthcare system. The latter may be associated with litigation. The lack of a reliable stent registry and recall system seems to be a problem the world over.

So, what can we look forward to?

The use of coated stents appears promising. Although far from perfect, this concept is the most likely to improve the morbidity of the conventional stents. The other innovation on the horizon is the biodegradable stent. Surely, this will be the most reliable method of avoiding the problem of the forgotten stent.

Perhaps, the combination of these two ideas – drug-eluting biodegradable stents will have to be harnessed into clinical use. It will be quite difficult to avoid the use of the conventional JJ stents altogether but surely, they will become more bio-compatible, tailor-made (perhaps by 3D printing) stents to suit the anatomy of the patient and thus reduce some of the morbidity.

Albert Einstein once said: "Learn from yesterday, live for today, hope for tomorrow. The important thing is not to stop questioning."

I think this sums the future of any human endeavour and is very appropriate for the future of urological stents.

Index

Ureteric Stenting, First Edition. Edited by Ravi Kulkarni.
© 2017 John Wiley & Sons Ltd. Published 2017 by John Wiley & Sons Ltd.